Sports Injuries in the Foot and Ankle

Editor
ANISH R. KADAKIA

CLINICS IN
SPORTS MEDICINE

www.sportsmed.theclinics.com

Consulting Editor
MARK D. MILLER

October 2015 • Volume 34 • Number 4

ELSEVIER

1600 John F. Kennedy Boulevard • Suite 1800 • Philadelphia, Pennsylvania, 19103-2899

http://www.theclinics.com

CLINICS IN SPORTS MEDICINE Volume 34, Number 4
October 2015 ISSN 0278-5919, ISBN-13: 978-0-323-40104-3

Editor: Jennifer Flynn-Briggs
Developmental Editor: Donald Mumford

Clinics in Sports Medicine (ISSN 0278-5919) is published quarterly by Elsevier Inc., 360 Park Avenue South, New York, NY 10010-1710. Months of issue are January, April, July, and October. Business and Editorial Offices: 1600 John F. Kennedy Blvd., Ste. 1800, Philadelphia, PA 19103-2899. Customer Service Office: 3251 Riverport Lane, Maryland Heights, MO 63043. Periodicals postage paid at New York, NY and additional mailing offices. Subscription prices are $340.00 per year (US individuals), $540.00 per year (US institutions), $165.00 per year (US students), $385.00 per year (Canadian individuals), $666.00 per year (Canadian institutions), $235.00 (Canadian students), $470.00 per year (foreign individuals), $666.00 per year (foreign institutions), and $235.00 per year (foreign students). Foreign air speed delivery is included in all Clinics subscription prices. All prices are subject to change without notice. **POSTMASTER:** Send address changes to Clinics in Sports Medicine, Elsevier Health Sciences Division, Subscription Customer Service, 3251 Riverport Lane, Maryland Heights, MO 63043. Customer Service (orders, claims, online, change of address): Elsevier Health Sciences Division, Subscription Customer Service, 3251 Riverport Lane, Maryland Heights, MO 63043. **Tel: 1-800-654-2452 (U.S. and Canada); 314-447-8871 (outside U.S. and Canada). Fax: 314-447-8029. E-mail: journalscustomerservice-usa@elsevier.com (for print support); journalsonlinesupport-usa@ elsevier.com (for online support).**

Reprints. For copies of 100 or more of articles in this publication, please contact the Commercial Reprints Department, Elsevier Inc., 360 Park Avenue South, New York, NY 10010-1710. Tel.: 212-633-3874; Fax: 212-633-3820; E-mail: reprints@elsevier.com.

Clinics in Sports Medicine is covered in MEDLINE/PubMed (Index Medicus) Current Contents/Clinical Medicine, Excerpta Medica, and ISI/Biomed.

Contributors

CONSULTING EDITOR

MARK D. MILLER, MD
S. Ward Casscells Professor, Head, Division of Sports Medicine, Department of Orthopaedic Surgery, University of Virginia, Charlottesville, Virginia; Team Physician, James Madison University, Harrisonburg, Virginia

EDITOR

ANISH R. KADAKIA, MD
Editor in Chief, Journal of Orthopedic Surgery and Research; Director, Foot and Ankle Fellowship; Associate Professor, Department of Orthopedic Surgery, Northwestern University–Feinberg School of Medicine, Northwestern Memorial Hospital, Chicago, Illinois

AUTHORS

DOMINIC S. CARREIRA, MD
Sports Medicine and Orthopedics, Broward Health Medical Center, Fort Lauderdale, Florida

JULIET CLUTTON, MBBS, MRCS
Research Fellow, Cardiff Regional Foot and Ankle Unit, University Hospital of Wales, Cardiff, United Kingdom

J. CHRIS COETZEE, MD
Twin Cities Orthopedics, Edina, Minnesota

MINTON TRUITT COOPER, MD
Assistant Professor, Department of Orthopaedic Surgery, University of Virginia, Charlottesville, Virginia

WILLIAM HODGES DAVIS, MD
OrthoCarolina Foot and Ankle Institute, Charlotte, North Carolina

JOHN KENT ELLINGTON, MD
OrthoCarolina Foot and Ankle Institute, Charlotte, North Carolina

NORMAN ESPINOSA, MD
Institute for Foot and Ankle Reconstruction Zurich, Zurich, Switzerland

ERIC FERKEL, MD
Southern California Orthopaedic Institute, Van Nuys, California

ERIC GIZA, MD
Associate Professor, Department of Orthopaedic Surgery, University of California Davis, Sacramento, California

BEAT HINTERMANN, MD
Department of Orthopaedic Surgery, Kantonsspital Baselland, Liestal, Switzerland

MUNIER HOSSAIN, FRCS (Orth), MSc (Orth Eng), MSc (Oxon)
Senior Foot and Ankle Fellow, Cardiff Regional Foot and Ankle Unit, University Hospital of Wales, Cardiff, United Kingdom

ANISH R. KADAKIA, MD
Editor in Chief, Journal of Orthopedic Surgery and Research; Director, Foot and Ankle Fellowship; Associate Professor, Department of Orthopedic Surgery, Northwestern University–Feinberg School of Medicine, Northwestern Memorial Hospital, Chicago, Illinois

MARKUS KNUPP, MD
Department of Orthopaedic Surgery, Kantonsspital Baselland, Liestal, Switzerland

WILLIAM AARON KUNKLE, DO
Sports Medicine and Orthopedics, Broward Health Medical Center, Fort Lauderdale, Florida

PATRICK LÖTSCHER, MD
Department of Orthopaedic Surgery, Kantonsspital Baselland, Liestal, Switzerland

TAMARA HORN LANG, PhD
Department of Orthopaedic Surgery, Kantonsspital Baselland, Liestal, Switzerland

KATHLEEN LYONS, MBBS
Consultant Radiologist, Sports Medicine Department, Spire Cardiff Hospital, Cardiff, United Kingdom

NICOLA MAFFULLI, MD, MS, PhD, FRCS(Orth)
Department of Musculoskeletal Disorders, School of Medicine and Surgery, University of Salerno, Salerno, Italy; Department of Musculoskeletal Disorders, Centre for Sports and Exercise Medicine, Mile End Hospital, Barts and the London School of Medicine and Dentistry, Mary University of London, London, United Kingdom

LYNDON W. MASON, MB BCh, MRCS (Eng), FRCS (Tr&Orth)
Consultant Orthopaedic Surgeon, Foot and Ankle Unit, University Hospital Aintree, Liverpool, United Kingdom

MARC A. MAURER, MD
Institute for Foot and Ankle Reconstruction Zurich, Zurich, Switzerland

MARCO MENDOZA, MD
Department of Orthopedic Surgery, Northwestern University–Feinberg School of Medicine, Northwestern Memorial Hospital, Chicago, Illinois

PATRICK MICHELIER, BS
University of California Davis School of Medicine, Sacramento, California

ANDREW P. MOLLOY, MBChB, MRCS (Ed), FRCS (Tr&Orth)
Consultant Orthopaedic Surgeon, Foot and Ankle Unit, University Hospital Aintree; Honorary Senior Lecturer, Liverpool University, Liverpool, United Kingdom

FRANCESCO OLIVA, MD, PhD
Department of Orthopaedic and Traumatology, School of Medicine, University of Rome "Tor Vergata," Rome, Italy

ANTHONY PERERA, MBChB, MFSEM, FRCS (Orth)
Orthopaedic Foot and Ankle Surgeon, Cardiff Regional Foot and Ankle Unit, University Hospital of Wales; Sports Medicine Department, Spire Cardiff Hospital, Cardiff, United Kingdom

PHINIT PHISITKUL, MD
Clinical Associate Professor, Department of Orthopaedics and Rehabilitation, University of Iowa Hospital and Clinics, Iowa City, Iowa

MARK RIDGEWELL, MBBS, FFSEM, MSc (SEM)
Consultant Sports Physician, Sports Medicine Department, Spire Cardiff Hospital, Cardiff, United Kingdom

BRENT ROSTER, MD
Missoula Bone and Joint, Missoula, Montana

CHAMNANNI RUNGPRAI, MD
Fellow, Department of Orthopaedics and Rehabilitation, University of Iowa Hospital and Clinics, Iowa City, Iowa; Lecturer, Department of Orthopaedics, Phramongkutklao Hospital and College of Medicine, Bangkok, Thailand

JEFFREY D. SEYBOLD, MD
Twin Cities Orthopedics, Edina, Minnesota

PAUL J. SWITAJ, MD
Department of Orthopedic Surgery, Northwestern University–Feinberg School of Medicine, Northwestern Memorial Hospital, Chicago, Illinois

JOSHUA N. TENNANT, MD, MPH
Assistant Professor, Department of Orthopaedics, University of North Carolina School of Medicine, Chapel Hill, North Carolina

ALESSIO GIAI VIA, MD
Department of Orthopaedic and Traumatology, School of Medicine, University of Rome "Tor Vergata," Rome, Italy

ROGER WALKER, DO
Sports Medicine and Orthopedics, Broward Health Medical Center, Fort Lauderdale, Florida

LUKAS ZWICKY, MSc
Department of Orthopaedic Surgery, Kantonsspital Baselland, Liestal, Switzerland

Contents

> Management of acute Achilles tendon rupture is controversial. Although in
> the past open surgery was considered the gold standard, recent studies
> have shown improved outcomes with nonoperative management, leading
> to an increase in popularity of this treatment option. Percutaneous tech-
> niques have gained attention and seem to offer excellent results. In addi-
> tion, as with many other orthopedic conditions, significant concerns and
> questions exist as to whether or not chemoprophylaxis is indicated in
> these patients.

> Tendinopathy of the Achilles tendon involves clinical conditions in and
> around the tendon and it is the result of a failure of a chronic healing
> response. Although several conservative therapeutic options have been
> proposed, few of them are supported by randomized controlled trials.
> The management is primarily conservative and many patients respond
> well to conservative measures. If clinical conditions do not improve after
> 6 months of conservative management, surgery is recommended. The
> management of chronic ruptures is different from that of acute ruptures.
> The optimal surgical procedure is still debated. In this article chronic Achil-
> les tendon disorders are debated and evidence-based medicine treatment
> strategies are discussed.

> Peroneal tendon pathology is often found in patients complaining
> of lateral ankle pain and instability. Conditions encountered include
> tendinosis; tendinopathy; tenosynovitis; tears of the peroneus brevis,
> peroneus longus, and both tendons; subluxation and dislocation; and
> painful os peroneum syndrome. Injuries can be acute as a result
> of trauma or present as chronic problems, often in patients with pre-
> disposing structural components such as hindfoot varus, lateral liga-
> mentous instability, an enlarged peroneal tubercle, and a symptomatic
> os peroneum. Treatment begins with nonoperative care, but when

surgery is required, reported results and return to sport are in general very good.

Syndesmotic injuries may occur as an isolated ligamentous disruption or with associated malleolar fractures. It is imperative these injuries be identified and managed properly to prevent any long-term dysfunction and morbidity. There are multiple surgical interventions that can be used for the treatment of acute and chronic syndesmotic injuries. Obtaining and maintaining an anatomic reduction is the key to long-term success when treating syndesmotic injuries.

Ankle ligament injuries are among the most frequent reasons for emergency consultations of athletes. A majority of these can be treated conservatively; however, up to 40% develop chronic ankle instability requiring surgical reconstruction to restore functionality.

Osteochondral defects, impingement, and instability of the ankle are common injuries in athletes. In this article, we review these diagnoses and their treatment options, with a focus on arthroscopic approaches. The treatment options continue to evolve, supported by innovation and outcome studies. In this article, we describe the advantages and disadvantages of both open and arthroscopic treatments using published evidence.

Injuries to the foot are common in the athletic population, accounting for approximately 16% of sporting injuries. The bony and ligamentous structures around the first and second tarsometatarsal (TMT) joints, or Lisfranc joint complex, are the most commonly involved in injuries to the midfoot because of the limited static and dynamic stability of this region. The appropriate management of Lisfranc or TMT joint injuries in athletes is controversial, with multiple classification schemes and treatment methods and little evidence-based guidelines to deliver appropriate care. This article reviews the current diagnosis and management principles for TMT injuries in the athletic population.

A turf toe injury encompasses a wide spectrum of traumatic problems that occur to the first metatarsophalangeal joint. Most of these injuries are mild and respond well to nonoperative management. However, more severe injuries may require surgical management, including presence of diastasis or retraction of sesamoids, vertical instability, traumatic hallux valgus deformity, chondral injury, loose body, and failed conservative treatment.

Os trigonum syndrome with disease of the flexor hallucis longus tendon, so-called stenosing flexor tenosynovitis, is a common cause of posterior ankle impingement. Conservative treatment is the recommended first line of treatment, with secondary treatment options of either open or arthroscopic os trigonum excision with flexor hallucis longus retinaculum release. The arthroscopic approaches have gained popularity in the past decade because of less scarring, less postoperative pain, minimal overall morbidity, and earlier return to activities. However, comprehensive understanding of the anatomy of the posterior ankle is crucial to warrant successful outcomes and minimizing complications.

Posterior tibial tendon dysfunction can be a difficult entity to treat in the athletic population. Understanding the deformity components allows the physician to maximize nonoperative intervention with orthotics and physical therapy. Not all patients improve with nonoperative treatment, and surgical intervention can be successful in minimizing symptoms. Although return to full athletic activity is not universally possible, an active lifestyle is possible for many after surgical reconstruction.

Stress fractures of the foot and ankle may be more common among athletes than previously reported. A low threshold for investigation is warranted and further imaging may be appropriate if initial radiographs remain inconclusive. Most of these fractures can be treated conservatively with a period of non–weight-bearing mobilization followed by gradual return to activity. Early surgery augmented by bone graft may allow athletes to return to sports earlier. Risk of delayed union, nonunion, and recurrent fracture is high. Many of the patients may also have risk factors for injury that should be modified for a successful outcome.

Posterior tarsal tunnel syndrome is the result of compression of the posterior tibial nerve. Anterior tarsal tunnel syndrome (entrapment of the deep peroneal nerve) typically presents with pain radiating to the first dorsal web space. Distal tarsal tunnel syndrome results from entrapment of the first branch of the lateral plantar nerve and is often misdiagnosed initially as plantar fasciitis. Medial plantar nerve compression is seen most often in running athletes, typically with pain radiating to the medial arch. Morton neuroma is often seen in athletes who place their metatarsal arches repetitively in excessive hyperextension.

CLINICS IN SPORTS MEDICINE

THE CLINICS ARE AVAILABLE ONLINE!
Access your subscription at:
www.theclinics.com

Foreword

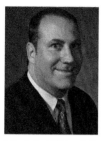

Mark D. Miller, MD
Consulting Editor

You should always put your best foot forward. Well, that is what this issue of *Clinics in Sports Medicine* has done, as I will elucidate in this foreword. Dr Anish R. Kadakia has done a superb job in putting together this treatise on sports foot and ankle. We have all seen how debilitating seemingly minor injuries to the ankle and foot can be. And, as I am sure you are aware, ankle sprains are the most common injury in sports. Therefore, this is a timely and important issue. Dr Kadakia, who is an excellent foot and ankle surgeon himself, includes a thorough review of tendon injuries, ankle sprains (to include high ankle sprains), arthroscopy, traumatic injuries, turf toe, overuse injuries, and entrapment neuropathies in this issue of *Clinics in Sports Medicine*. No one needs to tell him to step it up!

Mark D. Miller, MD
University of Virginia
James Madison University
400 Ray C. Hunt Drive, Suite 330
Charlottesville, VA 22908-0159, USA

E-mail address:
MDM3P@hscmail.mcc.virginia.edu

Clin Sports Med 34 (2015) xiii
http://dx.doi.org/10.1016/j.csm.2015.07.002
0278-5919/15/$ – see front matter © 2015 Published by Elsevier Inc.

sportsmed.theclinics.com

Preface

Sports Injuries in the Foot and Ankle

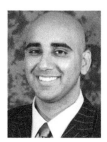

Anish R. Kadakia, MD
Editor

The focus on maintaining an active lifestyle has expanded the number of injuries that historically occurred primarily in collegiate and professional athletes. In addition, the intensity at which high school and intramural sports are played has increased, resulting in a higher demand on the foot and ankle for this population as well. Many injuries in the foot and ankle result in significant disability for the recreational and professional athlete. Both operative and nonoperative sports medicine physicians are at the frontline when dealing with many of the conditions discussed in this *Clinics in Sports Medicine*. This active patient population expects minimal downtime while maximizing their ability to return to play. Our aim was to provide an up-to-date review of foot and ankle sports–related topics to achieve these goals for our patients.

The authors in this issue of *Clinics in Sports Medicine* are experts in dealing with sports-related injuries and pathology of the foot and ankle. By sharing the knowledge and experience of our colleagues, each of us can expand our ability to understand and treat these conditions. I would like to commend the authors on the tremendous time and effort that they put forth in preparation of their articles. I also would like to thank everyone at Elsevier for their help in putting this issue together, and express my sincere

Clin Sports Med 34 (2015) xv–xvi
http://dx.doi.org/10.1016/j.csm.2015.07.001
0278-5919/15/$ – see front matter © 2015 Published by Elsevier Inc.
sportsmed.theclinics.com

appreciation to Mark Miller for allowing me to participate in this issue. I sincerely hope that you enjoy this issue and that the authors' efforts assist in the treatment of your patients.

Anish R. Kadakia, MD
Northwestern University–
Feinberg School of Medicine
Northwestern Memorial Hospital
259 East Erie
13th Floor
Chicago, IL 60611, USA

E-mail address:
kadak259@gmail.com

Acute Achilles Tendon Ruptures

Does Surgery Offer Superior Results (and Other Confusing Issues)?

Minton Truitt Cooper, MD

KEYWORDS

- Achilles tendon rupture • Operative repair of Achilles • Percutaneous tendon repair
- Functional rehabilitation

KEY POINTS

- Nonoperative management of Achilles ruptures has gained popularity in recent years because studies have shown improved results with functional rehabilitation in terms of re-rupture rates.
- Operative treatment includes open and percutaneous techniques, both of which have shown excellent results, although recent studies have shown decreased complication rates with percutaneous repair.
- Prophylaxis against thromboembolic events is controversial, and to date there is no strong evidence to support its use in patients with Achilles rupture.

INTRODUCTION

Despite being the strongest and largest tendon in the body, the Achilles tendon is the most frequently ruptured.[1–3] Acute ruptures of the Achilles tendon most commonly occur during high-impact sports, such as ball or racket games.[4–10] The mechanism of rupture has been divided into 3 categories[11,12]:

1. Weight bearing with the forefoot pushing off and the knee in extension (most common)
2. Sudden unexpected dorsiflexion of the ankle
3. Violent dorsiflexion of a plantarflexed foot

Several studies have shown a male preponderance of 75% to 80% of ruptures, with mean ages between 37 and 42 years.[7,9,10,13–17] One recent study[18] reported that 46% of ruptures occurred in women, a fact attributed to the popularity of netball in that

Department of Orthopaedic Surgery, University of Virginia, PO Box 801016, Charlottesville, VA 22908, USA
E-mail address: mtc2d@virginia.edu

Clin Sports Med 34 (2015) 595–606
http://dx.doi.org/10.1016/j.csm.2015.06.001
0278-5919/15/$ – see front matter © 2015 Elsevier Inc. All rights reserved.

region, which is played competitively almost exclusively by women. This finding raises the question of whether simply being male is a risk factor, or whether it is more related to participation in certain activities.

The incidence of rupture has been increasing for the last several decades. In Sweden from 1950 to 1979, the incidence was 9 per 100,000, primarily in individuals between 40 and 50 years of age.[7] At that time more than half of the injuries occurred during sport, with the most common being badminton and soccer. A study by Leppilahti and colleagues[6] found an incidence in Finland of 18 per 100,000 in 1994, with a younger peak age group of 39 to 40 years. Houshian and colleagues[4] found an even higher rate over a similar time period in Denmark. More recently, Huttunen and colleagues[5] found the incidence to have increased dramatically from 2001 to 2012. For men, the incidence increased from 47.0 to 55.2 per 100,000 person-years; in women it increased from 12.0 to 14.7 per 100,000 person-years over the same time interval. Although the highest incidence occurred in men aged between 40 and 59 years, the largest increase was in men more than 60 years of age (29.6 per 100,000 person-years in 2001 to 62.9 per 100,000 person-years in 2012). The incidence declined by 28% in men between 18 and 39 years of age over that time. Most of these studies attribute the increase in incidence of acute ruptures to the growing number of older individuals participating in high-impact athletics; tendons in younger individuals have higher tensile rupture stress and lower stiffness than older tendons.[19]

DIAGNOSIS ISSUES

However, 20% to 25% of acute Achilles tendon ruptures are misdiagnosed initially.[1,3,20] Nevertheless a thorough physical examination and history taking should lead to an expedient diagnosis.

Many patients report pain in the back of the ankle, and often the feeling that they had been kicked or struck in the back of the ankle. Most do not have the ability to bear full weight on the affected limb; however, a small percentage of patients present with little pain and the ability to ambulate.

Clinical examination in the acute setting typically shows edema, bruising, and often a palpable gap within the tendon approximately 3 to 5 cm proximal to its insertion. Many patients may be able to actively plantarflex the ankle using secondary muscles (flexor hallucis longus, flexor digitorum longus, posterior tibialis, and peroneal muscles). The Simmonds or Thompson test is performed by squeezing the calf with the patient in the prone position and the knee flexed. This test assesses the integrity of the soleus musculotendinous unit. When intact, plantarflexion occurs at the ankle primarily because of posterior bowing of the calf tendons.[21] When the tendon is ruptured, a positive test shows no plantarflexion of the ankle. This test has shown sensitivity of 0.96 and specificity of 0.93.[3]

The American Academy of Orthopaedic Surgeons clinical practice guidelines on Achilles tendon ruptures suggest that a detailed history and physical examination be performed and should include 2 of the following tests to establish the diagnosis: positive Thompson test, decreased ankle plantarflexion strength, presence of a palpable gap, increased passive ankle dorsiflexion with gentle manipulation.[22] Garras and colleagues[8] described a combination of 3 physical examination findings that led to 100% sensitivity for diagnosis of a complete rupture: a positive Thompson test; decreased ankle resting tension with the patient in the prone position and the knee flexed to 90° (Matles test), compared with the contralateral side (normal is 20°–30° of plantarflexion); and a palpable defect in the Achilles tendon.

Imaging

Plain radiographs are commonly obtained in the setting of acute injury. On the lateral plain film, several findings may be present. There may be loss of the normal configuration of the Kager triangle, deformation of the contours of the distal portion of the tendon, and abnormalities in the angle of the posterior skin surface. In addition, the lateral radiograph is critical in order to ensure that an avulsion of the insertion of the Achilles tendon has not occurred. In many of the insertional cases, preexisting tendinosis is present, which is a different clinical scenario from noninsertional rupture. Ultrasonography has been shown to be sensitive and accurate for diagnosing complete ruptures,[23] but it is operator dependent. MRI may be used to assist in the diagnosis of acute Achilles tendon ruptures when the clinical picture is inconclusive; however, Garras and colleagues[8] found that it was not as sensitive as clinical examination in diagnosing complete ruptures and delayed intervention by an average of 6.8 days.

TREATMENT

Treatment of acute Achilles tendon ruptures may be classified as either operative (either open or percutaneous) or nonoperative (cast immobilization or functional bracing). In the past, operative treatment was frequently more favored than nonoperative treatment, with the latter being reserved for sedentary patients, those with significant medical comorbidities, and those who simply chose not to have surgery. This preference was generally based on the reportedly high risk of rerupture with nonoperative treatment.[13,15,16,24–31] Rerupture rates have been found to be as high as 29% in those treated nonoperatively.[30] Recently, data suggest that nonoperative treatment has been gaining popularity.[5] In addition, miniopen and percutaneous techniques have become more common in recent years.

Nonoperative Treatment

Historically, nonoperative treatment of Achilles tendon ruptures has been associated with high rerupture rates,[13,15,16,24–31] which led many practitioners to favor operative treatment. These early studies reported on the outcomes of patients treated with long periods of cast immobilization. More recently, functional rehabilitation with nonsurgical management has gained attention, and at least 1 study has found that the percentage of patients treated in such a manner is increasing.[5] One of the first studies focusing on this type of treatment was performed by Saleh and colleagues[32] in 1992, in which all patients were treated nonoperatively, but were randomized to either early controlled motion or cast immobilization for 8 weeks. The patients in the early mobilization group regained motion and returned to activities more quickly than those who were casted, with only 1 rerupture out of 20 patients in the early mobilization group. Shortly thereafter, Thermann and colleagues[33] showed no difference between operative and nonoperative treatment using an aggressive early weight-bearing protocol. Typically, this type of treatment involves a brief period of immobilization in equinus, followed by functional bracing,[10,32–34] with a goal of minimizing weakness and stiffness. Multiple studies have shown improved tendon healing in humans and animals treated with early range of motion and controlled loading of the tendon.[32,35–39]

The author's preferred protocol for nonoperative treatment is similar to that described by Willits and colleagues,[10] focusing on early protected weight bearing and range of motion activities (**Table 1**).

Although it is becoming accepted that early range of motion is beneficial in nonoperative management, it is unclear how soon patients should begin bearing weight. In the study by Thermann and colleagues,[33] patients were allowed to bear weight within

Table 1 Rehabilitation program for nonoperative management of Achilles rupture	
Time from Presentation (wk)	**Activity**
0–2	Equinus cast in 15°–20° plantarflexion (posterior plaster splint if swelling severe). Non–weight bearing
2–4	Removable fixed ankle walker with 2.5-cm (1-inch) heel lift (4 separate 6-mm [0.25-inch] lifts stacked). Partial weight bearing with crutches, progress to full weight bearing between 3–4 wk. Patient may remove boot for active plantarflexion (unrestricted) and dorsiflexion to neutral
4–8	Patient continues full weight bearing in the boot. Remove 6-mm (0.25-inch) heel lift each week with goal of no lift in boot at 8 wk. May begin progressing dorsiflexion stretching and resisted plantarflexion at 6 wk
8–12	Discontinue boot after 1 wk of ambulating with no lift. Progress strengthening, range of motion, and proprioception under guidance of physical therapist

5 days of injury. A more recent study by Barfod and colleagues[40] randomized patients with acute ruptures treated nonoperatively to either immediate weight bearing or non–weight bearing for 6 weeks. Both groups were allowed early range of motion exercises. There was an overall rerupture rate of 9%, and the investigators were not able to find any statistically significant differences between the 2 groups in terms of rerupture, patient-reported outcomes, functional assessment, or return to work or sports.

Operative Management

As previously described, for many years operative management was favored for acute Achilles tendon ruptures, primarily because of the reported lower rates of rerupture but also in part because of a perception of earlier return to sport and improved long-term strength recovery. Although the differences in rerupture rates have focused on early and aggressive rehabilitation, it has also been suggested that primary repair may lead to better tendon healing.[41] By directly repairing the tendon, the surgeon is able to minimize the gap between the ends of the tendon, therefore leading to less scar formation and increased tendon healing through an intrinsic mechanism from within the tendon and epitenon, possibly leading to improved biomechanical strength of the healed tendon. In the past, operative treatment primarily consisted of direct open repair; however, recently there has been an increase in popularity of percutaneous or minimally invasive surgical techniques.

Open Repair

Direct open repair of the Achilles tendon has been considered the gold standard for treatment, leading to low rates of rerupture, which have typically been found to be between 1.7% and 5%.[9,13,15,24,41–43] In this procedure, a 6-cm incision is made over the medial or posteromedial border of the Achilles tendon. Dissection is carried down sharply through the paratenon, preserving it for direct repair. The ruptured tendon is identified and hematoma debrided. The tendon ends are identified, and most typically 1 or 2 #2 nonabsorbable sutures are placed in a locking fashion in each end of the stump (Krackow, Bunnell, or Kessler pattern). McCoy and Haddad[44] found no difference in repair strength between the different suture techniques, but they recommended that 2 sutures be placed in each end for a 4-strand repair, although in many cases a 4-strand repair is difficult to achieve and has not been proved to offer any clinical benefit. The sutures are secured with the foot in plantarflexion to bring the stumps into apposition, and the knots are secured. The contralateral limb may be prepped into the sterile field as well, so that it may be used for comparison to restore proper tension. Absorbable suture may then be used either circumferentially or intermittently to reinforce the repair. Reinforcement with tendon grafts or synthetic materials is not typically needed in the setting of an acute repair. Routine transfer of the flexor hallucis longus is not typically required. The paratenon is meticulously repaired, followed by skin closure. The ankle is splinted in approximately 15° to 20° of plantarflexion to maximize perfusion to the posterior soft tissue.

Percutaneous Repair

Percutaneous repair of the ruptured Achilles tendon was first described by Ma and Griffith[45] in 1977. Despite their promising results, percutaneous techniques have only more recently become more common. The aim of percutaneous or minimally invasive repair is to provide the surgical benefit of lower rerupture rate, while minimizing the rates of infections and soft tissue complications, which have found to be as high as 34.1% with open surgical repair.[24] Another cited benefit of percutaneous repair is cosmesis.[46] Although early studies showed a high risk of sural nerve injury,[47,48] techniques have been developed to decrease this complication.[49–51]

In their meta-analysis, Khan and colleagues[24] pooled the data of 2 trials comparing open and percutaneous repair. They found a statistically significant benefit of percutaneous surgery with regard to rerupture rate, complications other than rerupture, and infection.

The technique described by Carmont and Maffulli[52] is performed under local anesthesia. An 11 blade is used to make 4 longitudinal stab incisions medially and laterally 4 and 6 cm proximal to the rupture, and a 1-cm transverse incision directly over the defect. Small longitudinal incisions are also made medial and lateral to the tendon just proximal to its insertion. A Mayo needle is threaded with 2 double loops of suture and passed between the proximal stab incisions through the tendon. These sutures are then passed diagonally across the tendon and out the opposing stab incision. They are then passed out of the transverse incision over the rupture. Similarly, 2 double-looped sutures are passed through the distal stab incisions, and then out the transverse incision. The knots are secured with the foot in equinus.

Keller and colleagues[49] recently reported on 100 cases treated with a miniopen technique, with excellent results. A 2-cm incision is made medially 2 cm above the proximal stump of the ruptured tendon. The superficial fascia is incised, and the paratenon is left intact. The interval between the fascia and paratenon is developed and suture retrievers are positioned on either side of the distal stump. Three sutures are passed through the distal stump percutaneously, and the sutures are pulled out through the proximal incision. These sutures are then passed through the proximal stump and knots are secured. The investigators found only 2 reruptures, with no infections, no scar adhesions, and no sural nerve injuries. Mean time to return to work was 56 days and mean time to return to sport was 18.9 weeks. Ninety-eight percent of patients were satisfied with the procedure and there were no differences at a mean of 24 months in strength between the injured and uninjured limbs.

Comparisons

Twaddle and Poon[17] compared the results of operative treatment with nonoperative management with early range of motion. Patients were initially placed in a plaster cast in equinus for 10 days, then transitioned to a removable boot and instructed to participate in active range of motion exercises every hour. All patients in both groups were kept non–weight bearing for 6 weeks. No difference was found between the two groups in terms of range of motion, musculoskeletal function assessment index, or calf circumference, and the surgical group showed 10% rerupture (2 out of 20) compared with 4.5% (1 out of 22) in the nonsurgical group (all were caused by significant trauma).

In 2010, Willits and colleagues[10] published the results of a multicenter randomized trial comparing outcomes of open repair with nonoperative treatment using an accelerated functional rehabilitation. Their protocol was similar to the one described earlier, with range of motion exercises and protected weight bearing initiated at 2 weeks after injury. Of the patients treated nonoperatively, 3 of 72 patients (4.2%) experienced rerupture, which was similar to the operatively treated group. Aside from a significant difference in wound complications (favoring the nonoperative group), the only other significant difference between the two groups was a slight increase in plantarflexion strength at 240°/s at 1 and 2 years in those treated operatively.

Nilsson-Helander and colleagues[9] also performed a randomized study comparing nonoperative treatment with open surgical repair in 2010. Aside from surgical intervention, both groups were treated equivalently with an equinus cast for 2 weeks, followed by 6 weeks in an adjustable boot with gradual increase in dorsiflexion. Although they found no statistically significant differences between the two groups in terms of rerupture rate, functional outcome, or patient satisfactions, the nonoperative rerupture rate was 12%. Despite the short period of true cast immobilization, and what they describe as early mobilization, note that patients were kept non–weight bearing for 6 to 8 weeks in a boot to block dorsiflexion.

It is clear that the decision between operative and nonoperative treatment of acute Achilles ruptures depends in part on the weight given to different unfavorable outcomes. An expected-value decision analysis was performed in 1992 in an effort to determine whether operative or nonoperative treatment was superior for management of acute Achilles tendon ruptures.[53] At that time, nonoperative treatment led to a rerupture rate of 12.1%, compared with 2.2% with surgery. However, the probability of a moderate complication with surgery was 7.5%, compared with 0.3% with nonoperative treatment. Ultimately, based primarily on the patient's valuation of rerupture, they concluded that surgery was the optimal treatment.

According to the meta-analysis of Khan and colleagues,[24] all 4 included studies included favored surgery when the outcome was rerupture; however, when other complications, such as wound infection, sensory disturbance, or adhesions, were used as the unfavorable outcomes, all of the studies favored nonoperative treatment, and the pooled rate for other complications was 34.1% for surgery compared with 2.7% for the nonoperative group. Note that in all of the studies included in this analysis, the nonoperative cohorts were treated with lengthy immobilization.

More recently, Wilkins and colleagues[41] published a systematic review of randomized controlled trials comparing operative versus nonoperative management of acute Achilles tendon ruptures. They found 7 articles that met their criteria for inclusion.[9,10,13–17] Their pooled data found a significantly higher rate of rerupture in the nonoperative group (8.8% vs 3.2% for surgical) and an increased time to return to work in the nonoperative group. However, in the pooled surgical group, they found a higher rate of deep infection (2.36% vs 0%), a higher rate of noncosmetic scar complaints, as well as a higher rate of sural nerve disturbances.

One of the difficulties in interpreting such meta-analyses and systematic reviews comes from the diversity in treatment protocols. These protocols typically include older studies using long periods of cast immobilization in the analyses, leading to findings of high rerupture rates. Furthermore, there is no consistency in the definitions of functional or dynamic rehabilitation, which may include anything from immediate weight bearing, to partial early weight bearing, to complete non–weight bearing. Aside from the possible direct benefits of surgical repair, it is probable that the difference in postoperative protocols between the groups naturally biases the studies to favor the surgical group. This bias was summarized well by Twaddle and Poon,[17] who suggested that "it is possible that controlled early motion is the important factor in optimizing outcomes in patients with Achilles tendon rupture and that surgery makes no difference to the outcome apart from increasing the risk of local infection."[17]

In 2012, a meta-analysis comparing operative and nonoperative treatment of acute rupture found equivalent results with regard to rerupture rate when nonoperative protocols included early range of motion.[54] This analysis included newer studies published after 2004, a period when several studies showed improved results with nonoperative management, and more focused on functional rehabilitation. When all included studies were pooled and evaluated for rerupture rate, there was an absolute risk difference of 5.5% in favor of surgery. However, because of significant heterogeneity, a stratified analysis was performed by separating those studies that included early mobilization and prolonged immobilization in the nonoperatively treated groups. When including only studies that included early motion in the nonoperative protocols, surgery did not significantly reduce the risk of rerupture (absolute risk difference, 1.7%; $P = .45$). In contrast, surgery only significantly decreased the risk of rerupture by 8.8% ($P = .001$) compared with prolonged immobilization. In addition, there was a difference in the risk of other complications (including infection, skin necrosis, sural nerve damage, diminished ankle range of motion, deep vein thrombosis, and scar adhesion) of 15.8% in favor of nonsurgical treatment ($P = .016$). The investigators did not find any statistically significant difference between the treatments for strength or return to work.

One potential question that arises and requires further study is whether or not there is a maximal amount of time between injury and initiation of treatment within which nonoperative treatment may be successful. In this regard, studies have varied in the inclusion criteria, with inclusions ranging from 3 to 14 days.[9,10,55] It is possible that, by 14 days after injury, significant scar tissue can develop between the gapped ends of the tendon, preventing reapproximation with simply plantarflexing the foot. In cases of delayed presentation, it may be prudent to perform dynamic ultrasonography examination to verify that the tendon ends may be reapproximated with plantarflexion before initiating nonoperative treatment.

DEEP VEIN THROMBOSIS PROPHYLAXIS

As with many other orthopedic foot and ankle conditions, there are few data and no real consensus regarding prophylaxis of deep vein thrombosis during the management of acute Achilles tendon ruptures. The studies that do exist vary in the methods used to monitor the rates of deep vein thrombosis and pulmonary embolus and the incidences reported (**Table 2**).[56–61] Prospective studies in which patients were monitored with ultrasonography consistently showed much higher incidences of deep vein thrombosis than those that were performed retrospectively, essentially only reporting on patients with symptomatic thrombosis. Consistent within these studies is the finding that most deep vein thrombosis occurs in the veins distal to the knee, and pulmonary emboli are rare. In addition, in studies that have compared

Table 2
Studies that reported on incidence of deep vein thrombosis/pulmonary embolus in patients with acute Achilles tendon rupture

Author	Study Design	Treatment	Outcome
Patel et al,[60] 2012	Retrospective database review	Operative and nonoperative	0.43% DVT 0.34% PE No difference in operative vs nonoperative
Nilsson-Helander et al,[59] 2009	Prospective with ultrasonography surveillance	Randomized to operative vs nonoperative management	34% DVT 0.3% PE No difference between operative and nonoperative management
Healy et al,[56] 2010	Retrospective chart review	Cast immobilization	6.3% DVT
Lapidus et al,[57] 2007	Prospective study with ultrasonography surveillance	Operative, randomized to dalteparin vs placebo	34% DVT with dalteparin, 36% DVT with placebo
Saragas and Ferrao,[62] 2011	Retrospective chart review	Operative treatment	5.7% DVT
Makhdom et al,[58] 2013	Retrospective chart review	Operative treatment	23.5% DVT (one-third diagnosed preoperatively)

Abbreviations: DVT, deep vein thrombosis; PE, pulmonary embolus.

nonoperative and operative management,[10,59,60] no difference was found between the groups.

This is an area that requires further examination. At this time there is no conclusive evidence to suggest a benefit to chemoprophylaxis for deep vein thrombosis. In the only study that compared the rates of deep vein thrombosis in patients receiving prophylaxis and those receiving placebo,[57] no benefit was found in the prophylaxis group. However, it is therefore left up to the surgeon to consider patient risk factors and weigh the risks of apparently low incidences of symptomatic deep vein thrombosis and pulmonary embolism against the risks of chemoprophylaxis.

SUMMARY

There have been significant developments over the last 20 years in the management of acute Achilles tendon ruptures. In the past it was thought that operative management was far superior to nonoperative management because of the unacceptable risk of rerupture with nonoperative treatment, despite the known risks of open surgical treatment. With the advent of functional rehabilitation, as opposed to long periods of cast immobilization, the risk of rerupture with nonoperative treatment has been found to be comparable with that of operative treatment, with a decreased rate of other complications. In addition, recent studies have shown excellent results with percutaneous or minimally invasive techniques, at least comparable with, or superior to, those found with direct open repair. It is therefore reasonable to draw the conclusion that nonoperative management with functional rehabilitation (early range of motion and protected weight bearing), direct open repair, and percutaneous techniques are all appropriate forms of treatment of Achilles tendon rupture. Based on the body of literature at this point in time, a new set of questions needs to be answered:

1. Do certain subsets of patients benefit more from one form of treatment than another? A recent retrospective study attempted to address this question.[18] Men less than 40 years of age benefited significantly from surgical repair, with a rerupture rate of 18.1% with nonoperative treatment, whereas women more than 40 years of age were extremely unlikely to rerupture following nonoperative treatment (2%). While this study is weakened due to its retrospective nature and the fact that treatment groups were not randomized, it is the only study to the author's knowledge that has attempted to stratify patients in such a way. Further stratification of this nature is needed in randomized prospective studies.

2. When surgical repair is the treatment of choice, should open treatment be abandoned in favor of percutaneous or minimally invasive techniques? Advances in percutaneous treatments have led to safer procedures (particularly with regard to sural nerve injury) with low rerupture rates, minimal risk of infection, and excellent return of muscle function, so further randomized prospective studies are needed to definitively answer this question.

3. Is there a specific length of delay between injury and initiation of treatment, after which nonoperative management should no longer be considered an option? Wallace and colleagues[63] reviewed a large series of patients treated nonoperatively and did not find any significant increase in rerupture for those patients who presented after a delay of greater than 2 weeks.

4. Should chemoprophylaxis for deep vein thrombosis be instituted in patients with Achilles tendon ruptures? Although rates have been found to be high in studies in which ultrasonography was used routinely, proximal deep vein thrombosis and pulmonary embolus are rare occurrences, and no benefit has been shown for chemoprophylaxis.

REFERENCES

1. Maffulli N. Rupture of the Achilles tendon. J Bone Joint Surg Am 1999;81: 1019–36.
2. Maffulli N, Waterston SW, Squair J, et al. Changing incidence of Achilles tendon rupture in Scotland: a 15-year study. Clin J Sport Med 1999;9:157–60.
3. Maffulli N. The clinical diagnosis of subcutaneous tear of the Achilles tendon. A prospective study in 174 patients. Am J Sports Med 1998;26:266–70.
4. Houshian S, Tscherning T, Riegels-Nielsen P. The epidemiology of Achilles tendon rupture in a Danish county. Injury 1998;29:651–4.
5. Huttunen TT, Kannus P, Rolf C, et al. Acute Achilles tendon ruptures: incidence of injury and surgery in Sweden between 2001 and 2012. Am J Sports Med 2014; 42:2419–23.
6. Leppilahti J, Puranen J, Orava S. Incidence of Achilles tendon rupture. Acta Orthop Scand 1996;67:277–9.
7. Nillius SA, Nilsson BE, Westlin NE. The incidence of Achilles tendon rupture. Acta Orthop Scand 1976;47:118–21.
8. Garras DN, Raikin SM, Bhat SB, et al. MRI is unnecessary for diagnosing acute Achilles tendon ruptures: clinical diagnostic criteria. Clin Orthop Relat Res 2012;470:2268–73.
9. Nilsson-Helander K, Silbernagel KG, Thomee R, et al. Acute Achilles tendon rupture: a randomized, controlled study comparing surgical and nonsurgical

treatments using validated outcome measures. Am J Sports Med 2010;38: 2186–93.

10. Willits K, Amendola A, Bryant D, et al. Operative versus nonoperative treatment of acute Achilles tendon ruptures: a multicenter randomized trial using accelerated functional rehabilitation. J Bone Joint Surg Am 2010;92:2767–75.

11. Longo UG, Petrillo S, Maffulli N, et al. Acute Achilles tendon rupture in athletes. Foot Ankle Clin 2013;18:319–38.

12. Arner O, Lindholm A. Subcutaneous rupture of the Achilles tendon; as study of 92 cases. Acta Chir Scand Suppl 1959;116:1–51.

13. Cetti R, Christensen SE, Ejsted R, et al. Operative versus nonoperative treatment of Achilles tendon rupture. A prospective randomized study and review of the literature. Am J Sports Med 1993;21:791–9.

14. Metz R, Verleisdonk EJ, van der Heijden GJ, et al. Acute Achilles tendon rupture: minimally invasive surgery versus nonoperative treatment with immediate full weightbearing–a randomized controlled trial. Am J Sports Med 2008;36:1688–94.

15. Moller M, Movin T, Granhed H, et al. Acute rupture of tendon Achillis. A prospective randomised study of comparison between surgical and non-surgical treatment. J Bone Joint Surg Br 2001;83:843–8.

16. Nistor L. Surgical and non-surgical treatment of Achilles tendon rupture. A prospective randomized study. J Bone Joint Surg Am 1981;63:394–9.

17. Twaddle BC, Poon P. Early motion for Achilles tendon ruptures: is surgery important? A randomized, prospective study. Am J Sports Med 2007;35:2033–8.

18. Gwynne-Jones DP, Sims M, Handcock D. Epidemiology and outcomes of acute Achilles tendon rupture with operative or nonoperative treatment using an identical functional bracing protocol. Foot Ankle Int 2011;32:337–43.

19. Thermann H, Frerichs O, Biewener A, et al. [Biomechanical studies of human Achilles tendon rupture]. Unfallchirurg 1995;98:570–5 [in German].

20. O'Brien T. The needle test for complete rupture of the Achilles tendon. J Bone Joint Surg Am 1984;66:1099–101.

21. Scott BW, al Chalabi A. How the Simmonds-Thompson test works. J Bone Joint Surg Br 1992;74:314–5.

22. Chiodo CP, Glazebrook M, Bluman EM, et al. American Academy of Orthopaedic Surgeons clinical practice guideline on treatment of Achilles tendon rupture. J Bone Joint Surg Am 2010;92:2466–8.

23. Hartgerink P, Fessell DP, Jacobson JA, et al. Full- versus partial-thickness Achilles tendon tears: sonographic accuracy and characterization in 26 cases with surgical correlation. Radiology 2001;220:406–12.

24. Khan RJ, Fick D, Keogh A, et al. Treatment of acute Achilles tendon ruptures. A meta-analysis of randomized, controlled trials. J Bone Joint Surg Am 2005;87: 2202–10.

25. Nyyssonen T, Luthje P, Kroger H. The increasing incidence and difference in sex distribution of Achilles tendon rupture in Finland in 1987–1999. Scand J Surg 2008;97:272–5.

26. Wills CA, Washburn S, Caiozzo V, et al. Achilles tendon rupture. A review of the literature comparing surgical versus nonsurgical treatment. Clin Orthop Relat Res 1986;(207):156–63.

27. Lo IK, Kirkley A, Nonweiler B, et al. Operative versus nonoperative treatment of acute Achilles tendon ruptures: a quantitative review. Clin J Sport Med 1997;7: 207–11.

28. Popovic N, Lemaire R. Diagnosis and treatment of acute ruptures of the Achilles tendon. Current concepts review. Acta Orthop Belg 1999;65:458–71.

29. Wong J, Barrass V, Maffulli N. Quantitative review of operative and nonoperative management of Achilles tendon ruptures. Am J Sports Med 2002;30:565–75.
30. Inglis AE, Scott WN, Sculco TP, et al. Ruptures of the tendo achillis. An objective assessment of surgical and non-surgical treatment. J Bone Joint Surg Am 1976; 58:990–3.
31. Persson A, Wredmark T. The treatment of total ruptures of the Achilles tendon by plaster immobilisation. Int Orthop 1979;3:149–52.
32. Saleh M, Marshall PD, Senior R, et al. The Sheffield splint for controlled early mobilisation after rupture of the calcaneal tendon. A prospective, randomised comparison with plaster treatment. J Bone Joint Surg Br 1992;74:206–9.
33. Thermann H, Zwipp H, Tscherne H. [Functional treatment concept of acute rupture of the Achilles tendon. 2 years results of a prospective randomized study]. Unfallchirurg 1995;98:21–32 [in German].
34. McComis GP, Nawoczenski DA, DeHaven KE. Functional bracing for rupture of the Achilles tendon. Clinical results and analysis of ground-reaction forces and temporal data. J Bone Joint Surg Am 1997;79:1799–808.
35. Costa ML, MacMillan K, Halliday D, et al. Randomised controlled trials of immediate weight-bearing mobilisation for rupture of the tendo Achillis. J Bone Joint Surg Br 2006;88:69–77.
36. Gelberman RH, Woo SL, Amiel D, et al. Influences of flexor sheath continuity and early motion on tendon healing in dogs. J Hand Surg 1990;15:69–77.
37. Kangas J, Pajala A, Ohtonen P, et al. Achilles tendon elongation after rupture repair: a randomized comparison of 2 postoperative regimens. Am J Sports Med 2007;35:59–64.
38. Maffulli N, Tallon C, Wong J, et al. Early weightbearing and ankle mobilization after open repair of acute midsubstance tears of the Achilles tendon. Am J Sports Med 2003;31:692–700.
39. Mortensen HM, Skov O, Jensen PE. Early motion of the ankle after operative treatment of a rupture of the Achilles tendon. A prospective, randomized clinical and radiographic study. J Bone Joint Surg Am 1999;81:983–90.
40. Barfod KW, Bencke J, Lauridsen HB, et al. Nonoperative dynamic treatment of acute Achilles tendon rupture: the influence of early weight-bearing on clinical outcome: a blinded, randomized controlled trial. J Bone Joint Surg Am 2014; 96:1497–503.
41. Wilkins R, Bisson LJ. Operative versus nonoperative management of acute Achilles tendon ruptures: a quantitative systematic review of randomized controlled trials. Am J Sports Med 2012;40:2154–60.
42. Pajala A, Kangas J, Ohtonen P, et al. Rerupture and deep infection following treatment of total Achilles tendon rupture. J Bone Joint Surg Am 2002;84-A:2016–21.
43. Bhandari M, Guyatt GH, Siddiqui F, et al. Treatment of acute Achilles tendon ruptures: a systematic overview and metaanalysis. Clin Orthop Relat Res 2002;(400): 190–200.
44. McCoy BW, Haddad SL. The strength of Achilles tendon repair: a comparison of three suture techniques in human cadaver tendons. Foot Ankle Int 2010;31: 701–5.
45. Ma GW, Griffith TG. Percutaneous repair of acute closed ruptured Achilles tendon: a new technique. Clin Orthop Relat Res 1977;(128):247–55.
46. Del Buono A, Volpin A, Maffulli N. Minimally invasive versus open surgery for acute Achilles tendon rupture: a systematic review. Br Med Bull 2014;109:45–54.
47. Hockenbury RT, Johns JC. A biomechanical in vitro comparison of open versus percutaneous repair of tendon Achilles. Foot Ankle 1990;11:67–72.

48. Rowley DI, Scotland TR. Rupture of the Achilles tendon treated by a simple operative procedure. Injury 1982;14:252–4.

49. Keller A, Ortiz C, Wagner E, et al. Mini-open tenorrhaphy of acute Achilles tendon ruptures: medium-term follow-up of 100 cases. Am J Sports Med 2014;42:731–6.

50. Aibinder WR, Patel A, Arnouk J, et al. The rate of sural nerve violation using the Achillon device: a cadaveric study. Foot Ankle Int 2013;34:870–5.

51. Webb JM, Bannister GC. Percutaneous repair of the ruptured tendo Achillis. J Bone Joint Surg Br 1999;81:877–80.

52. Carmont MR, Maffulli N. Modified percutaneous repair of ruptured Achilles tendon. Knee Surg Sports Traumatol Arthrosc 2008;16:199–203.

53. Kocher MS, Bishop J, Marshall R, et al. Operative versus nonoperative management of acute Achilles tendon rupture: expected-value decision analysis. Am J Sports Med 2002;30:783–90.

54. Soroceanu A, Sidhwa F, Aarabi S, et al. Surgical versus nonsurgical treatment of acute Achilles tendon rupture: a meta-analysis of randomized trials. J Bone Joint Surg Am 2012;94:2136–43.

55. Young SW, Patel A, Zhu M, et al. Weight-bearing in the nonoperative treatment of acute Achilles tendon ruptures: a randomized controlled trial. J Bone Joint Surg Am 2014;96:1073–9.

56. Healy B, Beasley R, Weatherall M. Venous thromboembolism following prolonged cast immobilisation for injury to the tendo Achillis. J Bone Joint Surg Br 2010;92: 646–50.

57. Lapidus LJ, Rosfors S, Ponzer S, et al. Prolonged thromboprophylaxis with dalteparin after surgical treatment of Achilles tendon rupture: a randomized, placebo-controlled study. J Orthop Trauma 2007;21:52–7.

58. Makhdom AM, Cota A, Saran N, et al. Incidence of symptomatic deep venous thrombosis after Achilles tendon rupture. J Foot Ankle Surg 2013;52:584–7.

59. Nilsson-Helander K, Thurin A, Karlsson J, et al. High incidence of deep venous thrombosis after Achilles tendon rupture: a prospective study. Knee Surg Sports Traumatol Arthrosc 2009;17:1234–8.

60. Patel A, Ogawa B, Charlton T, et al. Incidence of deep vein thrombosis and pulmonary embolism after Achilles tendon rupture. Clin Orthop Relat Res 2012;470: 270–4.

61. Wysowski DK, Nourjah P, Swartz L. Bleeding complications with warfarin use - A prevalent adverse effect resulting in regulatory action. Arch Intern Med 2007;167: 1414–9.

62. Saragas NP, Ferrao PN. The incidence of venous thromboembolism in patients undergoing surgery for acute Achilles tendon ruptures. Foot Ankle Surg 2011; 17:263–5.

63. Wallace RG, Heyes GJ, Michael AL. The non-operative functional management of patients with a rupture of the tendo Achillis leads to low rates of re-rupture. J Bone Joint Surg Br 2011;93:1362–6.

Chronic Achilles Tendon Disorders

Tendinopathy and Chronic Rupture

Nicola Maffulli, MD, MS, PhD, FRCS(Orth)[a,b,*], Alessio Giai Via, MD[c], Francesco Oliva, MD, PhD[c]

KEYWORDS

- Achilles tendinopathy • Chronic Achilles tendon rupture • Neglected ruptures
- Mini-invasive surgery

KEY POINTS

- The management of Achilles tendinopathy is primarily conservative. Eccentric exercise and shock waves have proved to be effective.
- Surgery is recommended after 6 months of conservative treatment in nonresponder patients. Both open and mini-invasive surgical techniques have been described. Good results and lower rate of complications have been reported with minimally invasive Achilles tendon stripping and percutaneous longitudinal tenotomies.
- Neglected Achilles tendon ruptures have been reported up to 20% of cases. The diagnosis is more difficult, and management is technically more demanding than primary repair of acute rupture.
- Peroneus brevis tendon transfer is an effective surgical technique for neglected Achilles tendon rupture. If tendon gap is greater than 6 cm, a free gracilis autograft is indicated.

INTRODUCTION

Achilles tendinopathy (AT) occurs in athletic and sedentary people. The incidence in top level runners has been estimated between 7% and 9%,[1] and 30% of patients have a sedentary lifestyle.[2] The etiopathogenesis remains unclear. It is currently considered multifactorial and the interaction between intrinsic and extrinsic factors has been postulated.[3]

[a] Department of Musculoskeletal Disorders, School of Medicine and Surgery, University of Salerno, Via Allende, Baronissi, Salerno 84081, Italy; [b] Department of Musculoskeletal Disorders, Centre for Sports and Exercise Medicine, Mile End Hospital, Barts and the London School of Medicine and Dentistry, Mary University of London, 275 Bancroft Road, London E1 4DG, UK; [c] Department of Orthopaedic and Traumatology, School of Medicine, University of Rome "Tor Vergata", Viale Oxford 81, Rome 00133, Italy
* Corresponding author. Department of Musculoskeletal Disorders, School of Medicine and Surgery, University of Salerno, Via Allende, Baronissi, Salerno 84081, Italy.
E-mail address: n.maffulli@qmul.ac.uk

Clin Sports Med 34 (2015) 607–624
http://dx.doi.org/10.1016/j.csm.2015.06.010
0278-5919/15/$ – see front matter © 2015 Elsevier Inc. All rights reserved.

Changes in training pattern, poor technique, previous injuries, footwear, and environmental factors, such as training on hard, slippery, or slanting surfaces, are extrinsic factors that may predispose the athlete to AT.[3] Dysfunction of the gastrocnemius-soleus, age, body weight and height, pes cavus, marked forefoot varus, and lateral instability of the ankle have also been recognized as possible risk factors.[3] Fluoroquinolones and corticosteroids have been implicated as risk factors in tendinopathy. Ciprofloxacin causes enhanced interleukin-1b–mediated matrix metalloproteinase (MMP)-3 release, inhibits tenocyte proliferation, and, as corticosteroids, reduces the collagen and matrix synthesis.[4]

The Achilles tendon is not a static and inert tissue, and the tendon extracellular matrix (ECM) is a dynamic structure constantly remodeled, with rates of turnover depending on loading forces. ECM is the substrate to which cells adhere, migrate, and differentiate. It imparts information to cells and tissues by providing cell-binding motifs in its own proteins or by presenting growth factors and morphogens to the cells. Many studies currently advocate the importance of ECM for the homeostasis of connective tissue, and its physiologic and pathologic modifications seem the most important intrinsic factors involved in tendinopathies and tendon ruptures.[5] The turnover of ECM in normal tendon is mediated by MMPs,[6] in particular MMP-1, MMP-2, and MMP-3.[7] They are able to denature collagen type I. After tendon rupture, activity of MMP-1 increases, whereas a reduction of MMP-2 and MMP-3 have been showed.[8] An increase in MMP-1 activity and degradation of the collagen type I network is a potential cause of the weakening of the tendon and it may contribute to rupture. These findings may represent a failure of the normal matrix remodeling process. Transglutaminase (TGs) are also implicated in the formation of hard tissue development, matrix maturation, and mineralization.[9] Nine different TGs have been found in mammalians. TG2, also known as tissue TG, is widely distributed within many connective tissues, and it is implicated in organogenesis, tissue repair, and tissue stabilization. An animal model showed a reduction of TG2 protein expression in an injured supraspinatus tendon.[10] TG is important in maintaining the structural integrity of tendons thanks to its mechanical or cross-linking function in normal condition, and the fall of TG2 may mean the exhaustion of the reparative tendon's capabilities.

Metabolic diseases seem to play a role. The role of hormonal and metabolic diseases, such as diabetes mellitus,[11] hypercholesterolemia, and obesity, has been recently investigated.[12,13] The relationship between thyroid disorders and joint pain has been suspected since the late 1920s,[14] but it has not been systematically investigated. Thyroid hormones play an essential role in the development and metabolism of many tissues. Thyroxine (T4) is important for collagen synthesis and ECM metabolism. A recent study demonstrated that the thyroid hormones nuclear receptors are present on tenocytes, and that, in vitro, thyroid hormones enhance tenocytes growth and counteract apoptosis in healthy tenocytes isolated from tendon in a dose- and time-dependent manner.[15] Hypothyroidism causes accumulation of glycosaminoglycans in the ECM, which may predispose to tendinopathy and tendon ruptures. Diabetes mellitus is a chronic metabolic disease and patients with diabetes are prone to long-term complications that drastically reduce quality of life. The pathogenesis of diabetic complications is multifactorial and advanced glycation end-products (AGEs) play a central role.[16] Protein glycation is a spontaneous reaction that occurs in the presence of glucose, and it is directly proportional to the blood level of glucose. Glycated proteins can produce further reactions developing protein cross-linking. Collagen proteins are particularly susceptible to AGE formation, because of their long half-life, and this process may be involved in physiopathology of tendinopathy.[17] A recent animal study showed that AGE-related collagen cross-links alter biologic and mechanical properties of tendons.[18] The authors found that induction of AGEs inhibits sliding between collagen fibers, and that this matrix level change lies beneath reduced viscous properties of the tendon tissue. When a stretch is applied to a normal tendon, it responds with collagen fibril sliding more than with fiber stretch.[19] AGE tendons demonstrated a dominant fiber stretch relative to fiber sliding, a nearly complete removal of stress relaxation behavior, significantly altered failure stress, and a significantly altered yield behavior.[18] Thus, the formation of AGEs probably change the way tendon reacts to loading. Tendons try to compensate this loss of function by increasing collagen fiber stretch, which may have potentially important implications for predisposing to damage during everyday use.

THE ORIGIN OF PAIN

Although significant advances have been made in terms of understanding the pathologic changes in ECM and cells, relatively little is known about the role of neuronal regulation in tendinopathy, and the source of pain associated with mid-portion AT has not yet been clarified. The presence of pain in tendinopathy not only requires mechanical changes, but also alterations in the way the local cells and the peripheral nerves react to this change. Recent research identified the peripheral and central pain processing pathways as an important factor in the pathogenesis of painful human tendinopathy and changes in the peripheral neuronal phenotype may be the primary source of pain.[20] The term "peripheral neuronal phenotype" refers to specific characteristics of the peripheral nervous system including nerves, neuronal mediators, and receptors in peripheral tissue. Ectopic neural ingrowth has been clearly shown in some painful conditions, such as osteoarthritis,[21] degenerative spinal disease,[22] and rotator cuff tear,[23] and it has been postulated as a mechanism of pain generation. Even if the evidence of increased neural ingrowth in AT is weaker, Alfredson and colleagues[24] demonstrated increased ingrowth. A recent systematic review of literature showed that the peripheral neuronal phenotype is altered in tendinopathy.[20] The authors found strong evidence of an upregulation of the glutaminergic system in painful human tendinopathy and weaker, but still suggestive, evidence that changes in the peripheral neuronal phenotype were related to variations in pain symptomatology among patients. Glutamate levels have been shown to be increased in several painful musculoskeletal disorders.[25] It is a key metabolite and neurotransmitter involved in the transmission of pain. Glutamate NMDAR1 receptors have been frequently noted in morphologically altered tenocytes in tendon tissue proper and in the peritendinous connective tissue.[26] There is also some evidence for upregulation of the substance P/CGRP system, which has been implicated in pain generation in animal models and human disease.[20] The neuropeptides substance P and CGRP are also vasodilators and seem to have important roles in tissue healing.[27] Some studies also found an increased overall neural ingrowth in tendinopathy versus control.[24,28]

CLINICAL PRESENTATION AND DIAGNOSIS

Clinical history and examination are essential for diagnosis. AT is a clinical condition characterized by pain, swelling (diffuse or localized), and impaired performance of the Achilles tendon.[29] Tendinopathy of mid-portion of Achilles tendon accounts for 55% to 65% of all injuries, and in approximately 20% to 25% of cases an insertional AT can be diagnosed. Pain is the cardinal symptom of AT. It occurs at the beginning and a short while after the end of a training session. As the pathologic process progresses, pain may occur during the entire exercise session, and in severe cases it may interfere with activities of daily living. Clinical examination is the best diagnostic tool. Location of pain 2 to 6 cm above the insertion into the calcaneum and pain on palpation are reliable and accurate tests for diagnosis.[30] An evaluation of standing posture, balance, and anatomic mal-alignment is usually performed during clinical examination.

Plain radiography is used to diagnose associated or incidental bony abnormalities.[31] Ultrasound is an effective imaging method because it correlates well with the histopathologic findings despite being operator-dependent.[32] MRI studies should be performed only if the ultrasound scan remains unclear. MRI provides extensive information on the internal morphology of the tendon and the surrounding structures and is useful in evaluating the various stages of chronic degeneration and in differentiating between peritendinitis and tendinopathy. Areas of mucoid degeneration are shown on MRI as a zone of high signal intensity on T1- and T2-weighted images.[33]

MANAGEMENT OF ACHILLES TENDINOPATHY

The management of AT lacks evidence-based support, and patients are at risk of long-term morbidity with unpredictable clinical outcome.[31] The management is primarily conservative and many patients respond well to conservative measures. Eccentric exercise and shock waves have proved to be effective for the treatment of AT.[34]

However, conservative management is unsuccessful in 24% to 45.5% of patients, and surgery is recommended after 6 months of conservative management.[35] Long-standing AT is associated with poor postoperative results, with a greater rate of reoperation before reaching an acceptable outcome.[25] Frequency of surgery has been shown to increase with patient age, duration of symptoms, and occurrence of tendinopathic changes.[36,37] Both open and mini-invasive surgical techniques have been described for treatment of the mid-portion AT.

High Volume Injections

High-volume image-guided injections target the neurovascular bundles growing from the paratenon into the AT. High-volume image-guided injections produce local mechanical effects, causing the neovascularity to stretch, break, or occlude, and pain relief is explained by the destruction of these sensory nerves.[2] Denervation of the Achilles tendon by releasing the paratenon may be the most important part of this procedure. Several substances have been injected in and around tendons including normal saline, corticosteroids, and local anesthetic.[38,39] Platelet-rich plasma application did not show the expected benefits in Achilles tendon.[40] The injection is performed under ultrasound guidance to avoid intratendinous injections, which can be particularly harmful if corticosteroid is used. Patients are allowed to walk on the injected leg immediately, but they are strictly advised to refrain from high-impact activity for 72 hours. After this period, they are instructed to restart eccentric loading physiotherapy regime twice daily until they stop their sporting career. Good results have been reported with this technique at short-term follow-up.[41]

SURGERY FOR MID-PORTION ACHILLES TENDINOPATHY
Minimally Invasive Stripping for Chronic Achilles Tendinopathy

The patient is placed prone with the lower limb draped in the usual fashion and the ankles clear of the operating table. Four skin incisions are made. The first two incisions are 0.5 cm longitudinal incisions at the proximal origin of the Achilles tendon, just medial and lateral to the origin of the tendon. The other two incisions are also 0.5 cm long and longitudinal, but 1 cm distal to the distal end of the tendon insertion on the calcaneus. A mosquito is inserted in the proximal incisions (**Fig. 1**), and the

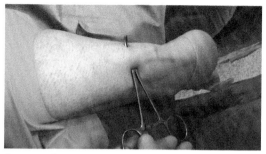

Fig. 1. A mosquito is inserted in the proximal incisions.

Achilles tendon is freed of the peritendinous adhesions. A #1 unmounted Ethibond (Ethicon, Somerville, NJ) suture thread is inserted proximally, passing through the two proximal incisions (**Fig. 2**). The Ethibond is retrieved from the distal incisions (**Fig. 3**), over the posterior aspect of the Achilles tendon. Using a gentle see-saw motion the Ethibond suture thread is made to slide posterior to the tendon (**Fig. 4**), which is stripped and freed from the fat of Kager triangle.

The procedure is repeated for the anterior aspect of the Achilles tendon. If necessary, using a #11 blade, longitudinal percutaneous tenotomies parallel to the tendon fibers are made. The subcutaneous and subcuticular tissues are closed in a routine fashion, and Mepore (Molnlycke Health Care, Gothenburg, Sweden) dressings are applied to the skin. A removable scotch cast support with Velcro straps can be applied if deemed necessary.

Postoperatively, patients are allowed to mobilize fully weight bearing. After 2 weeks patients start physiotherapy, focusing on proprioception, plantar flexion of the ankle, inversion, and eversion.

The rationale behind the present management modality is that the sliding of the suture breaks the neovessels and the accompanying nerve supply decreasing pain. Classically, open surgery has provided good results. However, wound complications can occur with these procedures. Minimal invasive technique reduces the risks of infection, is technically easy to master, and inexpensive. It may provide greater potential for the management of recalcitrant AT by breaking neovessels and the accompanying nerve supply to the tendon.[42] It can be associated with other minimally invasive procedures to optimize results.

Percutaneous Longitudinal Tenotomies

Percutaneous longitudinal tenotomy can be used when there is no paratenon involvement and when the intratendinous lesion is less than 2.5 cm long. The procedure can

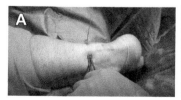 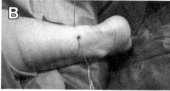

Fig. 2. (*A*) #1 Ethibond wire is inserted through the two proximal incisions. (*B*) The wire is passed the anterior aspect of the Achilles tendon.

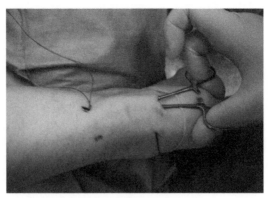

Fig. 3. The Ethibond is retrieved from the distal incisions.

be performed under ultrasound guidance that is able to confirm the precise location of intratendinous lesions and produced similar results to open procedures.[43]

Patients are operated as day cases. The patient lies prone on the operating table with the feet protruding beyond the edge, and the ankles resting on a sandbag. A bloodless field is not necessary. The tendon is accurately palpated, and the area of maximum swelling and/or tenderness marked, and checked again by ultrasound scanning. The skin and the subcutaneous tissues over the Achilles tendon are infiltrated with 10 to 15 mL of plain 1% lignocaine (Lignocaine Hydrochloride, Evans Medical Ltd, Leatherhead, England). A #11 surgical scalpel blade is inserted parallel to the long axis of the tendon fibers in the marked area in the center of the area of tendinopathy. The cutting edge of the blade points caudally and penetrates the whole thickness of the tendon (**Fig. 5**). Keeping the blade still, a full passive ankle plantar flexion movement is produced (**Fig. 6**). The scalpel blade is then retracted to the surface of the tendon, inclined 45° on the sagittal axis, and the blade is inserted medially through the original tenotomy (**Fig. 7**). Keeping the blade still, a full passive ankle flexion is produced. The whole procedure is repeated inclining the blade 45° laterally to the original tenotomy, inserting it laterally through the original tenotomy. Keeping the blade still, a

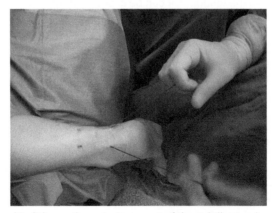

Fig. 4. The Ethibond is slid over the anterior aspect of the Achilles tendon with a gentle see-saw motion. The whole process is repeated over the posterior aspect of the tendon.

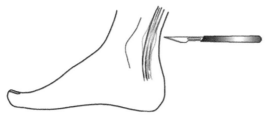

Fig. 5. A #11 scalpel blade inserted into the predetermined area with sharp edge pointing cranially.

full passive ankle flexion is produced. The blade is then partially retracted to the posterior surface of the Achilles tendon, reversed 180°, so that its cutting edge now points cranially, and the whole procedure repeated, taking care to dorsiflex the ankle passively. Preliminary cadaveric studies showed that a tenotomy 2.8 cm long on average is thus obtained through a stab wound in the main body of the tendon.[44] A Steri-Strip (3M Health Care, St Paul, MN, USA) can be applied on the stab wound. The wound is dressed with cotton swabs, and a few layers of cotton wool and a crepe bandage are applied. Active dorsiflexion and plantar flexion of the foot are encouraged early after surgery. Patients are allowed to walk using elbow crutches and weight bearing is allowed after 2 or 3 days as tolerated. Stationary bicycling and isometric, concentric, and eccentric strengthening of the calf muscles are started under physiotherapy guidance after 4 weeks. Swimming and water running are encouraged from the second week. Gentle running is started 4 to 6 weeks after the procedure, and mileage gradually increased.

We reported excellent and good results in 63% of athletes with unilateral AT treated with ultrasound-guided percutaneous longitudinal tenotomy after failure of conservative management, without experiencing significant complications.[43] This technique is simple, can be performed on an outpatient basis, requires minimal follow-up care, does not hinder further surgery if necessary, and should be considered in the management of chronic AT after failure of conservative management.[45]

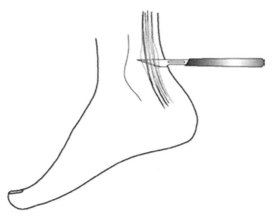

Fig. 6. The blade penetrating the whole thickness of the Achilles tendon and a full passive ankle dorsiflexion movement is produced.

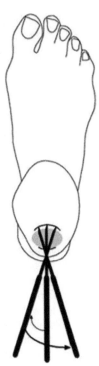

Fig. 7. The procedure is repeated with blade inclining 45° medial and 45° lateral to the original tenotomy.

Open Surgery

Under local with regional or general anesthesia, the patient is placed prone with the ankles clear of the operating table. A tourniquet is applied to the limb to be operated on. The limb is exsanguinated, and the tourniquet is inflated to 250 mm Hg. The incision is made on the medial side of the tendon to avoid injury to the sural nerve and short saphenous vein. The skin edge of the incision should be handled with extreme care because wound healing problems are serious problems. The paratenon is identified and incised. In patients with evidence of coexisting paratendinopathy, the scarred and thickened tissue is generally excised. Based on preoperative imaging studies, the tendon is incised sharply in line with the tendon fiber bundles. The tendinopathic tissue can be identified because it generally has lost its shiny appearance and it frequently contains disorganized fiber bundles that have more of a "crabmeat" appearance. This tissue is sharply excised (**Fig. 8**). The remaining gap can be repaired using a side-to-side repair, but we leave it unsutured. If significant loss of tendon tissue occurs during the débridement, a tendon augmentation or transfer can be considered, even if we rarely undertake this additional procedure. Then the subcutaneous tissues is sutured with absorbable material, the skin edges are juxtaposed with Steri-Strips, and a routine compressive bandage applied. The limb is immobilized in a below-knee synthetic weight-bearing cast with the foot plantigrade.

A period of initial splinting and crutch walking is generally used to allow pain and swelling to subside after surgery. After 14 days, the wound is inspected and motion exercises are initiated. The patient is encouraged to start daily active and passive

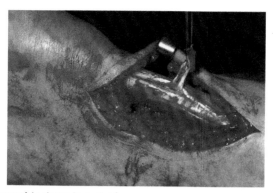

Fig. 8. The tendinopathic tissue is excised.

ankle range-of-motion exercises. The use of a removable walker boot is helpful during this phase. Weight bearing is not limited according to the degree of débridement needed at surgery, and early weight bearing is encouraged. However, extensive débridements associated with tendon transfers may require protected weight bearing for 4 to 6 weeks postoperatively. After 6 to 8 weeks more intensive strengthening exercises are started, gradually progressing to plyometrics and eventually running and jumping.

Successful results have been reported with this surgical procedure. A systematic review of literature showed successful results in more than 70% of cases,[45] but these relatively high success rates are not always observed in clinical practice, probably because of the poor method scores of many articles. Patients should be informed of the potential failure of the procedure, risk of wound complications, and at times prolonged recovery time. Possible complications of this surgical procedure are wound healing problems, infection, sural nerve injury, rupture of AT, and deep vein thrombosis.

CHRONIC ACHILLES TENDON RUPTURE

Achilles tendon ruptures are common injuries. Usually, they are not difficult to diagnose for experienced physicians, but it has been reported that the first examining physician can miss more than 20% of cases.[46] The diagnosis of chronic Achilles tendon rupture is more difficult than acute rupture. Although in acute tendon ruptures a gap is usually palpable, this gap may be absent in chronic ruptures because it is usually bridged by scar tissue. Active plantar flexion of the foot is usually preserved because of the action of tibialis posterior, the peroneal tendons, and the long toe flexors, but limp may be present. The calf squeeze test, first described by Simmonds[47] in 1957, but often credited to Thompson who redescribed it in 1962, is performed with the patient prone and the ankle clear of the edge of the examination table. The examiner squeezes the fleshy part of the calf, causing the deformation of the soleus and resulting in plantar flexion of the foot if the Achilles tendon is intact. The affected leg should be compared with the contralateral leg. The knee flexion test[48] is performed with the patient prone and ankles clear of the table. The patient is asked to actively flex the knee to 90°. During this movement the foot on the affected side falls into neutral or dorsiflexion and a rupture of the Achilles tendon can be diagnosed (**Fig. 9**). A false-positive may occur when there is neurologic weakness of the Achilles tendon.

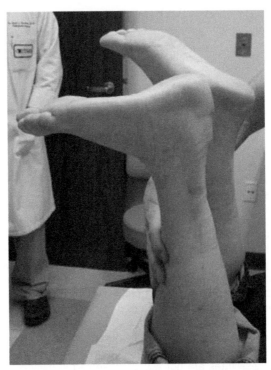

Fig. 9. The knee flexion test is performed with the patient prone and the knee flexed to 90° degrees.

Imaging is useful for diagnosis of Achilles tendon chronic ruptures. Plain lateral radiographs may reveal an irregular configuration of the fat-filled triangular space anterior to the Achilles tendon and between the posterior aspect of the tibia and superior aspect of the calcaneus (this space is known as the triangle of Kager). Ultrasonography of a chronic rupture usually demonstrates an acoustic vacuum with thick irregular edges. T1-weighted MRIs show disruption of signal within the tendon substance, whereas T2-weighted images show generalized high signal intensity.

MANAGEMENT OF CHRONIC ACHILLES TENDON RUPTURE

The management of chronic Achilles tendon tears is technically more demanding than primary repair of acute rupture because the tendon ends normally are retracted and the status of the surrounding soft tissues makes primary repair increasingly more difficult. Operative procedures for reconstruction of chronic Achilles tendon ruptures include flap tissue turn down using one and two flaps, local tendon transfer, autologous free tendon grafts, and allografts.[49–51] Complications, especially wound breakdown and infection, are frequent following open procedures. However, given the lack of prospective randomized trials and the small size of studies, a gold standard procedure is lacking. A less invasive peroneus brevis reconstruction technique using two para-midline incisions has been described. This technique allows reconstruction of the Achilles tendon preserving skin integrity over the site most prone to wound breakdown. Although not the authors' preference, the transfer of the flexor hallucis longus (FHL) has also been described in the treatment of chronic Achilles rupture.[52]

FHL is a strong, long tendon and allows bridging of large gaps. The muscle itself is able to produce force that supplements the strength exerted by the gastrocneus-soleus complex. We prefer not to use this tendon if the reconstruction is performed in running and sporting athletes, who necessitate being able to "grip" the ground in a powerful fashion, and therefore the loss of flexion of the interphalangeal joint of the hallux would be detrimental to performance. However, in patients where this feature is not of paramount importance, FHL transfer can be used with excellent results.[53,54] If the gap is greater than 6 cm despite maximal plantar flexion of the ankle and traction on the tendon stumps, peroneus brevis is not sufficient to fill the gap and ipsilateral hamstring tendon graft is indicated.[55]

Peroneus Brevis Tendon Transfer for Chronic Achilles Tendon Rupture

Under general anesthesia, the patient is placed prone with the ankles clear of the operating table. A tourniquet is applied to the limb to be operated on. The limb is exsanguinated, and the tourniquet is inflated to 250 mm Hg. Three skin incisions are made. The first incision is a 5-cm longitudinal incision, made 2 cm proximal and just medial to the palpable end of the residual tendon (**Fig. 10**). The second incision is 3 cm long and is also longitudinal. It is 2 cm distal and lateral to the distal end of the tendon rupture. Care is taken to prevent damage to the sural nerve, which lies 18.8 mm lateral to the tendon within proximity to the tendon insertion site and medial to the tendon 9.8 cm above the calcaneus, by making this incision as close as possible to the anterior aspect of the lateral border of the Achilles tendon. The third incision is a 2-cm longitudinal incision at the base of the fifth metatarsal (**Fig. 11**). The distal Achilles tendon

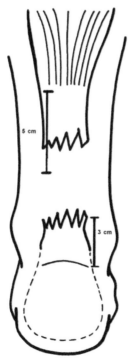

Fig. 10. The first incision is at the proximal end of the palpable tendon stump, as near as possible the medial border of the Achilles tendon. The second incision is lateral to the distal end of the tendon stump.

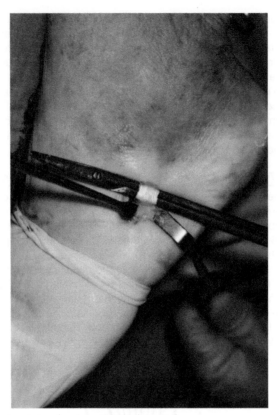

Fig. 11. Peroneus brevis tendon insertion is dissected.

stump is mobilized, freeing it of all the peritendinous adhesions, particularly on its lateral aspect. This allowed access to the base of the lateral aspect of the distal tendon close to its insertion. The ruptured tendon end is then resected back to healthy tendon and a #1 Vicryl locking suture is run along the free tendon edge to prevent separation of the bundles. The proximal tendon is mobilized from the proximal wound, any adhesions are divided, and further soft tissue release anterior to the soleus and gastrocnemius muscles allowed maximal excursion, minimizing the gap between the two tendon stumps. The ankle is then plantar flexed fully and the gap between the stumps is measured. If it is less that 6 cm, we bridge it using the peroneus brevis tendon.

The peroneus brevis tendon is identified through the incision on the lateral border of the foot at its insertion at the base of the fifth metatarsal. The tendon is exposed, and a #1 Vicryl locking suture is applied to the tendon end before release from the metatarsal base. The peroneus brevis tendon is identified at the base of the distal incision of the Achilles tendon after incision of the deep fascia overlying the peroneal muscles compartment. It is then withdrawn through the distal wound. This may take significant force because there may be tendinous strands between the two peroneal tendons distally. The muscular portion of the peroneus brevis is then mobilized proximally to allow increased excursion of the tendon of peroneus brevis.

A longitudinal tenotomy parallel to the tendon fibers is made through both stumps of the tendon. A clamp is used to develop the plane, from lateral to medial, in the distal stump of the Achilles tendon, and the peroneus brevis graft is passed through the tenotomy. With the ankle in maximal plantar flexion, a #1 Vicryl suture is used to suture the peroneus brevis to both sides of the distal stump. The peroneus brevis tendon is then passed beneath the intact skin bridge into the proximal incision and passed from medial to lateral through a transverse tenotomy in the proximal stump; it is further secured with #1 Vicryl. Finally, the peroneus brevis tendon is sutured back onto itself on the lateral side of the proximal incision (**Fig. 12**). The tourniquet is deflated.

The wounds are closed with subcuticular 2.0 Vicryl, and Steri-Strips are applied, taking care to avoid the risk of postoperative hematoma and to minimize wound breakdown. A below-knee weight bearing synthetic cast is applied with the foot in maximal plantar flexion.

Free Gracilis Tendon Graft for Chronic Rupture of the Achilles Tendon

A longitudinal incision about 3 to 5 cm long is performed 2 cm above the palpable gap, medial to the midline of the tendon. A second 3-cm longitudinal incision, 2 cm distal to the distal end of the rupture, lateral to the midline, is performed, taking care to prevent damage to the sural nerve. Through the proximal incision, the peritendinous adhesions are gently dissected and a partial resection of the proximal tendon stump is performed to expose the healthy portion of the tendon. The free tendon edge is sutured with a #1 Vicryl locking suture to prevent separation of the bundles. The soft tissues anterior to the soleus and gastrocnemius are released to better mobilize the proximal stump of the tendon and minimize the gap. The distal stump is mobilized. A loop of polyglyco-nate is used in a Krackow configuration to impose adequate traction to the proximal stump of the tendon. Moderate traction to the proximal stump is applied taking care

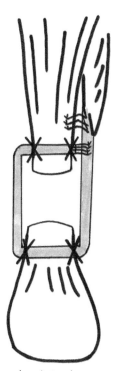

Fig. 12. Final suture of the peroneus brevis tendon.

to maintain the ankle in maximal plantar flexion. The ipsilateral semitendinosus tendon is harvested through a 2-cm transverse incision over the anteromedial aspect of the tibia in proximity to the pes anserinus insertion site. Once the two ends of the semitendinosus graft have been tubularized using a 1-0 Vicryl whipstitch, the graft is passed into the substance of the proximal stump of the Achilles tendon about 2 cm above the tendon end through a small incision and secured to the Achilles tendon at both the entry and exit points with a 3-0 Vicryl suture (**Fig. 13**). Then, the graft is delivered to the distal incision beneath the intact skin bridge and passed through a transverse tenotomy into the distal stump from the medial to the lateral side (**Fig. 14**). With the ankle in maximal plantar flexion, the semitendinosus tendon is sutured to the entry and exit points of the distal stump using a 3-0 Vicryl suture, and the reconstruction is tensioned with the ankle in maximum equinus. One extremity of the semitendinosus tendon graft is moved again to the proximal incision, beneath the intact skin bridge and passed into the proximal stump through a transverse tenotomy from medial to lateral. Similarly, the other extremity of the semitendinosus tendon is passed again into the distal stump from medial to lateral.

POSTOPERATIVE CARE

Patients are usually discharged on the day after surgery after having been taught to use crutches by an orthopedic physiotherapist. Thromboprophylaxis is provided. Patients are told to bear weight on the operated leg as able, but to keep it elevated as much as possible at home for the first 2 postoperative weeks. The cast is removed at the second postoperative week, and a synthetic anterior below-knee slab is applied with the foot in maximal equinus. Patients can graduate to full weight bearing as soon as comfort allows. A trained physiotherapist supervises the introduction of gentle mobilization exercises of the ankle, isometric contraction of the gastrocneus-soleus complex, and gentle concentric contraction of the calf muscles. Inversion and eversion of the ankle is also encouraged. At 6 weeks postoperatively, the patient is followed up and the anterior slab removed. Physiotherapists supervise gradual stretching and strengthening exercises. Cycling and swimming are started at 8 weeks postoperatively. Patients are allowed to return to their normal activities at the fifth postoperative month.

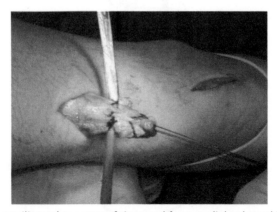

Fig. 13. The free gracilis tendon autograft is passed from medial to lateral into the proximal stump.

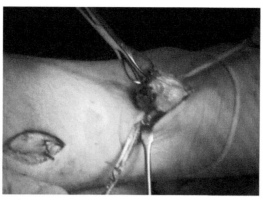

Fig. 14. The graft is delivered to the distal incision beneath the intact skin bridge and passed into the distal Achilles tendon stump.

OUTCOMES

Good results have been reported in 32 patients who underwent surgical reconstruction of chronic Achilles tendon tear using peroneus brevis tendon transfer.[56] At final follow-up, all patients were able to walk on tiptoes and to perform at least 10 single-legged heel lifts on the affected leg. No patient used a heel lift or walked with a visible limp and they returned to their preinjury working occupation. No reruptures have been reported. However, despite subjective patient satisfaction, the maximum calf circumference remained significantly decreased in the operated leg and the operated limb was significantly less strong than the nonoperated one.

The results of 26 patients who underwent minimally invasive semitendinosus autologous graft reconstruction for chronic ruptures to the Achilles tendon have been recently reported.[57] The average follow-up was 8.2 years. All patients returned to their preinjury working occupation, and 22 patients returned to their preinjury level of activity at a mean of 6.7 months after surgery. At final follow-up, the maximum calf circumference was significantly higher than preoperatively but significantly lower than the contralateral side, but the isometric plantar flexion strength in the operated leg was lower than in the uninjured one.

SUMMARY

Although AT has been extensively studied, there is a clear lack of properly conducted scientific research to clarify its cause, pathology, and natural history. The cause is currently considered multifactorial. However, the precise role that each predisposing factor plays has still to be understood. The management of AT lacks evidence-based support, and tendinopathy sufferers are at risk of long-term morbidity with unpredictable clinical outcome. Most patients respond to conservative measures, but if patients do not improve after 3 to 6 months of conservative management surgery is recommended. The surgical procedures are commonly successful, but patients should be informed of the potential failure of the procedure, risk of wound complications, and at times prolonged recovery time. The management of chronic Achilles tendon rupture is technically demanding because of tendon retraction, muscle atrophy, and the skin contracture that is frequently present around the tendon. Complications, such as wound breakdown and infection, are frequent following open procedures. Peroneus brevis reconstruction technique using two para-midline incisions is safe, less invasive, and reliable, and good results have been reported in recent literature. If the tendon gap is higher than 6 cm, a free gracilis autograft is indicated.

REFERENCES

1. Rompe JD, Furia JP, Maffulli N. Mid-portion Achilles tendinopathy: current options for treatment. Disabil Rehabil 2008;30:1666–76.
2. Ames PR, Longo UG, Denaro V, et al. Achilles tendon problems: not just an orthopaedic issue. Disabil Rehabil 2008;30:1646–50.
3. Maffulli N, Sharma P, Luscombe KL. Achilles tendinopathy: aetiology and management. J R Soc Med 2004;97:472–6.
4. Parmar C, Meda KP. Achilles tendon rupture associated with combination therapy of levofloxacin and steroid in four patients and a review of the literature. Foot Ankle Int 2007;28:1287–9.
5. Modesti A, Oliva F. All is around ECM of tendons!? Muscles Ligaments Tendons J 2013;3:1.
6. Dalton S, Cawston TE, Riley GP, et al. Human shoulder tendon biopsy samples in organ culture produce procollagenase and tissue inhibitor of metalloproteinases. Ann Rheum Dis 1995;54:571–7.
7. Choi HR, Kondo S, Hirose K, et al. Expression and enzymatic activity of MMP-2 during healing process of the acute suprasupinatus tendon tear in rabbits. J Orthop Res 2002;20:927–33.
8. Riley GP, Curry V, DeGroot J, et al. Matrix metalloproteinase activities and their relationship with collagen remodelling in tendon pathology. Matrix Biol 2002;21:185–95.
9. Tarantino U, Oliva F, Taurisano G, et al. FXIIIA and TGF-beta over-expression produces normal musculoskeletal phenotype in TG2-/-mice. Amino Acids 2009;36:679–84.
10. Oliva F, Zocchi L, Codispoti A, et al. Transglutaminases expression in human supraspinatus tendon ruptures and in mouse tendons. Biochem Biophys Res Commun 2009;20:887–91.
11. de Oliveira RR, Lemos A, de Castro Silveira PV, et al. Alterations of tendons in patients with diabetes mellitus: a systematic review. Diabet Med 2011;28:886–95.
12. Oliva F, Via AG, Maffulli N. Physiopathology of intratendinous calcific deposition. BMC Med 2012;10:95.
13. Oliva F, Berardi AC, Misiti S, et al. Thyroid hormones and tendon: current views and future perspectives. Concise review. Muscles Ligaments Tendons J 2013;3:201–3.
14. Duncan WS. The relationship of hyperthysoidism to joint conditions. JAMA 1928;91:1779.
15. Oliva F, Berardi AC, Misiti S, et al. Thyroid hormones enhance growth and counteract apoptosis in human tenocytes isolated from rotator cuff tendons. Cell Death Dis 2013;4:e705.
16. Ahmed N. Advanced glycation endproducts: role in pathology of diabetic complications. Diabetes Res Clin Pract 2005;67:3–21.
17. Reigle KL, Di Lullo G, Turner KR, et al. Non-enzymatic glycation of type I collagen diminishes collagen–proteoglycan binding and weakens cell adhesion. J Cell Biochem 2008;104:1684–98.
18. Li Y, Fessel G, Georgiadis M, et al. Advanced glycation end-products diminish tendon collagen fiber sliding. Matrix Biol 2013;32:169–77.
19. Screen HR. Investigating load relaxation mechanics in tendon. J Mech Behav Biomed Mater 2008;1:51–8.

20. Dean BJ, Franklin SL, Carr AJ. The peripheral neuronal phenotype is important in the pathogenesis of painful human tendinopathy: a systematic review. Clin Orthop Relat Res 2013;471:3036–46.
21. Ghilardi JR, Freeman KT, Jimenez-Andrade JM, et al. Neuroplasticity of sensory and sympathetic nerve fibers in a mouse model of a painful arthritic joint. Arthritis Rheum 2012;64:2223–32.
22. Freemont AJ, Peacock TE, Goupille P, et al. Nerve ingrowth into diseased intervertebral disc in chronic back pain. Lancet 1997;350:178–81.
23. Xu Y, Bonar F, Murrell GA. Neoinnervation in rotator cuff tendinopathy. Sports Med Arthrosc 2011;19:354–9.
24. Alfredson H, Ohberg L, Forsgren S. Is vasculo-neural ingrowth the cause of pain in chronic Achilles tendinosis? An investigation using ultrasonography and colour Doppler, immunohistochemistry, and diagnostic injections. Knee Surg Sports Traumatol Arthrosc 2003;11:334–8.
25. Kreiner F, Galbo H. Elevated muscle interstitial levels of pain inducing substances in symptomatic muscles in patients with polymyalgia rheumatica. Pain 2011;152: 1127–32.
26. Schizas N, Weiss R, Lian O, et al. Glutamate receptors in tendinopathic patients. J Orthop Res 2012;30:1447–52.
27. Carlsson O, Schizas N, Li J, et al. Substance P injections enhance tissue proliferation and regulate sensory nerve ingrowth in rat tendon repair. Scand J Med Sci Sports 2011;21:562–9.
28. Lian O, Dahl J, Ackermann PW, et al. Pronociceptive and antinociceptive neuromediators in patellar tendinopathy. Am J Sports Med 2006;34:1801–8.
29. Maffulli N, Khan KM, Puddu G. Overuse tendon conditions: time to change a confusing terminology. Arthroscopy 1998;14:840–3.
30. Hutchison AM, Evans R, Bodger O, et al. What is the best clinical test for Achilles tendinopathy? Foot Ankle Surg 2013;19:112–7.
31. Maffulli N, Testa V, Capasso G, et al. Surgery for chronic Achilles tendinopathy yields worse results in nonathletic patients. Clin J Sport Med 2006;16:123–8.
32. Maffulli N, Wong J, Almekinders LC. Types and epidemiology of tendinopathy. Clin Sports Med 2003;22:675–92.
33. Rompe JD, Nafe B, Furia JP, et al. Eccentric loading, shock-wave treatment, or a wait-and-see policy for tendinopathy of the main body of tendo Achilles: a randomized controlled trial. Am J Sports Med 2007;35:374–83.
34. Frairia R, Berta L. Biological effects of extracorporeal shock waves on fibroblasts. A review. Muscles Ligaments Tendons J 2011;1:138–47.
35. Sayana MK, Maffulli N. Eccentric calf muscle training in non-athletic patients with Achilles tendinopathy. J Sci Med Sport 2007;10:52–8.
36. Maffulli N, Binfield P, Moore D. Surgical decompression of chronic central core lesions of the Achilles tendon. Am J Sports Med 1999;27:747–52.
37. Paavola MK, Paakkala T, Pasanen M, et al. Long term prognosis of patients with Achilles tendinopathy. An observational 8-year follow-up study. Am J Sports Med 2000;28:634–42.
38. Loppini M, Maffulli N. Conservative management of tendinopathy: an evidence-based approach. Muscles Ligaments Tendons J 2012;1:134–7.
39. Chan O, O'Dowd D, Padhiar N, et al. High volume image guided injections in chronic Achilles tendinopathy. Disabil Rehabil 2008;30:1697–708.
40. de Vos RJ, Weir A, van Schie HT, et al. Platelet-rich plasma injection for chronic Achilles tendinopathy: a randomized controlled trial. JAMA 2010;303: 144–9.

41. Maffulli N, Spiezia F, Longo UG, et al. High volume image guided injections for the management of chronic tendinopathy of the main body of the Achilles tendon. Phys Ther Sport 2013;14:163–7.

42. Longo UG, Ramamurthy C, Denaro V, et al. Minimally invasive stripping for chronic Achilles tendinopathy. Disabil Rehabil 2008;30:1709–13.

43. Testa V, Capasso G, Benazzo F, et al. Management of Achilles tendinopathy by ultrasound-guided percutaneous tenotomy. Med Sci Sports Exerc 2002;34: 573–80.

44. Maffulli N, Testa V, Capasso G, et al. Results of percutaneous longitudinal tenotomy for Achilles tendinopathy in middle- and long-distance runners. Am J Sports Med 1997;25:835–40.

45. Tallon C, Coleman BD, Khan KM, et al. Outcome of surgery for chronic Achilles tendinopathy: a critical review. Am J Sports Med 2001;29:315–20.

46. Maffulli N. Clinical tests in sports medicine: more on Achilles tendon. Br J Sports Med 1996;30:250.

47. Simmonds FA. The diagnosis of the ruptured Achilles tendon. Practitioner 1957; 179:56–8.

48. Matles AL. Rupture of the tendo Achilles: another diagnostic sign. Bull Hosp Joint Dis 1975;36:48–51.

49. Hadi M, Young J, Cooper L, et al. Surgical management of chronic ruptures of the Achilles tendon remains unclear: a systematic review of the management options. Br Med Bull 2013;108:95–114.

50. Young JS, Sayana MK, McClelland D, et al. Peroneus brevis tendon transfer for delayed Achilles tendon ruptures. Tech Foot Ankle Surg 2005;4:143–7.

51. Young J, Sayana MK, Maffulli N, et al. Technique of free gracilis tendon transfer for delayed rupture of the Achilles tendon. Tech Foot Ankle Surg 2005;4:148–53.

52. Neufeld SK, Farber DC. Tendon transfers in the treatment of Achilles' tendon disorders. Foot Ankle Clin 2014;19:73–86.

53. Mahajan RH, Dalal RB. Flexor hallucis longus tendon transfer for reconstruction of chronically ruptured Achilles tendons. J Orthop Surg (Hong Kong) 2009;17: 194–8.

54. Oksanen MM, Haapasalo HH, Elo PP, et al. Hypertrophy of the flexor hallucis longus muscle after tendon transfer in patients with chronic Achilles tendon rupture. Foot Ankle Surg 2014;20:253–7.

55. Maffulli N, Ajis A, Longo UG, et al. Chronic rupture of tendo Achilles. Foot Ankle Clin 2007;12:583–96.

56. Maffulli N, Spiezia F, Longo UG, et al. Less-invasive reconstruction of chronic Achilles tendon ruptures using a peroneus brevis tendon transfer. Am J Sports Med 2010;38:2304–12.

57. Maffulli N, Del Buono A, Spiezia F, et al. Less-invasive semitendinosus tendon graft augmentation for the reconstruction of chronic tears of the Achilles tendon. Am J Sports Med 2013;41:865–71.

Peroneal Tendon Disorders

Brent Roster, MD[a],*, Patrick Michelier, BS[b], Eric Giza, MD[c]

KEYWORDS

- Peroneal tendon • Peroneus brevis • Peroneus longus • POPS
- Tendon subluxation/dislocation • Peroneal tendon tears • Peroneal tendoscopy

KEY POINTS

- Pathology of the peroneal tendons must be considered in the differential diagnosis of the patient with lateral ankle pain.
- Symptomatic peroneal tendon injuries can be the result of both acute and chronic processes.
- Peroneal tendon injuries can often be resolved with nonoperative treatment, but if that fails, surgical intervention is usually successful.
- Any surgical treatment of peroneal tendon pathology must address not only the peroneal tendons but also any predisposing structural or anatomic abnormalities for the highest chance of success.

ANATOMY OF THE PERONEAL TENDONS

Knowledge of the anatomy of the peroneal tendons and their associated structures and restraints is critical to understanding their patterns of injury and pathology.

The peroneus brevis originates from the lower two-thirds of fibula and intermuscular septum and runs immediately posterior to the lateral malleolus, superficial to the calcaneofibular ligament, anterior to the peroneus longus tendon, and superior to peroneal tubercle of the calcaneus.[1] Both the peroneus brevis and longus tendons traverse the posterior aspect of the fibula in the retromalleolar sulcus; an anatomic study revealed that this sulcus is concave in 82%, flat in 11%, and convex in 7%.[1] Retromalleolar sulcus shape has not been shown to be significantly correlated with peroneal tendon subluxation/dislocation.[2] It has been hypothesized that the pressure from the tendons is responsible for the sulcus in the distal fibula.[3,4] The peroneus brevis tendon has a flattened ovoid shape and inserts onto the styloid process on the base of the fifth metatarsal.[1]

[a] Missoula Bone & Joint, 2360 Mullan Road, Suite C, Missoula, MT 59808, USA; [b] University of California Davis School of Medicine, 4860 Y Street, Suite 3800, Sacramento, CA 95817, USA; [c] Department of Orthopaedic Surgery, University of California Davis, 4860 Y Street, Suite 3800, Sacramento, CA 95817, USA
* Corresponding author.
E-mail address: brentroster@gmail.com

Clin Sports Med 34 (2015) 625–641
http://dx.doi.org/10.1016/j.csm.2015.06.003
0278-5919/15/$ – see front matter © 2015 Elsevier Inc. All rights reserved.

sportsmed.theclinics.com

The peroneus longus originates from the upper two-thirds of fibula, the head of the fibula, the tibiotalar intermuscular septum, and the lateral condyle of the tibia.[1] The tendon travels along the posterior aspect of the peroneus brevis tendon, inferior to the peroneal tubercle on the lateral wall of the calcaneus, and then turns medially around the lateral border of the cuboid in the cuboid notch toward the first metatarsal.[1] In a cadaver study, the peroneal tubercle was present in 90% of specimens; its shape was described as flat in 43%, prominent in 29%, concave in 27%, and tunnel shaped in 1%.[5] The os peroneum is a fibrocartilaginous sesamoid in the tendon on the peroneus longus; it is fully ossified in 20% of feet and exists in the tendon at the point where it wraps around cuboid in the cuboid tunnel, at the lateral border of the calcaneus, or at the calcaneocuboid articulation.[1,6] The os peroneum provides an increased mechanical advantage, which allows the peroneus longus to plantarflex the first ray. At the point where it articulates with the cuboid, it is anchored into the cuboid notch by 2 medial and 2 lateral ligaments.[1] Just proximal to the cuboid and distal to the peroneal tubercle on the calcaneus is the calcaneal peroneal facet, a well-developed cartilage-covered area with which the peroneus longus tendon articulates.[6]

The peroneus longus and brevis tendons share a synovial sheath starting 2.5 to 3.5 cm proximal to the tip of the fibula and then separate into their own, separate sheaths at the level of the peroneal tubercle. In 15% of patients, the shared peroneal tendon sheath communicates with the ankle or subtalar joint through which synovial fluid can pass.[1] The peroneus brevis has a long musculotendinous junction that may extend inferior to the ankle joint and occupy space in tendon sheath, leading to pathologic conditions such as tenosynovitis, superior peroneal retinaculum (SPR) damage, and chronic tears.[1] The peroneus longus tendon runs in a second peroneal sheath, the plantar peroneal tunnel, as it travels anteromedial toward its insertion on the base of the first metatarsal and medial cuneiform.[1]

The tendons lie laterally to the subtalar joint line and function to plantarflex the ankle and evert the foot. Almost 28% of hindfoot eversion power comes from the peroneus brevis and 35% of power comes from the peroneus longus.[1] In addition, the peroneus brevis is the primary abductor of the forefoot, while the peroneus longus also plantarflexes the first metatarsal.[1] Both muscles are active stabilizers in inversion-supination ankle sprains, and the peroneus longus is a passive stabilizer of the ankle during inversion-supination.[7] At 15° to 25° of plantarflexion, the tendons are perched along the distal fibula and prone to injury with inversion.[8,9] Both muscles are innervated by the superficial peroneal nerve proximally in leg and get their blood supply from the posterior peroneal artery.[1] Both tendons have a hypovascular zone where they wrap around the tip of the fibula, with the peroneus longus tendon having an additional hypovascular zone at the cuboid notch; not surprisingly, these are common areas of injury.[1] The peroneus quartus is an anomalous muscle that exists in 6.6% to 22% of subjects. This muscle originates from the peroneus brevis and travels through the shared tendon sheath to insert onto the peroneal tubercle and has been implicated in several peroneal tendon disorders.[1] This muscle is the most common accessory muscle found in the ankle.

There are multiple stabilizers of the peroneal tendons as they wrap around the lateral malleolus that serve to counteract the forces that would work to sublux or dislocate the tendons anteriorly during plantarflexion. The SPR extends from the posterolateral surface of the fibula 2 cm above its tip to the lateral wall of the calcaneus and/or Achilles and helps to confine the peroneal tendons within the retrofibular groove (**Fig. 1A**).[1] The calcaneal component of the SPR runs parallel to the calcaneofibular component of the lateral ankle ligament complex.[1] The calcaneofibular ligament, which lies deep to the tendons, also helps to stabilize the tendons in the retromalleolar groove.[10] The

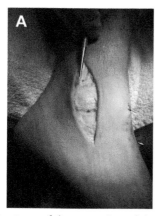
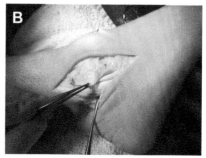

Fig. 1. Anatomy of the constraints of the peroneal tendons. (*A*) Freer elevator is underneath the SPR and within the shared peroneal sheath. The knee is toward the top of the picture, and the foot is to the bottom right. (*B*) The SPR has been divided and the peroneal sheath opened; the peroneus brevis and longus tendons are visible posterior to the fibula. The fibrocartilaginous ridge is grasped and should be protected during approach to this region.

inferior peroneal retinaculum secures the tendons to their respective sides of the peroneal tubercle.[11] Finally, a fibrocartilaginous ridge is located along the posterolateral border of the distal fibula, which acts to deepen the retrofibular/retromalleolar groove by 2 to 4 mm and also functions as a bumper to prevent subluxation; it has been shown to be more important than the fibular shape in securing the peroneal tendons (see **Fig. 1**B).[1]

PATHOPHYSIOLOGY/MECHANISM OF INJURY

Injury to peroneal tendons can cause pain and is commonly found in conjunction with lateral ligamentous instability. In patients undergoing surgery for chronic lateral ankle instability, 77% had peroneal tenosynovitis, 54% had an attenuated peroneal retinaculum, and 25% had a peroneus brevis tear.[12] Peroneal tendon tears can be the result of acute trauma or chronic conditions. At 15° to 25° of plantarflexion, the tendons are perched along the distal fibula and prone to injury with inversion.[8,9] Anatomic and biomechanical factors can cause chronic wearing leading to inflammation and possible thickening of the tendon and tendon sheath and eventual rupture or tears (**Fig. 2**).[1]

Subluxation/Dislocation

One common injury pattern is traumatic subluxation and dislocation of the peroneal tendons (**Fig. 3**A). First described in snow skiing, it has subsequently been described in numerous sports. The forced dorsiflexion with concurrent firing of the peroneal muscles during sudden stopping or hitting moguls in skiing makes these athletes vulnerable to injury.[4,13] In multiple positions of the ankle, forceful contraction of the peroneal tendons can overcome the soft tissue constraints holding the tendons in their retromalleolar groove.[14] Dorsiflexion tightens the peroneal tendons and creates an anteriorly directed force; eversion of the subtalar joint increases the force on the SPR, and inversion tightens the calcaneofibular ligament and pushes the tendons against the retinaculum.[14] Whatever the exact mechanism, it is the disruption in the restraining tissues of the peroneal tendons that leads to injury. At the time of injury,

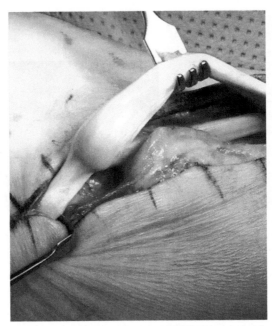

Fig. 2. Stenosis at the inferior peroneal retinaculum leading to proximal enlargement of the peroneus brevis tendon.

the ligaments and bony structures may also be affected, resulting in lateral ankle instability, fracture of the lateral process of the talus, rupture of the Achilles tendon, and ankle or calcaneus fracture.[14] It has been estimated that 30% of patients undergoing surgery for ankle instability have concomitant peroneal tendon pathology.[15]

Peroneal tendon dislocations are classified into 4 grades. In Grade I, the SPR is lifted off the fibula subperiosteally. In Grade II, the fibrocartilaginous ridge is elevated off the fibula. In Grade III, the SPR is avulsed off the fibula with a small cortical fragment attached (see **Fig. 3**B). In Grade IV, the SPR ruptures off its posterior attachment on the calcaneus and/or Achilles tendon.[1,13,16] In addition, cases of distal peroneus longus dislocations have been reported because of rupture of the inferior peroneal

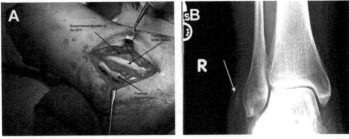

Fig. 3. Traumatic peroneal tendon dislocation. (*A*) Surgical photograph depicting a traumatic dislocation; the SPR has been disrupted, and the peroneus brevis has dislocated anteriorly out of the retrofibular groove and is lying on the lateral border of the distal fibula. The peroneus longus in this case remained in the retrofibular groove. Close inspection reveals subperiosteal traumatic elevation of the SPR (Grade 1). (*B*) Fleck sign (*yellow arrow*), pathognomonic of an acute peroneal tendon dislocation, Grade 3.

retinaculum, causing the peroneus longus tendon to dislocate superior to the peroneal tubercle.[17]

Tears of the Peroneus Brevis

Peroneus brevis tears often result from the damage caused by repeated subluxation. The sharp posterolateral edge of the fibula can create a small hole in the tendon as it repeatedly subluxes over the ridge (**Fig. 4**A). This hole most often extends into a longitudinal tear 2.5 to 5 cm in length.[4] Occasionally, a bucket handle tear can occur in which the peroneus longus acts as a wedge between the 2 split ends of the peroneus brevis.[15] Tears also result from mechanical wear at the tip of the fibula where there is increased pressure and relative hypovascularity; this may also cause inflammation, which further decreases normal movement of the tendon.[1] When there is decreased space in the retromalleolar groove, this force is increased, which also increases the risk for tearing. Factors that can cause a decreased space include local inflammation, a low-lying peroneus brevis muscle belly (see **Fig. 4**B), and the presence of a peroneus quartus muscle (see **Fig. 4**C, D).[1] The presence of a peroneus quartus muscle has been reported to double the risk for a peroneus brevis tear.[1] These volume effects can also increase SPR laxity, which in turn can increase the risk for subluxation.[4] Tears of the peroneus brevis can also occur at its insertion such as when the base of the fifth metatarsal is fractured during an inversion injury.[15] In addition, in rare instances, an anomalous os vesalianum can cause pain over the base of the fifth metatarsal.[18]

Tears of the Peroneus Longus

Peroneus longus tears are less common than peroneus brevis tears. These tears can occur in isolation or in conjunction with peroneus brevis tears. Tears commonly occur

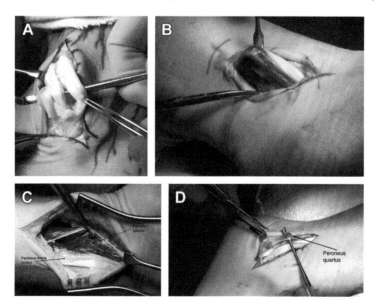

Fig. 4. Peroneus brevis tears and abnormalities found in the peroneal sheath. (*A*) Complex chronic tear of the peroneus brevis tendon; note the hypertrophy of the tendon and multiple longitudinal tears. (*B*) Low-lying peroneus brevis muscle belly; the muscle belly extends down past the level of the distal fibula. (*C*) Example of a very large peroneus quartus. The muscle belly is clearly distinct from that of the peroneus brevis. (*D*) Another example of a peroneus quartus. The muscle belly in this example is much smaller and is more typical.

at the tip of the distal fibula, at the peroneal tubercle, or at the os peroneum.[4] The peroneus longus can be divided into 3 zones: Zone A from the from of the tip of the malleolus to the peroneal tubercle, Zone B from the peroneal tubercle to the inferior retinaculum, and Zone C from the inferior retinaculum to the cuboid notch.[15,19] Most tears of the peroneus longus occur in Zone C.[15] Similar to peroneus brevis tears, tears of the longus can occur from chronic stress and degeneration as well as from acute inversion injuries and forced eversion of a supinated foot.[4] Hindfoot varus and cavovarus foot deformities have been implicated in propensity for injury.[4] Conversely, chronic peroneus longus rupture can be associated with the development of a cavovarus deformity.[15]

Painful Os Peroneum Syndrome

A term that has been used to describe many of the locations and causes of peroneal tendon injury is painful os peroneum syndrome (POPS).[6] POPS can include an acute or chronic os peroneum fracture (**Fig. 5**) or diastasis of a multipartite os peroneum with possible callus formation; attrition or partial rupture of the peroneus longus tendon, either distal or proximal to the os peroneum; and a large peroneal tubercle that entraps the peroneus longus or os peroneum.[6] In one study, 29% of specimens had a prominent tubercle.[5] There is one case report in the literature of the peroneal tubercle completely encasing the peroneal tendons.[20] Callus formation in the healing of a fractured or injured os peroneum can create stenosis, resulting in tenosynovitis of the peroneus longus tendon.[6] In addition, reports of calcific tendonitis of the peroneus longus may be the result of this callus formation.[6]

Concomitant Peroneus Brevis and Longus Tears

Although longitudinal ruptures are more common, particularly in regard to chronic dislocation and subluxation, there are reports of transverse ruptures of both peroneus tendons. These ruptures more commonly result from acute injuries and occur distal to the os peroneum, but can occur elsewhere, including at the musculotendinous junction.[21] A case report described the development of lateral compartment syndrome following a rupture at this junction.[22]

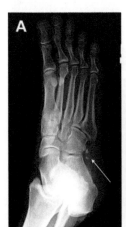
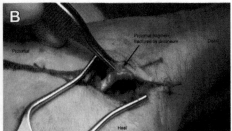

Fig. 5. Case example of a fractured os peroneum. (*A*) Radiograph depicting a fracture of an os peroneum (*yellow arrow*). Note the jagged cortical margins and diastasis of the fragments. (*B*) Surgical exposure and findings.

WORKUP OF PERONEAL TENDON DISORDERS
History and Physical Examination

It is important to consider a peroneal tendon injury in each patient who presents with lateral ankle pain. A thorough and complete history and physical examination should be performed. Injuries to the peroneal tendons and associated structures can be acute or chronic. Patients often complain of chronic lateral ankle pain and may report a history of ankle sprain, ankle fracture, calcaneus fracture, or other injuries. Peroneal tendonitis may present with a gradual onset of pain and posterolateral ankle swelling.[23] Patients with peroneal tendon subluxation often complain of a painful clicking sensation. Peroneus brevis tears are often characterized by persistent swelling along the course of the peroneals, whereas peroneus longus tears can present with pain in or around the cuboid groove and extending into the plantar aspect of the foot near its insertion.[23,24] Patients may also not complain of pain but rather a feeling of instability. Use of ciprofloxacin and other fluoroquinolones has been associated with tendon rupture and should be included in the history.[23]

Inspection and palpation with active firing of the tendons are important parts of the physical examination. Warmth and swelling along the course of the peroneal tendons should be identified, which can indicate peroneal tendonitis. Assessment of hindfoot and forefoot alignment is paramount because a varus hindfoot can predispose the peroneals to injury.[25] Palpation along the course of the peroneals should be performed, and any areas of tenderness should be noted; in some cases, one may be able to feel thickening of the tendon. Strength testing of the peroneals should be performed; weakness, pain, or both with resisted ankle eversion and/or resisted plantarflexion of the first ray may indicate pathology. Ligamentous stability should be assessed. Peroneal subluxation is tested by flexing the knee and having the patient actively plantarflex and dorsiflex the ankle with resisted eversion. The test yields positive result when the peroneal tendons can be felt or seen to subluxate anterior to the lateral malleolus. Intrasheath subluxation should be suspected if the tendons are noted to translate relative to one another without truly subluxating anterior to the lateral malleolus. Sobel and colleagues[6] described the peroneal compression test, which can be used to evaluate for peroneus brevis tendonitis; to perform this test, the foot is everted and dorsiflexed while manual pressure is placed against the fibular groove. Pain elicited with this maneuver is considered a positive result of test.

Imaging

Imaging workup of a patient with lateral ankle pain and a suspected peroneal tendon injury should begin with radiographs. Weight-bearing radiographs of the symptomatic foot and ankle should be acquired. Abnormal findings specific to peroneal tendon pathology may include an avulsion of the base of the fifth metatarsal, a fleck avulsion off the distal fibula (indicating traumatic subluxation or dislocation of the peroneal tendons out of the fibular groove because of injury to the SPR, see **Fig. 3**B), hypertrophy of the peroneal tubercle, or the presence of an os peroneum.[25] A Harris heel view helps with assessing hindfoot alignment and is best for evaluating peroneal tubercle hypertrophy as well as the retromalleolar groove.[24] Plain radiographs may also reveal a fractured os peroneum (see **Fig. 5**A) or distracted bipartite or multipartite os. It may be necessary to obtain contralateral foot and ankle imaging for comparison.

Ultrasonography is another imaging modality that can be used to evaluate the peroneal tendons. This modality is noninvasive and inexpensive, does not expose the patient to radiation, and can also be used in dynamic evaluation of the tendons.[26] It should be noted, however, that ultrasonography is operator dependent and can be time consuming. Ultrasonography can also be used for injection of the peroneal tendon sheath; accuracy of up to 100% has been reported.[27] Ultrasonography is an ideal test to determine the presence of intrasheath peroneal tendon subluxation.

MRI provides the most detailed evaluation of peroneal tendon pathology. MRI is useful in that it provides 3-dimensional assessment of the anatomy and allows one to evaluate the tendons, muscles, ligaments, and bone in the area of interest. Several MRI studies specifically aimed at the peroneal tendons have been published. Normal tendons typically have homogenous signal intensity on T1-and T2-weighted and short tau inversion recovery (STIR) images; tenosynovitis, tendinosis, or tendon tear may be associated with increased signal intensity on T2-weighted or STIR imaging or loss of signal homogeneity, as well as thickening of the tendons.[10,25] It is important to recognize that a thin area of high signal intensity surrounding the peroneal tendons within the tendon sheath on T2-weighted imaging and STIR is normal, but a large amount of fluid may indicate tenosynovitis.[10] Findings associated with longitudinal split tears of the peroneus brevis include a chevron-shaped peroneus brevis, partial enveloping of the peroneus longus (**Fig. 6**), increased signal intensity in the tendon on T2-weighted images, increased signal intensity in the fibular groove, a flat peroneal groove, a lateral fibular spur, and abnormal lateral ligaments; findings that may be seen but have not been statistically correlated on MRI to be associated with brevis tears include flattening of the peroneus brevis, subluxation of the tendons, abnormal SPR, and the presence of a peroneus quartus.[10,28] Peroneus longus tears can be associated with loss of homogeneity on MRI, discontinuity of the tendon, increased signal along the lateral calcaneal wall, a hypertrophied peroneal tubercle, and fracture of or increased signal within an os peroneum.[23] MRI can also reveal injuries to the SPR, intrasheath subluxation of the tendons (a reversal of their normal position relative to one another), and ganglion cysts.[10]

Although MRI is a powerful imaging tool, it should be noted that its findings are not always correlated with clinically relevant pathology. A study by Giza and colleagues[29] comparing clinical examination of patients with positive findings of peroneal tendon

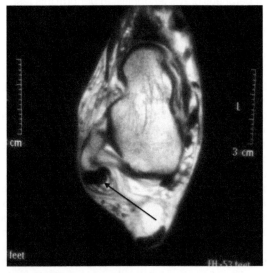

Fig. 6. Axial T1 MRI cut showing enveloping of the peroneus longus tendon (*arrow*) by the peroneus brevis tendon, suggesting a longitudinal peroneus brevis tear.

pathology on MRI reported a positive predictive value of MRI of only 48%, that is, incidental findings of peroneal pathology on MRI are not uncommon and clinical correlation is required. Conversely, studies have been published that suggest that MRI underestimates the extent of the pathology. Finally, one must consider the magic angle effect of MRI imaging of tendons; this is a phenomenon that causes increased intratendinous T1 signal as a tendon curves obliquely into the plane of imaging, and if not recognized, it can lead to false-positive interpretation of the MRI.[28] Given the moderate sensitivity and specificity of MRI in determining peroneal tendon pathology, a detailed history and physical examination is critical in this patient population.

NONOPERATIVE TREATMENT

Treatment of most peroneal tendon disorders begins with nonoperative treatment, which is often successful depending on the pathology. This treatment includes the use of nonsteroidal antiinflammatory drugs (NSAIDs), ice, physical therapy, and periods of immobilization in a boot or cast. Ankle bracing may improve symptoms for some. Use of a lateral wedge orthosis can also be helpful in that it unloads the peroneal tendons. A steroid or NSAID injection into the tendon sheath can be both diagnostic and therapeutic, but steroid injections should be used judiciously.[25] A recent study of 408 patients using ultrasound-guided platelet-rich plasma injections for the treatment of tendinopathy included 23 patients with peroneal tendon pathology; the investigators reported a statistically significant improvement in both functional outcomes scores and measurement of tendinopathy.[30]

OPERATIVE TREATMENT

Operative treatment is reserved for patients in whom conservative management has failed and symptoms persist. Surgical intervention should be focused on treating the tendon pathology as well as any underlying disorder, such as lateral ligamentous instability, varus hindfoot, prominent peroneal tubercle, presence of a low-lying peroneus brevis muscle belly, or peroneus quartus.[23,25] Failure to incorporate this thought into the surgical plan may lead to suboptimal outcomes and ultimately, recurrence.

Peroneal Tendonitis and Tendinosis

Tendonitis and tendinosis of the peroneal tendons are generally the result of repetitive and/or prolonged activity, but they can also be the result of trauma in the form of fractures or sprain.[25] This spectrum of disorders can be seen in patients of all ages and activity groups but are commonly seen in dancers, runners, and those with chronic ankle instability.[24] Anatomic factors such as an enlarged peroneal tubercle, low-lying brevis muscle, and presence of a peroneus quartus can lead to stenosis within the tendon sheath and ultimately, development of these conditions.[31] Surgical treatment of this spectrum of pathologic conditions involves synovectomy and debridement, with concurrent treatment of any underlying disorders. Traditional treatment includes open debridement, but tendoscopy is becoming more popular and widely used.[32–34]

Preferred surgical technique for treatment
Dr Giza prefers the following technique.

Open debridement/synovectomy The patient is positioned toward the end of the table in the lateral decubitus position on a bean bag, and appropriate antibiotics are given. A tourniquet is placed on the upper part of the thigh of the operative extremity. A stack of blankets is placed underneath the operative ankle, and all bony prominences on the well leg are padded. The leg is prepared and draped in the usual sterile manner and exsanguinated, and the tourniquet is inflated. A curvilinear incision is made around the distal tip of the fibula just posterior to the fibula and in line with the peroneal tendons. Careful dissection is taken down to the level of the tendon sheath, and any branches of the sural or superficial peroneal nerves are protected. The peroneal tendon sheath is then longitudinally opened sharply with a scalpel, taking care to leave a cuff of tissue on the posterior fibula for later closure/repair and to not disturb the fibrocartilaginous ridge. The tendons are inspected, and a tenosynovectomy is performed (**Fig. 7**). Tears of 30% or less of the tendon are resected, as are diseased areas of tendinosis. If a low-lying peroneus brevis muscle or peroneus quartus muscle is encountered, it is resected. If a prior ankle fracture was treated with posterolateral antiglide plating, this hardware can easily be removed. Split tears of the tendons are resected using the above-mentioned criteria, and the tendon is then tubularized using 2-0 nonabsorbable suture. Up to 50% of the inferior peroneal retinaculum can be opened to facilitate tendon gliding distally. If a prominent peroneal tubercle is present, this can be shaved down or removed. The retinaculum and tendon sheath are then closed with 2-0 nonabsorbable suture, and the skin is closed in layers. A splint is applied.

Peroneal tendoscopy The patient is positioned toward the end of the table in the lateral decubitus position on a bean bag, and appropriate antibiotics are given (**Fig. 8**A). A tourniquet is placed on the upper part of the thigh of the operative extremity. A stack of blankets is placed underneath the operative ankle ending at the level of the medial malleolus so that the foot can be inverted and everted during the case, and all bony prominences on the well leg are padded. The leg is prepared and draped in the usual sterile manner and exsanguinated, and the tourniquet is inflated.

Bony landmarks are as follows: fibula, fifth metatarsal base, peroneus brevis/longus, and the peroneal tubercle. Three portals are used: superior, middle, and inferior (see **Fig. 8**B). The tendon sheath is then injected with saline (see **Fig. 8**C). The 2.7- or 1.9-mm 30° arthroscope is first introduced into the middle portal, looking superiorly (see **Fig. 8**D). A probe is placed in the superior portal, and the tendons are assessed. Next, the scope is placed into the superior portal, and while looking inferiorly, the tendons as well as the fibular groove can be examined. Synovitis and tears can be debrided using a shaver in the middle portal. The arthroscope is the moved to the

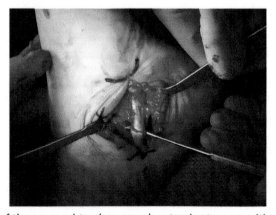

Fig. 7. Exposure of the peroneal tendons reveals extensive tenosynovitis.

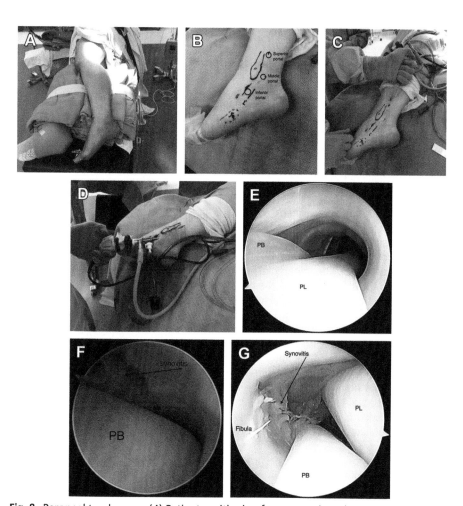

Fig. 8. Peroneal tendoscopy. (*A*) Patient positioning for peroneal tendoscopy. The patient is in the lateral decubitus position, with the ankle positioned on a stack of towels, taking care to place the towel stack at the level of the ankle joint and not beyond it. (*B*) Portal locations for peroneal tendoscopy. Circles indicate portal position; 5th, base of the fifth metatarsal; B, peroneus brevis tendon; F, fibula; L, peroneus longus tendon. (*C*) Injection of the peroneal tendon sheath. (*D*) Arthroscope in the inferior portal, looking proximally. (*E*) View of the peroneal tendons traversing the shared peroneal tendon sheath; PB, peroneus brevis; PL, peroneus longus. (*F*) Example of tenosynovitis (*arrow*) associated with the peroneus brevis tendon (PB); this can easily be debrided using the shaver. (*G*) Another arthroscopic picture showing the peroneus longus, peroneus brevis, and synovitis.

middle portal, looking inferiorly. The separate fibrocartilaginous tunnels at the level of the peroneal tubercle and inferior peroneal retinaculum can then be examined, and any pathology treated as necessary (see **Fig. 8**E–G).

Tendon Subluxation and Dislocation

Many different techniques have been reported to treat symptomatic peroneal tendon subluxation and/or dislocation. Depending on the mechanism of subluxation/dislocation, open and endoscopic reconstruction or repair of the SPR, augmentation/repair of the fibrocartilaginous ridge, repair of an avulsion fracture, and either endoscopic or open fibular groove deepening have all been described.[14,17,35–43] The goals of surgery for subluxation/dislocation are as follows: restoring the periosteum and SPR to the lateral fibula, reestablishing the fibrocartilaginous rim, and securely repairing the SPR with enough space for uninhibited tendon gliding. Groove deepening is rarely necessary in acute repair but may be indicated in more chronic cases because it has been noted to decrease the pressure within the retromalleolar groove. However, there is no clinical evidence to demonstrate the superiority of concomitant groove deepening compared with no groove deepening with regard to clinical outcome or recurrence in the setting of chronic tendonitis or tendinosis.

Preferred technique for treatment

The technique preferred by the senior author is described in the following paragraphs.

Patient positioning, incision, and exposure is the same as described for open treatment of tendonitis/tendinosis. Active eversion/inversion is performed and subluxation/dislocation confirmed. The superficial peroneal retinaculum is closely examined and is often found to be attenuated from the peroneal tendons subluxating/dislocating anteriorly over the fibula. The fibrocartilaginous ridge is closely examined as well and the type of injury, if present, is noted. The periosteal layer along with the fibrocartilaginous corner is then elevated anteriorly off the fibula, and the distal fibula is roughened with a curette or rasp (**Fig. 9**A). Suture anchors are then placed into the fibula, and a pants over vest repair of the SPR is performed with the foot in slight eversion (see **Fig. 9**B). A Freer elevator is placed in the tendon sheath during this repair to ensure that the tendons are not trapped in the repair and also to prevent overtightening. A 2-0 nonabsorbable suture is used to augment this repair and to close the remainder of the tendon sheath. The foot and ankle are then reexamined to confirm that no further dislocation/subluxation occurs, and the wound is closed as described earlier. A splint is placed.

In cases of chronic instability, a groove-deepening procedure can be performed before the repair of the SPR and fibrocartilaginous rim. The exposure is the same as above (**Fig. 10**A). To perform the groove deepening, the most distal 3 cm of the posterior fibula are addressed. An inverted U-shaped osteotomy is made with a sagittal saw after first making drill holes in line with the planned saw cuts (see **Fig. 10**B). This area of bone is then impacted with a tamp to a depth of approximately 3 to 4 mm (see **Fig. 10**C). The SPR and fibrocartilaginous rim and periosteum are then

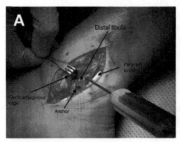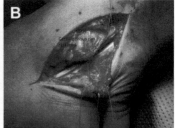

Fig. 9. Treatment of acute or chronic peroneal tendon dislocation/subluxation. (*A*) The fibrocartilaginous ridge has been elevated anteriorly off of the fibula, subperiosteally, and protected. Two suture anchors are placed in the distal fibula. (*B*) The fibrocartilaginous ridge and associated SPR are repaired in a pants-over-vest manner.

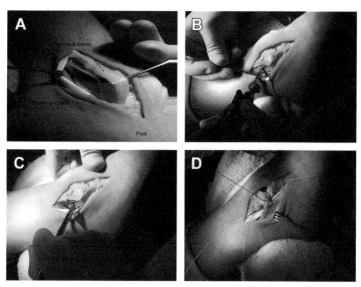

Fig. 10. Groove-deepening procedure. (*A*) The peroneal tendons are exposed, taking care to not disrupt the fibrocartilaginous ridge. Note in this case a low-lying peroneus brevis muscle belly and some flattening of the peroneus brevis tendon. (*B*) The peroneal tendons have been retracted posteriorly and protected. The inverted U-shaped osteotomy has been drawn out on the posterior border of the fibula, and a sagittal saw is used to cut the bone. (*C*) Once the cuts have been performed, a tamp is used to depress this segment of bone, thereby deepening the retrofibular groove. (*D*) The SPR and the fibrocartilaginous ridge are repaired in a pants-over-vest manner. In this case, a lateral ligament stabilization procedure is being performed in conjunction with the groove deepening.

repaired with suture anchors or sutured as described above, and the tendons are then examined for stability (see **Fig. 10**D).

Peroneal Tendon Tears

Tears of the peroneus longus tendon are more rare than those of the peroneus brevis, and concomitant tears of both are even less common.[8,31,44–47] Chronic tears are more commonly seen than a traumatic rupture. Complete ruptures can lead to recurrent sprains, pain, instability, and in the case of peroneus longus ruptures, eventual development of a cavovarus foot deformity.[24,31] Partial tears of the peroneus brevis are most commonly seen in the area of the retromalleolar sulcus, whereas peroneus longus tears are more often observed near the peroneal tubercle or distal to the os peroneum in the cuboid tunnel.[23]

In general, partial tears of 30% to 50% or less can be treated with debridement and tubularization. In cases of acute rupture, an end-to-end repair can be attempted. Chronic complete ruptures or tears encompassing greater than 50% of the tendon can be treated with side-to-side anastomosis of the diseased tendon to the healthy or intact one (**Fig. 11**), or with a Pulvertaft weave.[5,31] Both tendon transfers as well as allograft reconstruction of complete ruptures have been described, with good results.[21,48,49]

Painful Os Peroneum Syndrome

Surgical treatment of POPS generally involves open debridement of the tendon and tenosynovectomy. An incision is made along the course of the peroneus longus to

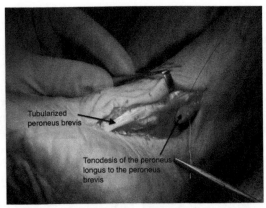

Fig. 11. Treatment of peroneal tendon tears. In this case, the peroneus brevis has been debrided and tubularized. The peroneus longus was beyond repair; the diseased portion was removed, and the proximal portion was then tenodesed to the peroneus brevis in a side-to-side repair. The distal end of the longus tendon is tenodesed distally to the brevis tendon as well.

the level of the lateral border of the foot. The os peroneum is carefully shelled out, and the tendon debrided and/or repaired via tubularization or an end-to-end repair, depending on the size of the defect. If greater than 50% of the tendon has been compromised, tenodesis of the longus tendon to the peroneus brevis is generally recommended.[8,24,25] An enlarged peroneal tubercle should be shaved down or removed and the tendon sheath left open to prevent stenosis.

Postoperative Protocol

After surgery, the leg is immobilized for a period of 2 weeks in a short leg splint. The sutures are removed at the end of 2 weeks, and the leg is then placed into either a removable walking boot or an Aircast brace. The patient is allowed to begin full weight bearing as tolerated at this time and is referred to physical therapy, with no resisted eversion until 6 weeks after surgery. At 6 weeks, the patient is weaned out of the boot or brace and allowed to begin more vigorous activities and resisted eversion exercises.

OUTCOMES/RETURN TO SPORT

In general, reported operative outcomes in terms of pain improvement and return to activity are very good in patients with peroneal tendon tears. Demetracopoulos and colleagues[50] reported on the long-term outcomes of debridement and primary repair of peroneal tendon tears in 34 patients; at final follow-up, there was a significant improvement in both pain and functional outcomes scores and 94% had returned to normal sporting activities. Similarly, Saxena and Cassidy[51] reported an 87% rate of return to sport in their series of 49 operatively treated peroneal tendon tears, with a mean return time of 3.49 months. Other reported rates of return to sport and satisfaction of patients with peroneal tendon tears treated surgically range from 46% to 98%.[52–54]

Outcomes of surgery for peroneal subluxation and recurrent dislocation are also very good. A series of 31 patients treated with SPR repair reported 100% return to sport at an average of approximately 3 months; patients with associated tendon tears took longer.[55] Another study comparing retinaculum repair with and without fibular groove deepening showed similar improvements in pain and functional scores, as well as an average time to return to sport of 3 months in both groups.[56]

SUMMARY

Peroneal tendon injuries are diverse in their presentation, chronicity, pathology, and severity of symptoms. A careful history and thorough physical examination are crucial for correct diagnosis. A combination of imaging modalities including radiographs, MRI, and sometimes ultrasonography can be used, as can diagnostic and therapeutic injections. Nonoperative treatment should be attempted first, but when surgical intervention is planned, thoughtful consideration to and correction of any underlying factors that predispose the patient to peroneal tendon injury must be included for the highest odds of success.

REFERENCES

1. Altchek DW, DiGiovanni CW, Dines JS, et al. Foot and ankle sports medicine. Philadelphia: LippinCott Williams & Wilkins; 2013.
2. Adachi N, Fukuhara K, Kobayashi T, et al. Morphologic variations of the fibular malleolar groove with recurrent dislocation of the peroneal tendons. Foot Ankle Int 2009;30(6):540–4.
3. Myerson M, Quill GE Jr. Late complications of fractures of the calcaneus. J Bone Joint Surg Am 1993;75(3):331–41.
4. Cerrato RA, Myerson MS. Peroneal tendon tears, surgical management and its complications. Foot Ankle Clin 2009;14(2):299–312.
5. Hyer CF, Dawson JM, Philbin TM, et al. The peroneal tubercle: description, classification, and relevance to peroneus longus tendon pathology. Foot Ankle Int 2005;26(11):947–50.
6. Sobel M, Pavlov H, Geppert MJ, et al. Painful os peroneum syndrome: a spectrum of conditions responsible for plantar lateral foot pain. Foot Ankle Int 1994; 15(3):112–24.
7. Ziai P, Benca E, von Skrbensky G, et al. The role of the peroneal tendons in passive stabilisation of the ankle joint: an in vitro study. Knee Surg Sports Traumatol Arthrosc 2013;21(6):1404–8.
8. Baumhauer JF, Nawoczenski DA, DiGiovanni BF, et al. Ankle pain and peroneal tendon pathology. Clin Sports Med 2004;23(1):21–34.
9. Bassett FH 3rd, Speer KP. Longitudinal rupture of the peroneal tendons. Am J Sports Med 1993;21(3):354–7.
10. Lee SJ, Jacobson JA, Kim SM, et al. Ultrasound and MRI of the peroneal tendons and associated pathology. Skeletal Radiol 2013;42(9):1191–200.
11. Bluman EM, DiGiovanni C, Greisberg J. Foot and ankle. In: Murphy K, editor. Philadelphia: Elsevier Mosby; 2007. p. 211.
12. DIGiovanni BF, Fraga CJ, Cohen BE, et al. Associated injuries found in chronic lateral ankle instability. Foot Ankle Int 2000;21(10):809–15.
13. Oden RR. Tendon injuries about the ankle resulting from skiing. Clin Orthop Relat Res 1987;(216):63–9.
14. Brage ME, Hansen ST Jr. Traumatic subluxation/dislocation of the peroneal tendons. Foot Ankle 1992;13(7):423–31.
15. Squires N, Myerson MS, Gamba C. Surgical treatment of peroneal tendon tears. Foot Ankle Clin 2007;12(4):675–95, vii.

16. Eckert WR, Davis EA Jr. Acute rupture of the peroneal retinaculum. J Bone Joint Surg Am 1976;58(5):670–2.

17. Staresinic M, Bakota B, Japjec M, et al. Isolated inferior peroneal retinaculum tear in professional soccer players. Injury 2013;44(Suppl 3):S67–70.

18. Dorrestijn O, Brouwer RW. Bilateral symptomatic os vesalianum pedis: a case report. J Foot Ankle Surg 2011;50(4):473–5.

19. Brandes CB, Smith RW. Characterization of patients with primary peroneus longus tendinopathy: a review of twenty-two cases. Foot Ankle Int 2000;21(6):462–8.

20. Lalli TA, King JC, Santrock RD. Complete encasement of the peroneal tendons by the peroneal tubercle. Orthopedics 2014;37(7):e649–52.

21. Borton DC, Lucas P, Jomha NM, et al. Operative reconstruction after transverse rupture of the tendons of both peroneus longus and brevis. Surgical reconstruction by transfer of the flexor digitorum longus tendon. J Bone Joint Surg Br 1998; 80(5):781–4.

22. Slabaugh M, Oldham J, Krause J. Acute isolated lateral leg compartment syndrome following a peroneus longus muscle tear. Orthopedics 2008;31(3):272.

23. Selmani E, Gjata V, Gjika E. Current concepts review: peroneal tendon disorders. Foot Ankle Int 2006;27(3):221–8.

24. Heckman DS, Gluck GS, Parekh SG. Tendon disorders of the foot and ankle, part 1: peroneal tendon disorders. Am J Sports Med 2009;37(3):614–25.

25. Philbin TM, Landis GS, Smith B. Peroneal tendon injuries. J Am Acad Orthop Surg 2009;17(5):306–17.

26. Molini L, Bianchi S. US in peroneal tendon tear. J Ultrasound 2014;17(2):125–34.

27. Muir JJ, Curtiss HM, Hollman J, et al. The accuracy of ultrasound-guided and palpation-guided peroneal tendon sheath injections. Am J Phys Med Rehabil 2011;90(7):564–71.

28. Major NM, Helms CA, Fritz RC, et al. The MR imaging appearance of longitudinal split tears of the peroneus brevis tendon. Foot Ankle Int 2000;21(6):514–9.

29. Giza E, Mak W, Wong SE, et al. A clinical and radiological study of peroneal tendon pathology. Foot Ankle Spec 2013;6(6):417–21.

30. Dallaudiere B, Pesquer L, Meyer P, et al. Intratendinous injection of platelet-rich plasma under US guidance to treat tendinopathy: a long-term pilot study. J Vasc Interv Radiol 2014;25(5):717–23.

31. Clarke HD, Kitaoka HB, Ehman RL. Peroneal tendon injuries. Foot Ankle Int 1998; 19(5):280–8.

32. Sammarco VJ. Peroneal tendoscopy: indications and techniques. Sports Med Arthrosc 2009;17(2):94–9.

33. Cychosz CC, Phisitkul P, Barg A, et al. Foot and ankle tendoscopy: evidence-based recommendations. Arthroscopy 2014;30(6):755–65.

34. van Dijk CN, Kort N. Tendoscopy of the peroneal tendons. Arthroscopy 1998; 14(5):471–8.

35. Roth JA, Taylor WC, Whalen J. Peroneal tendon subluxation: the other lateral ankle injury. Br J Sports Med 2010;44(14):1047–53.

36. Ogawa BK, Thordarson DB. Current concepts review: peroneal tendon subluxation and dislocation. Foot Ankle Int 2007;28(9):1034–40.

37. Mason RB, Henderson JP. Traumatic peroneal tendon instability. Am J Sports Med 1996;24(5):652–8.

38. Karlsson J, Eriksson BI, Sward L. Recurrent dislocation of the peroneal tendons. Scand J Med Sci Sports 1996;6(4):242–6.

39. Ferran NA, Oliva F, Maffulli N. Recurrent subluxation of the peroneal tendons. Sports Med 2006;36(10):839–46.

40. Oliva F, Del Frate D, Ferran NA, et al. Peroneal tendons subluxation. Sports Med Arthrosc 2009;17(2):105–11.
41. Vega J, Batista JP, Golano P, et al. Tendoscopic groove deepening for chronic subluxation of the peroneal tendons. Foot Ankle Int 2013;34(6):832–40.
42. Jerosch J, Aldawoudy A. Tendoscopic management of peroneal tendon disorders. Knee Surg Sports Traumatol Arthrosc 2007;15(6):806–10.
43. Guillo S, Calder JD. Treatment of recurring peroneal tendon subluxation in athletes: endoscopic repair of the retinaculum. Foot Ankle Clin 2013;18(2):293–300.
44. Pelet S, Saglini M, Garofalo R, et al. Traumatic rupture of both peroneal longus and brevis tendons. Foot Ankle Int 2003;24(9):721–3.
45. Redfern D, Myerson M. The management of concomitant tears of the peroneus longus and brevis tendons. Foot Ankle Int 2004;25(10):695–707.
46. Verheyen CP, Bras J, van Dijk CN. Rupture of both peroneal tendons in a professional athlete. A case report. Am J Sports Med 2000;28(6):897–900.
47. Wind WM, Rohrbacher BJ. Peroneus longus and brevis rupture in a collegiate athlete. Foot Ankle Int 2001;22(2):140–3.
48. Jockel JR, Brodsky JW. Single-stage flexor tendon transfer for the treatment of severe concomitant peroneus longus and brevis tendon tears. Foot Ankle Int 2013;34(5):666–72.
49. Mook WR, Parekh SG, Nunley JA. Allograft reconstruction of peroneal tendons: operative technique and clinical outcomes. Foot Ankle Int 2013;34(9):1212–20.
50. Demetracopoulos CA, Vineyard JC, Kiesau CD, et al. Long-term results of debridement and primary repair of peroneal tendon tears. Foot Ankle Int 2014; 35(3):252–7.
51. Saxena A, Cassidy A. Peroneal tendon injuries: an evaluation of 49 tears in 41 patients. J Foot Ankle Surg 2003;42(4):215–20.
52. Steel MW, DeOrio JK. Peroneal tendon tears: return to sports after operative treatment. Foot Ankle Int 2007;28(1):49–54.
53. Grasset W, Mercier N, Chaussard C, et al. The surgical treatment of peroneal tendinopathy (excluding subluxations): a series of 17 patients. J Foot Ankle Surg 2012;51(1):13–9.
54. Dombek MF, Lamm BM, Saltrick K, et al. Peroneal tendon tears: a retrospective review. J Foot Ankle Surg 2003;42(5):250–8.
55. Saxena A, Ewen B. Peroneal subluxation: surgical results in 31 athletic patients. J Foot Ankle Surg 2010;49(3):238–41.
56. Cho J, Kim JY, Song DG, et al. Comparison of outcome after retinaculum repair with and without fibular groove deepening for recurrent dislocation of the peroneal tendons. Foot Ankle Int 2014;35(7):683–9.

Acute and Chronic Injuries to the Syndesmosis

Paul J. Switaj, MD[a], Marco Mendoza, MD[a], Anish R. Kadakia, MD[b],*

KEYWORDS

- Syndesmosis • Tibiofibular • Chronic syndesmosis • Syndesmotic • Disruption
- High ankle sprain

KEY POINTS

- Stable syndesmotic injuries do not require surgical stabilization and can be treated with protected weight bearing. Advanced imaging demonstrating an intact deltoid ligament with preservation of the interosseous ligament and posterior inferior tibiofibular ligament is associated with a stable injury.
- Unstable syndesmotic injuries require operative stabilization. The use of a suture button device may be appropriate in the setting of a length-stable fibula.
- Use of a suture button device in the setting of a Maisonneuve injury may not provide sufficient coronal and sagittal stability and should be used with caution in these cases.
- Anatomic reduction of the syndesmosis is critical to providing improved outcomes, and direct visualization should be considered in addition to obtaining a contralateral lateral radiograph to assess the reduction.
- Chronic syndesmotic diastasis requires restoration of the mortise and can be performed with graft reconstruction or arthrodesis. The use a graft has been successful in limited clinical series and may offer stability without limiting the motion of the fibula and theoretically may improve function and decrease the risk of ankle arthritis compared with syndesmotic fusion.

ANATOMY OF THE SYNDESMOSIS

Understanding of the anatomy of the normal syndesmosis is essential in both interpretation of diagnostic imaging and therapeutic management.

Distal Tibiofibular Joint

A syndesmosis is defined as a fibrous joint in which 2 adjacent bones are linked by a strong membrane or ligaments. The distal tibiofibular joint comprises the convex

[a] Department of Orthopedic Surgery, Northwestern University–Feinberg School of Medicine, Northwestern Memorial Hospital, 676 North Saint Clair, 13th Floor, Chicago, IL 60611, USA;
[b] Department of Orthopedic Surgery, Northwestern University–Feinberg School of Medicine, Northwestern Memorial Hospital, 259 East Erie, 13th Floor, Chicago, IL 60611, USA
* Corresponding author.
E-mail address: kadak259@gmail.com

Clin Sports Med 34 (2015) 643–677
http://dx.doi.org/10.1016/j.csm.2015.06.009
0278-5919/15/$ – see front matter © 2015 Elsevier Inc. All rights reserved.
sportsmed.theclinics.com

medial aspect of the distal fibula and the concave lateral aspect of the distal tibia, known as the incisura fibularis. Direct contact facets, which are very small and covered with articular cartilage, between the distal tibia and the fibula, are present in approximately three-quarters of patients.[1]

The size and shape of the incisura fibularis play an important role in ankle injury, and have been investigated using cadavers and computed tomography (CT). The anterior tibial tubercle is typically larger than the posterior tubercle and prevents forward translation of the distal fibula. In 97% of normal cases, the fibula is situated either anteriorly or centrally in the tibial incisura.[2] This posterior joint space width is significantly wider than the central and anterior joint spaces.[2] The axis of the distal tibiofibular joint was found to be, on average, 32° externally rotated in relation to the transmalleolar axis.[3]

Significant variance in this bony anatomy exists between individuals.[4] However, there is minimal difference between ankles of the same person, with tibiofibular intervals not varying by more than 2.3 mm and the rotation of the fibula not varying by more than 6.5°.[4] Because of significant anatomic variation between individuals, using a patient's contralateral ankle for comparison provides a precise definition of normal tibiofibular relationships.

Ligamentous Structures

The distal tibiofibular syndesmosis consists of 3 distinct ligaments that act to statically stabilize the distal tibiofibular joint.[5–7]

Anterior tibiofibular ligament

This multilayered ligament extends obliquely from the anterolateral tubercle of the distal tibia on average 5 mm above the articular surface to the longitudinal tubercle located on the anterior border of the lateral malleolus. The inferior fibers can be viewed arthroscopically as they cover the anterolateral corner of the ankle and anterolateral dome of the talus.

Posterior tibiofibular ligament

This ligament consists of a deep and superficial component. The superficial portion extends obliquely from the lateral malleolus to a broad attachment on the posterolateral tibia tubercle. The deep component is the transverse ligament, which is sometimes referred to as a separate ligament. This portion is thick and strong and originates from the round posterior fibular tubercle, inserting on the lower part of the posterior border of the tibial articular surface. This deep portion is more transverse and acts as a labrum, deepening the tibial articular surface.

Tibiofibular interosseous membrane and ligament

This membrane spans most of the length of the lower leg between the tibia and fibula. The ligament is a pyramidal thickening of the distal membrane that terminates just superior to the anterior tibiofibular ligament (AITFL) and posterior tibiofibular ligament (PITFL), helping stabilize the talocrural joint during loading.

Blood Supply

The vascular supply to the syndesmosis has been examined in a singular study. The posterior branch of the peroneal artery is the predominant blood supply to the posterior syndesmotic ligaments. The anterior branch of the peroneal artery, which is the predominant blood supply to the anterior ligaments, perforated the interosseous membrane on average 3 cm proximal to the ankle joint. Thus, this vascular supply would be at considerable risk of insult with a syndesmotic injury, which could explain why syndesmotic injuries are associated with slower healing rates than other ankle ligament injuries.[8]

BIOMECHANICS OF SYNDESMOSIS

The understanding of ankle biomechanics is critical to the formulation of rational treatment plans for syndesmotic pathology. Ankle motion requires rotation and translation of the fibula at the level of the syndesmosis.[9] Dorsiflexion of the ankle results in an average of 2.5° of external rotation of the fibula, whereas plantarflexion results in less than 1° of internal rotation.[9] In normal individuals, external rotation force causes external rotation, medial translation, and posterior displacement of the fibula through the syndesmosis.[10] The intact syndesmosis prevents lateral fibular translation during weight bearing, enabling the fibula to bear 10% to 17% of the weight-bearing load during gait.[11] In anatomic specimens, the relative importance of the individual syndesmotic ligaments to syndesmotic stability was found to be 42% for the transverse ligament and PITFL complex (33% and 9%, respectively), 35% for the AITFL, and 22% for the interosseous ligament.[12] Disruption of the syndesmotic complex disrupts the articular congruity and places increased weight-bearing forces to the tibiotalar articulation, resulting in a nonphysiologic increase in external rotation of the talus.[13] The talar shift results in decreased tibiotalar contact surface,[14,15] which may lead to secondary degeneration of the joint.

Injury Mechanisms

A variety of mechanisms individually or combined can cause syndesmosis injury. The patient often poorly recalls the mechanism, which is in contrast to the classic inversion ankle sprain. The most common mechanisms, individually and particularly in combination, are external rotation and hyperdorsiflexion.[16] Injuries to the syndesmotic complex can occur in isolation or with associated fractures. They can occur with any type of fracture but are most commonly associated with pronation-external rotation and supination-external rotational (SER) fractures and proximal fibular fractures (Maisonneuve injuries),[17,18] although the exact mechanism of these fractures have been called into question in recent years.[19]

ACUTE SYNDESMOTIC INJURIES
Epidemiology

Although injuries to the ankle are extremely common, injuries to the syndesmotic complex are uncommon, comprising 1% to 10% of all ankle sprains.[20–22] The incidence is poorly defined but has been reported to be 6445 syndesmotic injuries per year in the United States when using emergency room and inpatient data. This rate will most likely continue to increase, especially given the expanding utilization of MRI and a heightened awareness in sports medicine. The highest rate of injury was found in patients aged 18 to 34 years.[23] The injuries may occur more frequently in athletes, with 2 studies reporting that greater than 20% of acute ankle sprains in athletes demonstrate syndesmotic disruption.[22,24] Sports at a considerable risk involve immobilization of the ankle in a boot, such as skiing and hockey,[25–28] and in collision sports, such as football, wrestling, rugby, and lacrosse.[29–32]

Diagnosis

The diagnosis of syndesmotic injury is based on the mechanism of injury, manifesting symptomology, a thorough physical examination, and radiographic findings. Importance must be placed on each one of those facets to make the correct diagnosis.

Isolated Syndesmotic Injuries

Clinical evaluation

In the absence of fracture, patients with syndesmotic injuries typically complain of persistent pain on weight bearing or an unusually long period of recovery after the initial injury. The clinical history should include the mechanism of injury, delineation of any prior ankle injuries, and direct location of pain. Any history of an eversion mechanism should prompt the physician toward consideration of a syndesmotic injury.

Physical examination

Physical examination findings include tenderness and swelling over the anterolateral aspect of the syndesmosis.[33–36] This finding is distinctly different in quality from the contralateral lower extremity. The patient may have reduced passive dorsiflexion.[37] Tenderness of the deltoid ligament may also be noted. In patients with complaints of instability, physical examination may denote a normal anterior drawer and inversion stress test, increasing suspicion of a syndesmotic injury over a lateral ankle sprain. In addition, the proximal fibula can be palpated to assess for a Maisonneuve-type injury. The physical examination can be performed 5 days after injury without compromising diagnostic accuracy and causing less discomfort to the patient.[38,39]

Stress tests are also useful in the diagnosis of syndesmotic injuries. Pain, rather than fibular translation, should be the outcome measure of these tests, because very small amounts of displacement are actually conferred by the physical examination maneuvers.[40] The external rotation stress test can be performed either by sitting while placing the knee in 90° of flexion and applying an external rotatory force on the foot or standing with a single limb stance on the affected side and then rotating the body externally[41,42] (**Fig. 1**). This test causes the greatest amount of displacement of the fibula when biomechanically analyzed.[40] A positive test result occurs if pain if reproduced in the syndesmosis.[30,41] The squeeze test involves compressing the proximal fibula to the tibia above the level of the calf, which may separate the bones distally.[43] The test result is positive if pain is elicited in the distal tibiofibular joint[29] (**Fig. 2**). The crossed legged stress test entails crossing the injured leg over the non-injured legged in the seated position followed by applying a downward pressure to the knee of the injured leg.[44] The fibula translation test places an anterior-to-posterior force on the fibula, and the result is considered positive if this translation causes pain at the level of the syndesmosis.[42] Lastly, the stabilization test is performed by tightly taping circumferentially just proximal to the ankle joint to stabilize the syndesmosis. The test result is positive if the patient has less pain with activities such as standing, walking, and jumping after the taping.[45]

The reliability and accuracy of these specialty tests are limited, and these tests should be used in conjunction with further imaging and/or arthroscopy.[46,47] The external rotation stress and the squeeze test demonstrated high specificity, but low sensitivity, when using MRI to confirm the diagnosis.[48,49] Intrarater reliability was high for the squeeze, Cotton, dorsiflexion range of motion, and external rotation tests. Interrater reliability was good for the external rotation tests and fair-to-poor for other tests.[50,51] Thus, the physical examination should always be used in accordance with the clinical history, as the clinician cannot rely on a single test to make the diagnosis. If an injury is suspected, additional diagnostic tests should be considered before making a final diagnosis.

Initial radiographic evaluation

Plain radiographs Typically, anteroposterior (AP), lateral, and mortise views of the ankle are used to evaluate the integrity of the distal tibiofibular joint and to assess

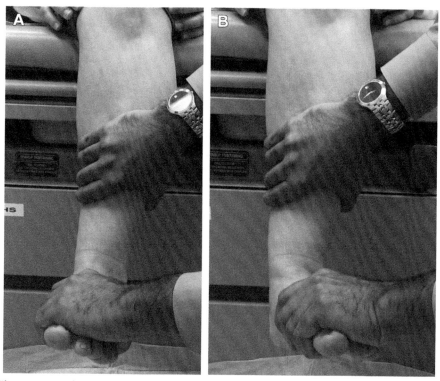

Fig. 1. External rotation stress test for evaluation of a syndesmotic injury. One hand is placed at the mid-calf to stabilize the leg. The foot is then grasped and taken from internal rotation (*A*) to maximum external rotation (*B*). Pain with external rotation indicates syndesmotic injury.

for fractures. Views of the proximal tibia and fibula are obtained if a Maisonneuve injury is suspected (**Fig. 3**). Occasionally, an avulsion fracture at the posterior tibial tubercle can be seen on the lateral view.[41]

When attempting to define abnormal radiographic relationships, it is important to try to describe the normal appearance. Harper and Keller[52] first described the normal relationships of the distal tibiofibular syndesmosis in 12 normal cadavers 1 cm proximal to the plafond. The tibiofibular clear space (TFCS) on the AP and mortise views should normally be less than 6 mm. The tibiofibular overlap (TFO) should normally be greater than 6 mm on the AP view and greater than 1 mm on the mortise view. The medial clear space (MCS) should be less than or equal to the superior joint space. Measurements on lateral radiographs to assess the syndesmosis have not been well defined. Croft and colleagues[53] showed with high reliability that 40% of the tibia was anterior to the fibula at 1 cm above plafond. However, the rotation of the limb can significantly influence each of these measurements[54] except for the TFCS on the AP view.[55]

Recent studies have found great variability in the radiographic measurements of normal patients.[54,56] A study in patients without known clinical or radiographic evidence of abnormality found that the mean TFCS was 4.6 mm on the AP view and 4.3 mm on the mortise view, whereas the mean TFO was 8.3 mm on the AP view and 3.5 mm on the mortise view. It was also demonstrated that a lack of overlap on the mortise view may represent a normal variant.[56] MRI studies have demonstrated that the TCFS and TFO did not correlate with syndesmotic injury, and MCS greater

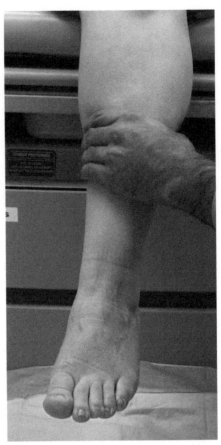

Fig. 2. Squeeze test to assess for syndesmotic injury. Pain distally at the syndesmosis with medial/lateral compression at the mid-calf is suggestive of injury.

than 4 mm may correlate with disruption of deltoid and tibiofibular ligaments.[57,58] Thus, relying solely on these measurements may result in both failure to treat and over-treatment of patients. Therefore, because of the variability among different individuals, comparison views of the contralateral extremity and advanced imaging are an important diagnostic tool for confirmation of clinical suspicion of syndesmosis disruption.[56] Although plain weight bearing radiographs can show abnormalities, frank diastasis without fracture or applied stress is a rare occurrence.[54,55,59] External rotation stress or gravity stress views may be used to confirm latent diastasis.[13,60] Late disruption is best visualized on the lateral radiographs, with posterior displacement of the fibula.[13]

Computed tomography Owing to the questionable reliability of plain radiographic parameters and the difficulty in detecting subtle injuries, advanced imaging is frequently used. The recent literature has investigated the normal anatomic morphology as visualized on CT scan, focusing on the axial cuts.[35] CT is more sensitive than radiography for detecting mild diastasis.[61] Fibular malrotation is still difficult to assess, because there has been no standardized method for measurement.[62,63] Knops and colleagues[62] investigated multiple measurement methods for rotational malreduction and found the angle between the tangent of the anterior tibial surface and the bisection of the vertical midline of the fibula at the level of the incisura to be fairly reliable and

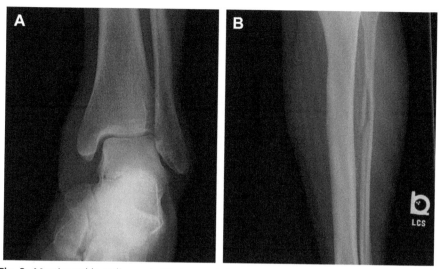

Fig. 3. Mortise ankle radiograph (*A*) does not demonstrate significant radiographic abnormality. A thorough examination noted pain within the proximal leg and a full length tib/fib radiograph demonstrates the presence of a proximal fibula fracture (*B*). This finding is highly suggestive of a Maisonneuve injury.

accurate. Just as with plain radiography, CT imaging has demonstrated variability in the anatomy of the syndesmosis between individuals.[64] Thus, bilateral imaging can be extremely useful.[65,66] Even after plain radiographs have demonstrated diastasis of the syndesmosis, CT scan can be a useful adjunct on the bony anatomy to guide surgical planning.

MRI In the setting of nondiagnostic radiographs, the use of MRI is superior to obtain the diagnosis of a syndesmotic injury, especially on the T1 and T2 axial images[67] **(Fig. 4)**. MRI has excellent sensitivity, specificity, positive predictive value, negative predictive value, and accuracy at diagnosing syndesmotic disruption.[68] In a series of 78 patients, Han and colleagues[69] reported MRI to be 90% sensitive and 94.8% specific in diagnosing syndesmotic injury, using arthroscopic findings as a definitive diagnostic standard. In a similar study by Oae and colleagues,[70] MRI demonstrated 100% sensitivity and 94% specificity for AITFL disruption and 100% specificity and sensitivity for PITFL injury. MRI can be used to grade the injury and may be useful in predicting the time of disability, with involvement of the PITFL possibly signifying a more severe injury.[71] Although MRI is sensitive and specific for syndesmotic injuries using standard protocol at 3.0 T,[68] it is not predictive for instability because it is a static test.[49] In addition, injury to the tibiofibular syndesmosis has a significant association with several secondary findings on MRI, including anterior talofibular ligament injury and osteochondral lesions.[72,73]

Classification

Multiple classification systems have been described.[31,45,74] Most use clinical findings and plain radiographic interpretation, but no current classification uses anatomic location or MRI findings. There is a general agreement that there are 3 grades of injury (I–III). Grade I injuries have a stable syndesmosis with normal results on radiographs and may manifest with mild clinical symptoms and tenderness at the distal tibiofibular joint. Grade II indicates complete AITFL and interosseous ligament (IOL) disruption.

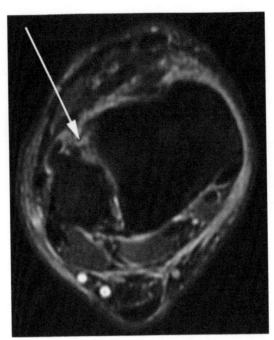

Fig. 4. Axial T2 fat-saturated image of a patient with a complete tear of the AITFL. Note the complete absence of the ligament in the anterior aspect of the tibiofibular joint space (*white arrow*).

Radiograph results are normal, and the provocative test results are positive. Unfortunately, there is no consensus regarding the stability of this injury pattern. The authors' preference for this injury depends on the status of the deltoid ligament. In the setting of an injury to the deltoid, stabilization of the syndesmosis is performed. If the deltoid ligament appears intact based on MRI, then conservative treatment in a controlled ankle motion (CAM) walker is initiated. Grade III injuries represent complete disruption of the AITFL, PITFL, IOL, and deltoid ligament. The distal tibiofibular joint is unstable and requires operative stabilization.

Syndesmotic Injuries with Associated Fractures

Fractures of the malleoli should increase clinical suspicion for syndesmotic injury. Although syndesmotic instability has been shown to occur more commonly in pronation-external rotational ankle fractures with high fibular fractures (36%–60%),[75,76] it also occurs in 17% to 45% of unstable SER ankle fractures with lower fibula fractures.[65,77–81] Multiple studies have attempted to predict syndesmotic disruption based on fracture pattern. Syndesmotic injury has been positively correlated with transverse fractures of the medial malleolus and bimalleolar fractures.[82] Choi and colleagues[83] found that in SER patterns, fracture height (distance between the lowest point of the fracture and the plafond) greater than 7 mm and MCS greater than 4.5 mm were significant preoperative factors associated with syndesmotic injury. The presence of a posterior malleolar fracture is the equivalent of a bony disruption of the PITFL (**Fig. 5**). Therefore, the authors advocate either direct fixation of the posterior malleolus or syndesmotic stabilization in this setting. Although not all patients do poorly without fixation, late posterolateral subluxation of the talus is extremely difficult to treat and should be avoided if possible. Fixation of the posterior malleolus in the

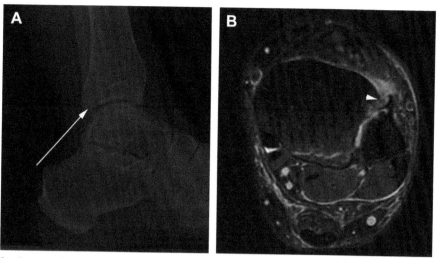

Fig. 5. Lateral radiograph (*A*) of a patient with a history of an ankle sprain with a subtle finding of a posterior malleolar fracture (*arrow*). MRI was performed to evaluate the syndesmosis with evidence of complete disruption of the AITFL (*arrowhead*) with fluid within the syndesmosis itself (*B*). Patient was appropriately treated with open reduction and internal fixation.

setting of a Weber B fibular fracture typically mitigates the need for additional syndesmotic fixation presuming all other bony fixation has been completed. However, in the setting of a Weber C fibular fracture, rotational stability to the fibula may not be restored with fixation of the posterior malleolus, and additional stabilization of the syndesmosis with either a screw or suture button device is considered.

Because plain radiographic findings are often inadequate for diagnosing syndesmotic disruptions in malleolar fractures and injuries can happen across all fracture patterns,[57,65,79] the diagnosis depends on thorough intraoperative assessment. This evaluation can be performed using an external rotation test or Cotton hook test under fluoroscopy.[84] In the external rotation stress, the tibia is stabilized and an external rotation force is applied to the medial aspect of the forefoot and lateral aspect of the hindfoot. Fluoroscopy is used to evaluate for MCS widening. The hook, or lateral stress, test uses a bone hook applied to the lateral malleolus to assess for greater than 2 mm of lateral movement of the lateral malleolus.[85] There is evidence to suggest that assessment of the fibula on the lateral radiograph may improve both the accuracy of the hook test[86] as well as the external rotation test.[13] The fibula demonstrates maximal motion in the sagittal plane with disruption of the syndemosis that is increased with concomitant deltoid disruption that lends more strength to the argument that anterior/posterior stress testing of the fibula is superior to isolated coronal plane stress testing. Pakarinen and colleagues[84] prospectively compared these 2 intraoperative tests with a standardized 7.5-Nm external rotation stress test as a reference. Although tests showed excellent interobserver agreement and specificity, both also had poor sensitivity. A prospective cohort study showed that widening with stress external rotation was significantly greater than with lateral fibular stress and appreciable on standard fluoroscopic views.[87] However, these results must be taken in the context of biomechanical evidence to suggest that the hook test with a 100 N force and visualization of widening of the TFCS is superior in differentiating syndesmotic disruption from isolated deltoid ligament injury in a Weber B ankle fracture model.[88,89] Thus, even if the external rotation stress may demonstrate significant widening, this may represent a deltoid ligament injury based on biomechanical data; this underlies the point that the clinician needs to use all available techniques to accurately diagnose a syndesmotic injury.

Lastly, as noted previously, due to individual anatomic differences, using a patient's contralateral ankle for comparison provides a precise definition of their normal tibiofibular relationships under stress examination.[66]

Role of Arthroscopy

The role of arthroscopy in the treatment of acute syndesmotic injuries is an ever-evolving field with little support in the literature. Its primary role at present is to diagnose syndesmotic instability and other intra-articular pathology.[72,90] Takao and colleagues[91] showed that in operative ankle fractures, arthroscopy confirmed 100% of cases of disruption that had been identified on preoperative plain radiographs and identified 12 additional patients with instability. A subsequent study revealed that compared with arthroscopy for diagnosis of syndesmosis disruption, MRI had 100% sensitivity and 93.1% specificity, showing 2 false-positive cases.[92]

CONSERVATIVE TREATMENT

There is limited quality literature available to help the clinician make a decision in terms of operative versus nonoperative treatment. Conditions with clinical evidence of syndesmotic injury without radiographic abnormality on static images and stress tests can be treated nonoperatively (grades I and II). MRI evidence of an intact deltoid ligament with isolated injury to the AITFL without involvement of the PITFL does not warrant surgical intervention in the opinion of the authors.

When an appropriate diagnosis is made, nonsurgical treatment of stable injury patterns has shown good results[30,31] and consists of a 3-phase approach.[93] The optimal rehabilitation program for these injuries is unknown, because there is no high-quality literature to direct the surgeon. A typical program includes a short period of non–weight bearing, followed by restoration of mobility, strength, and function and lastly advanced sports-specific training. An orthopedic device, most commonly a CAM walker, to limit external rotation is often used. The length of restricted weight bearing and advancement of activities depend on the clinical symptoms, injury severity, and the patient's functional presentation.[45] Rest, elevation, compression, anti-inflammatory medications, and appropriate use of therapeutic modalities such as electric stimulation and massage should be incorporated into the treatment regimen. After 4 to 6 weeks, transition to a lace-up ankle brace is initiated with more aggressive physical therapy as the patient can tolerate. The lace-up brace may be used for a further 6 weeks to minimize symptoms.

A systematic review evaluated 6 studies regarding conservative treatment of syndesmotic injuries.[25,29–31,36,41,94] These studies involved sprains without diastasis on radiographic examination. When compared with lateral ankle sprains, all studies showed prolonged recovery in the syndesmotic sprain group, with a resultant delayed return to play. Return to play is challenging, and is typically based on a functional testing evaluation and physical examination. One study in National Hockey League players showed a mean time to return to play of 45 days versus 1.4 days for lateral ankle sprains.[25] More severe injuries, as determined by MRI involvement of the IOL and PITFL, were positively correlated with increased numbers of missed games and practices.[71] The number of missed competitions also correlated with the interosseous tenderness length[30] and a squeeze test with positive results.[30,71] Although syndesmotic injury is most predictive of persistent symptoms in the athletic population,[95] with correct diagnosis, function is typically good after the initial recovery period.

In syndesmotic injuries associated with malleolar fractures, those with resultant incongruity of the ankle mortise require surgical treatment. Proper intraoperative assessment is paramount and was discussed in the prior section.

SURGICAL TREATMENT

Patients with persistent symptoms despite conservative treatment or with higher-grade injuries with tibiofibular diastasis benefit from operative treatment. Athletes with grade III injuries treated operatively demonstrated similar long-term outcomes when compared with nonsurgical patients.

Most syndesmotic injuries that occur with malleolar fractures require surgical stabilization. There is some debate as to whether syndesmotic fixation is always necessary in SER-type ankle fractures. As bony injuries heal anatomically, the ligamentous injuries may heal at their proper length after malleolar reduction. In 2 small prospective randomized studies of SER ankle fractures, there was no difference in functional outcomes scores or radiologic findings in stress-positive ankles with and without syndesmotic fixation at 1-[77] and 4-year[96] follow-up. In addition, the recent literature has investigated deltoid ligament repair instead of syndesmotic repair in bimalleolar equivalent ankle fractures and found comparable subjective, functional, and radiographic outcomes at mid-term follow up.[97]

However, to prevent potential chronic instability and late arthrosis, the syndesmosis disruption is typically addressed. In the settings of fibular fracture with deltoid disruption, anatomic reduction of the ankle mortise relies on the fibula to hold the talus in proper alignment. The presence of a syndesmotic injury prevents the fibula from facilitating proper alignment of the mortise, leading to recurrent talar translation. Thordarson and colleagues[98] have shown that a 50% increase in pressure in the lateral half of the tibiotalar joint occurs with only 2 mm of lateral talar translation.

Reduction Techniques

Once the decision has been made to proceed to address the syndesmotic injury surgically, the first step is reduction of the distal tibiofibular joint. When applicable, fibular length must be assessed and corrected appropriately to facilitate anatomic reduction of the syndesmosis.[99]

Clamp placement

The syndesmosis is most commonly reduced with use of reduction clamps to compress across the tibia and fibula (**Fig. 6**). If choosing to reduce the syndesmosis with a clamp application, it is important to consider clamp trajectory and force. A cadaveric study demonstrated small, but significant, overcompression and external rotation displacement of the fibula when clamps were placed at 15° and 30° of angulation in the axial plane, relative to the anatomic axis of the syndesmosis.[100] Another cadaveric study showed that placing a clamp in the neutral anatomic axis reduced the syndesmosis most accurately, although minimal overcompression was observed.[101] The authors use a clamp in some situations; however, they have used manual reduction and stabilization using the thumb to generate the reduction force. This is an emerging technique that may decrease the risk of malreduction associated with a clamp. Once the syndesmosis is felt to be reduced, a K-wire may be placed along the syndesmotic axis to stabilize the position of the fibula. The use of a clamp at this point allows further reduction of the syndesmosis in the coronal plane without risking sagittal malalignment.

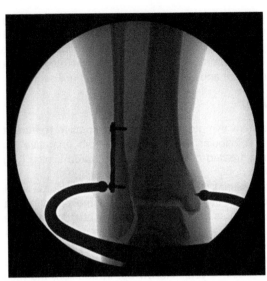

Fig. 6. Intraoperative photograph demonstrating placement of a large reduction clamp to reduce the syndesmosis. The clamp should be placed at the level of the ankle joint with the foot held in neutral.

Assessment of reduction

Once a reduction is attempted, the next important step is the assessment of the reduction.

Assessment may be attempted indirectly via radiographic imaging. Unfortunately, the same inaccuracies in diagnosing injuries using plain radiographs in the preoperative setting exist when assessing the reduction in the operative setting. A cadaveric study suggested that a 30° external malrotation of the fibula may result when using TFCS, TFO, and posterior subluxation to assess reduction.[102]

Because of these difficulties, surgeons have attempted to compare the injured side with a normal contralateral extremity.[103,104] Although substantial variation in ankle anatomy exists between individuals, there is little variation between contralateral ankles of a single individual.[4] A cadaveric study using perfect lateral radiographs showed that anterior displacement and greater than 5 mm translation were accurately detected and that fluoroscopic comparisons to the normal ankle were helpful in determining reduction.[104] In a clinical study, Summers and colleagues[105] used uninjured contralateral ankle radiographs as a template for reduction and demonstrated anatomic reduction on intraoperative CT scan in 17 of 18 of patients.

Other investigators have suggested the use of intraoperative CT scan to improve the reduction.[106–108] Franke and colleagues[108] used this technology in a consecutive series and altered the surgical outcome in 32.7% of cases, improving reduction of the distal tibiofibular joint in 30.7% of the total cases. Other studies have shown that intraoperative CT reduced their posterior malreduction rate but not the anterior malreduction rate.[107] Thus, although intraoperative 3-dimensional imaging increases cost and exposes the patient to additional radiation, it provides an intraoperative assessment that can improve reduction.

The reduction can also be assessed directly via open reduction of the syndesmosis. Studies have demonstrated improved accuracy of the reduction with direct visualization of the incisura, although 15% to 16% still demonstrated incongruity on postoperative CT scan.[109,110] Direct repair of the deltoid ligament is Dr Kadakia's preference when treating syndesmotic injuries, which may improve the reduction of the fibula within the incisura fibularis. A combination of direct visualization of the syndemosis and incisura along with primary repair of the superficial component of the deltoid ligament may minimize the risk of iatrogenic malreduction.

Fixation Construct and Placement

Once a reduction is obtained and maintained, the syndesmosis must be stabilized. There are numerous studies evaluating the technical aspects of syndesmotic fixation. The next step is choosing an implant for fixation.

Screw composition, size, number, and cortices engaged

The traditional method, and the most common current practice,[111] is stainless steel screw fixation, although other screw compositions have demonstrated satisfactory results.[112,113] The composition of the screw has not been shown to differ in biomechanical testing nor does it significantly influence the radiographic or clinical outcomes; this is true in regards to bioabsorbable screws[114–116] and titanium screws.[117] Bioabsorbable screws may offer slightly increased range of motion[118] and obviate subsequent hardware removal but have a higher incidence of foreign body reactions.[118]

If choosing a stainless steel screw, fixation can be achieved with 3.5- or 4.5-mm screws. There is biomechanical evidence to suggest that the 4.5-mm screw provides more resistance to shear stress,[119] although other studies showed no biomechanical difference.[120,121] Once the screw size is selected, there has been no difference in radiographic or functional outcomes in tricortical and quadricortical screws.[117,122–125] Two screws or locking plate fixation provides stronger mechanical fixation,[13,126] without translating into improved clinical outcomes.[99,127,128] Multiple screws are typically considered in Maisonneuve injuries, in obese patients, or in severely osteoporotic bone to increase construct stability.[129] If screw fixation is chosen, the authors' preference is a 3.5-mm tricortical screw if the fibula is fixated.

Dynamic fixation

Dynamic fixation with suture-button fixation has been widely studied.[130–144] A hole is drilled through the fibula and tibia, and then a suture is passed through and secured on both ends via a metallic button. Systematic reviews of low levels of clinical evidence have demonstrated similar functional outcomes, with quicker return to work and less frequent need for implant removal. A single suture button device has demonstrated lack of sagittal stability compared with a screw and must be considered when choosing this implant. A prospective, randomized control trial demonstrated better clinical and radiographic outcomes with a dynamic device, with improved maintenance of reduction and lower reoperation rate.[131] Despite the increased cost of the implant, the decreased need for hardware removal may confer cost-effectiveness to this technique. Lastly, one can consider hybrid fixation with a screw and suture button construct for severe diastasis or large athletes.

Implant placement

Once a reduction is obtained and maintained and an implant is selected, the implant must be placed.

There is conflicting biomechanical evidence regarding placement of the implant relative to the tibiotalar joint. One study showed that a screw placed 2.0 cm above the tibiotalar joint resulted in less syndesmotic widening than a screw placed 3.5 cm above the joint,[145] whereas another showed that fixation 3 to 4 cm above the joint may have biomechanical advantages.[146] Clinical evidence has not demonstrated significantly different radiographic or clinical outcomes in transsyndesmotic or suprasyndesmotic fixation.[147] Screw placement more than 4.1 cm above the joint negatively influences patient outcomes, likely due to decreased stability at this level or by slight bending of the fibula on insertion, causing widening at the mortise.[148]

All evidence regarding orientation of the fixation is from cadaveric and anatomic studies. Anatomically, the fibula sits posteriorly in the tibia, and screws should therefore be directed 30° anteriorly.[149] This position corresponds to a line from the lateral cortical apex of the fibula to the anterior half of the medial malleolus.[150] Aberrant screw placement may cause malreduction.[100] Furthermore, the screw should be inserted parallel to the ankle joint in the coronal plane to prevent any proximal migration.

The sagittal position of the ankle while the implant is being placed has been debated. An older cadaveric study suggested that dorsiflexion of the ankle may be restricted if the ankle is not in a maximally dorsiflexed position during fixation.[151] However, more recent literature does not support this.[152,153] Thus, it is the surgeon's choice in determining the position of the ankle during fixation. However, in the setting of a posterior malleolar fracture, the authors do not recommend dorsiflexion to minimize iatrogenic posterior translation of the fibula.

Posterior Malleolar Fixation and Anterior Tibiofibular Ligament Reconstruction

There has been much interest in the role of the posterior malleolar fracture in regards to syndesmotic stability. Syndesmotic injuries are not infrequently associated with a fracture of the posterior malleolus. When there is a posterior malleolar fracture, the PITFL is reliably intact and attached to the posterolateral fragment.[154] Subsequently, malreduction of this component may result in malreduction of the syndesmosis with resultant posterolateral subluxation of the fibula. Fixation of this fragment alone confers increased stability to the syndesmosis[154] and equivalent functional outcomes in small series when compared with syndesmotic screw fixation.[155] This method of syndesmotic stabilization would also obviate removal of screw fixation from the syndesmosis and may allow for earlier weight bearing as a result of bony healing as opposed to ligamentous healing. In addition, there is some limited evidence that repair or reconstruction of the AITFL restores the stability, allows for early return to functional activities, and obviates syndesmotic screw fixation.[156]

Postoperative Protocol

Return to sports can be expected as early as 4 weeks after rigid fixation of an isolated fibula fracture and up to 8 to 10 weeks after stabilization of a bimalleolar equivalent fracture with deltoid repair. Syndesmosis fixation can take up to 4 to 6 months before successful return to sport.

Outcomes and Complications

Satisfactory outcomes can be expected with syndesmotic fixation, even in high-level athletes.[78,127,157,158] There exist a variety of factors that can influence a patient's surgical outcome. Failure to diagnose the syndesmotic injury has been found to be a common cause of reoperation.[159] Thus, it is important for the surgeon to have a high incidence of suspicion for injury and assess for disruption appropriately.

Injury factors

There is literature indicating that syndesmotic injuries associated with trimalleolar fractures have significantly lower outcomes than unimalleolar or bimalleolar fractures.[148,160] When compared with all operative ankle fractures not requiring syndesmotic fixation, those requiring stabilization had worse American Orthopedic Foot and Ankle Society (AOFAS) scores in function and pain and worse Short Musculoskeletal Functional Assessment (SMFA) scores at 12 months.[161] Litrenta and colleagues[162] found similar findings in SER-IV ankle fractures, with small clinical differences in SMFA and bother index but not in the AOFAS score. However, conflicting evidence was presented by Kortekangas and colleagues[163] in SER-IV ankle fractures, who showed no clinical or radiographic differences at 4- to 6-year follow-up in patients with syndesmotic injury compared with patients with a stable syndesmosis. This lack of significant difference was also seen by Kennedy and colleagues[164] in Weber C ankle fractures. Worse functional results have been demonstrated in ankle fractures that were dislocated on initial presentation.[165]

Patient factors

There is evidence demonstrating that increasing age negatively affects outcome.[148,160] Although diabetes mellitus and smoking did not show an effect on loss of syndesmosis reduction, obese patients were 12 times more likely to lose reduction than were patients with a normal body mass index[166] and had poorer functional outcomes.[123] Wukich and Kline[167] found that patients with complicated diabetes were 3.4 times more likely to have soft-tissue and bony complications than patients with uncomplicated diabetes, without considering specifically syndesmotic injuries.

Surgeon factors

As discussed previously, there have been no major differences in functional or radiographic outcomes between 1 and 2 screws, tricortical and quadricortical screws, or screws of varying compositions. The literature on dynamic fixation is evolving, with the recent high-level literature suggesting improved outcomes without the need for hardware removal.[131]

The most pertinent, technical aspect of surgical treatment is the accuracy of the reduction. This aspect has been shown to be the most important independent predictor of clinical outcomes and vital in avoiding posttraumatic arthrosis.[14,15,78,123,132,165] It involves first correctly diagnosing the injury, then establishing an anatomic reduction of the syndesmosis and the fibula if there is a fracture.[159] In a prospective evaluation with minimum 2-year follow-up, Sagi and colleagues[109] found that malreduced syndesmotic injuries had significantly worse functional outcome scores than those with anatomic reductions.

Malreduction Despite the focus on syndesmotic injuries and the importance placed on anatomic restoration, malreduction is still commonplace. The literature has shown syndesmotic malreductions to occur in as many as 25.5% to 52% of patients.[66,75,76,102,109,110] The malpositioning is often in the sagittal plane with anterior displacement and internal rotation.[108–110] Predictors of malreduction have been investigated, but no significant factors could be elucidated.[168]

Given the high rates of malreduction several strategies were noted for improving the accuracy of reduction, including recent evidence that accuracy in reduction can be improved using direct visualization of the reduction,[109,110] contralateral radiographs as a template,[103,105] and intraoperative CT scan.[106–108] In Maisonneuve injuries, a small series demonstrated improved syndesmotic reduction with open reduction and internal fixation of the proximal fibular fracture.[169] Despite all those techniques, there is still difficulty in obtaining and maintaining an anatomic reduction. Because of this, dynamic implants have been investigated in malreduced cadaveric models and have been shown to mitigate clamp-induced malreduction in the coronal and sagittal planes.[144]

By improving the reduction, the surgeon can hopefully maximize patient outcomes and minimize need for secondary interventions.

Hardware-related complications

The syndesmosis is a dynamic articulation, and screw insertion provides a static means of stabilization. This nonphysiologic intervention, theoretically, may result in some degree of functional incapacity and abnormal ankle motion.[170,171]

Syndesmotic screws are typically left in place 12 weeks to allow for ligamentous healing.[172,173] The authors prefer screw retention for 4.5 months to decrease the risk of syndesmotic failure after screw removal. Whether or not it is necessary to remove the intact screw remains a subject of debate. As patients increase their weight bearing, this causes increased shear stresses that can result in screw breakage.[161] If this screw breakage, or removal, occurs before ligamentous healing, it can result in loss of reduction.[158,174,175] One study found that 3.5-mm screws were more likely to break than 4.0- or 4.5-mm screws but without any increased loss of reduction.[176]

A survey demonstrated that 65% of respondents from the Orthopaedic Trauma Association and AOFAS routinely removed syndesmotic screws.[111] However, there is evidence to suggest that patients with retained syndesmotic screws have no functional or radiographic deficits when compared with those with screws removed[78,161,177–179] or with broken screws that are retained.[158,178–180] However, when comparing retained broken screws with retained intact screws, there are studies to suggest that screw removal, or hardware failure, may allow the distal tibiofibular joint to return to normal function and improve functional outcomes. Hamid and colleagues[178] showed that patients with retained broken screws had higher AOFAS scores than patients with intact screws or removed screws. Manjoo and colleagues[181] demonstrated similar results and also showed that there was no benefit in screw removal in patients with loose or fractured screws. Song and colleagues[182] used CT scans to find that 8 of 9 malreductions of the syndesmosis showed adequate reduction once the screw was removed.

It is important to thoroughly consider the literature, because complications can occur with screw removal, with Schepers and colleagues[174] demonstrating a 9.2% wound infection rate and 6.6% rate of recurrent diastasis. In conclusion, there is no high-quality evidence to support the absolute need for routine removal of the syndesmotic screw. Removal may be reserved for intact screws that cause hardware irritation or reduced range of motion after 4 to 6 months or have known malreduction of the syndesmosis.

Dynamic fixation of the syndesmosis has been reported to have cases of infection, skin irritation, and granulomatous tissue formation necessitating secondary intervention.[143] These complications may occur at a lower rate in the new generation of implants that do not have as large of a knot as the original implant, but this has yet to be shown in the literature.

Authors' approach to fixation

Given the lack of direct evidence to determine which mode of fixation is superior, the authors have developed a treatment algorithm based on sagittal stability.

The deltoid ligament is treated with open repair in all cases of preoperative incongruity of the mortise on nonstress radiographs. In the setting of stress-only widening of the mortise, the deltoid is not repaired as in these cases; the authors have noted that the deep component of the deltoid is torn without complete rupture of the superficial deltoid ligament. Repair of the deltoid is associated with improved reduction of the syndesmosis and decreases sagittal plane instability.

In the setting of a Weber B fracture without a posterior malleolar fracture, a suture button device is used to stabilize the syndesmosis given the minimal sagittal instability in these fractures as the IOM is typically intact.

In the setting of a Weber B fracture with a posterior malleolar fracture, the posterior malleolar fracture is reduced and stabilized if amenable to fixation. The authors are aggressive in fixation of all posterior malleolar fractures to directly restore the integrity of the PITFL without additional syndesmotic stabilization. However, if the posterior malleolus is reduced and not amenable to fixation, then rigid fixation with a screw is performed to ensure sagittal stability.

Weber C fractures typically involve greater soft-tissue injury relative to a Weber B fracture with sagittal stability compromised in most cases. Without the presence of a posterior malleolar fracture, a suture button device is used if the deltoid ligament is repaired. If the deltoid ligament is not repaired, sagittal instability is not minimized, and therefore, rigid fixation with a screw or 2 suture button devices is used. Given the cost of 2 suture button devices, the use of a screw is used in the authors' practice.

Weber C fractures with a posterior malleolar fracture are best treated with fixation of the posterior malleolus if possible to restore the anatomy of the incisura. Unlike a Weber B with a posterior malleolar fracture, disruption of the AITFL and IOL occurs in most cases. Therefore, a suture button device is used to restore rotational and coronal stability. If the posterior malleolus cannot be fixated, then rigid fixation is used as discussed earlier.

In the setting of a Maisonneuve injury, fixation of the fibula is difficult and may be associated with injury of the peroneal nerve and is not routinely advocated. In this setting, isolated use of suture button devices may not be provide sufficient sagittal or axial stability despite providing coronal stability and are therefore not used in isolation for this injury. However, given the improved reduction that has been noted with the use of a suture button device, a hybrid construct with a suture button device and a 3.5-mm tricortical screw over a 4-hole plate is used. Traction is placed on the fibula with a reduction clamp to help restore fibular length with temporary stabilization performed with a 0.062 K-wire. A 4-hole plate is chosen with the most distal hole at the level of the tibiotalar joint. The plate is fixed to the fibula using the proximal and distal screw holes. A large reduction clamp is placed with gentle compression to ensure fibular reduction in this setting. The suture button device is placed initially followed by placement of the transsyndesmotic screw (**Fig. 7**).

Routine hardware removal is no longer performed unless the patient is noted to be symptomatic.

CHRONIC SYNDESMOTIC INJURIES

Chronic syndesmotic injuries are defined as persistent widening of the tibiofibular joint 3 months after the initial injury[11] and may occur secondary to malreduction or missed diagnosis. Chronic diastasis of the distal tibiofibular joint is a cause of persistent pain and dysfunction after a rotational ankle injury. Widening and chronic instability of the distal tibiofibular syndesmosis has been shown to be associated with poor outcomes and the development of osteoarthritis.[93,109,183–187] The distal tibiofibular instability is treated with various reconstruction techniques, including tightening with advancement or transposition, autograft substitution, and arthrodesis. Most reconstructions include anatomic restoration of length and rotation of the fibula in addition to addressing the soft-tissue hypertrophy and its mechanical impaction in the ankle joint.

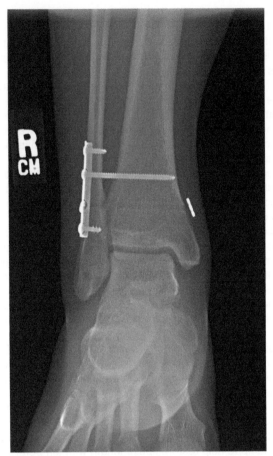

Fig. 7. Postoperative standing AP radiograph of a patient treated with Dr Kadakia's preferred method of a 4-hole plate with 1 syndesmotic screw and 1 suture button. Removal of the screw can be performed at 4.5 months without any concern for fracture of the fibula. Although rare, the complication can lead to significant disability if it occurs. At present, the author no longer performs routine removal of hardware.

DIAGNOSIS
Clinical Evaluation and Physical Examination

Similar methods are used for the diagnosis of chronic injuries to the syndesmosis. Again, the clinician must have a high index of suspicion for the injury and use numerous physical examination techniques and radiographic modalities to make an accurate diagnosis.

Radiographic Evaluation

Plain radiographs
Just as in acute syndesmotic injuries, plain radiography are the first step in imaging evaluation. In the setting of a chronic syndesmotic injury, many patients present with abnormal diastasis of the syndesmosis along with lateral talar translation and an increased MCS (**Fig. 8**). In this scenario, the increase in the forces on the lateral tibiotalar joint is greater than in either condition alone. In addition, instability may be

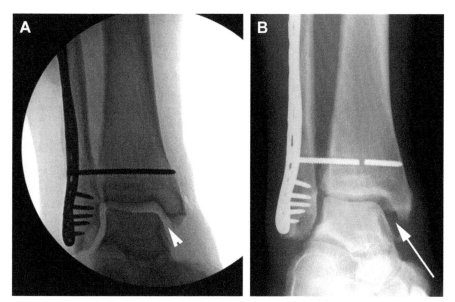

Fig. 8. Early failure of the syndesmotic fixation in a patient who had a concomitant fibular fracture. Appropriate intraoperative reduction and fixation was obtained (*A*) with reduction of the medial clear space (*arrowhead*). With failure of the syndesmosis in the postoperative period (*B*), the loss of syndesmotic stability results in lateral talar translation with an increased medial clear space (*arrow*).

evaluated by dynamic stress evaluation.[42,69,91,92] Instability is present if there is 2 mm or more of widening after an external rotatory stress is applied to the ankle in a neutral position.

CT scan is often more useful in a chronic setting when assessing for associated bony injury, fracture healing, and presence of arthritis. CT is used preoperatively to assess fibular length, degenerative changes within the syndesmosis or tibiotalar joint, presence and location of a synostosis, a malreduced posterior malleolar fracture, and presence of osteochondral lesions[188] (**Fig. 9**). Given anatomic variations, bilateral ankle CT scans are vital to allow the surgeon to compare angular measurements to detect latent diastasis.[189]

MRI may also be obtained to aid in diagnosis and assess for intra-articular pathology and is sensitive, specific, and accurate in the diagnosis of chronic syndesmotic injury.[69] A recent publication noted that, in the presence of positive physical examination findings, a high-intensity signal seen on coronal MRI that resembles the Greek letter λ was sensitive (75%) and specific (85%) for a latent syndesmotic injury with greater than 2 mm of diastasis as seen on arthroscopy.[49]

Arthroscopy

Ankle arthroscopy is a useful tool in the diagnosis of chronic disruption of the distal tibiofibular syndesmosis allowing direct visualization of the disrupted anatomy. Arthroscopic assessment allows for debridement of fibrous tissue interposed in the distal tibiofibular joint as well as concomitant osteochondral defects and synovitis (**Fig. 10**). In a prospective randomized trial of 20 patients, Han and colleagues[69] showed no statistical difference in AOFAS scores in patients treated with arthroscopic debridement with or without screw fixation. These findings were supported by a

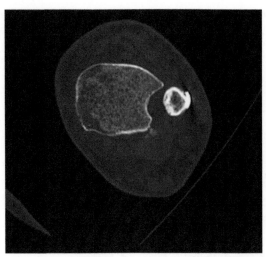

Fig. 9. CT scan of a patient demonstrating clear anterior and lateral malreduction of the fibula.

previous trial by Olgivie-Harris and Reed[42] suggesting that patients' symptoms were secondary to hypertrophied soft tissue within the joint and not instability. Arthroscopic debridement is best used in the setting of normal findings on radiographs without bony abnormality or as an adjunct to a reconstructive procedure. The authors use a suture button device in addition to arthroscopic debridement in these cases to maximize syndesmotic stability. Isolated arthroscopic debridement is contraindicated in the presence of frank diastasis, as the underlying deformity cannot be corrected with arthroscopy alone.

SURGICAL TREATMENT
Reconstruction

Reconstructive techniques depend on the integrity of the distal tibiofibular ligaments, with the goal of restoring the normal anatomy between the distal tibia and fibula in

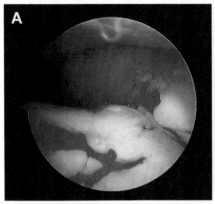
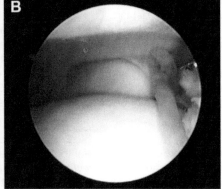

Fig. 10. Arthroscopic view of a patient with chronic syndesmotic instability with an associated osteochondral defect (*A*). Note the significant synovitis and hypertrophic tissue emanating from the syndesmosis. This image is in contrast to a normal appearance (*B*) of the syndesmosis in a patient who had intra-articular fibrous scar after a low ankle sprain.

addition to stabilizing the talus within the mortise. In the setting of a continuous AITFL, bone block advancement has been demonstrated to be a viable option. In a prospective study, Wagener and colleagues[190] osteotomized and mobilized the insertion of the AITFL with a 1 × 1-cm bone block. A gutter directed medial and proximal to the original insertion was then made in the tibia. After application of maximal compression to the mortise with a pelvic clamp, the bone block was advanced into the gutter and stabilized with screw fixation. The bone block was supplemented with a tetracortical syndesmotic screw. Follow-up demonstrated improved average AOFAS scores (75–92) in 12 patients treated greater than 2 years after initial injury with an average follow-up of 25 months.

When the AITFL is ruptured or attenuated, reconstructive surgery using local graft or free autogenous substitute may be used. Grass and colleagues[34] used a split peroneus longus tendon autograft with a tricortical transfixation screw in a series of 16 patients. At an average follow-up of 16 months, 15 of 16 patients reported pain relief and stated they would undergo the surgery again. Hamstring autograft is another alternative that has been performed with encouraging results.[33] This technique described by Morris and colleagues[33] anatomically reconstructed the AITFL and the interosseous ligament using 2 tunnels. The first tunnel was directed from slightly posterolateral to the fibula to slightly anterior in the tibia. The second tunnel was placed anterior to the fibula below the level of and parallel to the first tunnel. The graft was then passed medial to lateral through tunnel 1 and finally looped over the fibula into tunnel 2. The graft was secured medially and laterally with 15-mm interference screws. Visual analog pain scores improved from 73 preoperatively to 19 postoperatively. No preoperative AOFAS scores were recorded preoperatively; however, the average postoperative AOFAS score was 85.4. The graft used in this technique was 7 to 8 mm in diameter compared with the previously described peroneus graft, which was only 3.5 mm in diameter.

Lui[191] described a minimally invasive triligamentous reconstruction using 3 tunnels. The first tunnel connects the anterior and posterior tubercle of the distal tibia, followed by a second tunnel joining the fibular insertions of the AITFL and PITFL. The third and final tunnel is made over the lateral malleolus and directed posteromedially above and toward the tibial tunnel. The peroneus longus tendon is then harvested and passed through the posterior half of the tibial tunnel exiting the third fibular tunnel reconstructing the interosseous ligament. The opposite end of the graft is passed anteriorly through the fibular tunnel reconstructing the PITFL. Finally, the 2 ends are sutured to each other and inserted into the anterior half of the tibial tunnel to reconstruct the AITFL. No long-term follow-up or outcomes were recorded.

Moravek and Kadakia[188] used a double-limbed hamstring allograft reconstruction of the syndesmosis in 6 patients. In contrast to the previously described methods, this technique primarily reconstructs the IOL and is augmented with suture button fixation, which obviates a second procedure for hardware removal. The surgical algorithm is presented in **Box 1**. A single tunnel directed at a 30° angle (posterior to anterior) was drilled from the fibula to the anteromedial tibia. A semitendinosis allograft is first passed medial to lateral and fixed medially with a biotenodesis screw. The free end is then passed over the fibular bridge and fixed over the medial aspect of the tibia. Next, the remaining graft is finally sewn to itself over a medial tibia bone bridge and augmented with a fibular locking plate due to the high stress placed on the fibula during graft tensioning to prevent iatrogenic fracture (**Fig. 11**). Although this was not the initial technique used, following a late stress fracture, the technique was modified. A suture button device is additionally used to decrease the stress on the allograft during the initial phase of healing (**Figs. 12** and **13**). No long-term follow-up was available;

Box 1
Surgical algorithm for the treatment of chronic syndesmotic diastasis

1. Hardware removal of prior fibular and syndesmotic fixation if present
2. Debridement of the syndesmosis and/or excision of synostosis
3. Posterior malleolar osteotomy if preoperative CT indicates a malunion
4. Transection of the deltoid ligament or medial malleolar osteotomy if malunion is present
5. Debridement of medial ankle joint gutter
6. Oblique lengthening fibular osteotomy if a shortened fibula is present
7. Reduction of the syndesmosis with a large tong clamp
8. Suture button fixation proximal to the proposed graft site
9. Doubled allograft reconstruction of the syndesmosis
10. Removal of the reduction clamp with assessment of syndesmotic reduction and stability
11. Imbrication of the deltoid ligament or reduction and fixation of medial malleolar osteotomy

---

however, all patients reported they would undergo surgical intervention again. Before graft placement, the syndesmosis was debrided and fibular and posterior malleolar nonunions were corrected to facilitate an anatomic reduction of the mortise.

Arthrodesis

An alternative to syndesmotic reconstruction particularly in the setting of existing syndesmotic arthritis is arthrodesis. Arthrodesis has proven results that ensure long-term stability of the distal tibiofibular joint provided that successful union occurs. However, this eliminates the normal motion of the syndesmosis that may lead to abnormal load to the talar articular surface with resultant risk of long-term ankle arthrosis. Incorrect positioning in both the sagittal and coronal planes may result in further abnormal forces to the talar articular surface. Despite the theoretic concerns regarding the abnormal talar constraints with resultant risk of arthritis, there is some evidence to suggest the contrary.[11,192,193] Olson and colleagues[193] described debriding the distal tibiofibular joint and stabilizing the arthrodesis with two 3.5-mm cortical screws placed in a lag fashion through 4 cortices. At an average follow-up of 41 months, mean AOFAS scores

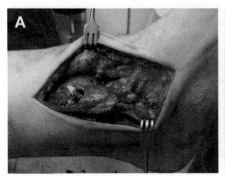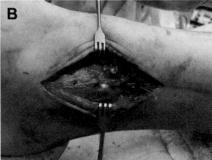

Fig. 11. Final appearance of the graft medially (*A*) and laterally (*B*).

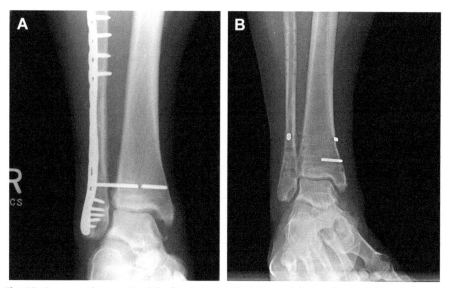

Fig. 12. Preoperative mortise (*A*) of a patient with failure of the syndesmotic fixation status post open reduction and internal fixation. The 6-month postoperative weight bearing radiograph (*B*) demonstrates stable reduction of the syndesmosis and medial clear space.

increased from 37 ± 15 to 87 ± 11. Again, all associated deformities were corrected such as fibular malunions and equinus contractures. The investigators noted an increase in the Kellgren and Moore grade of arthritis in 2 of the 10 patients, with 1 of the 2 patients having a normal ankle preoperatively. These results supported earlier findings by Pena and

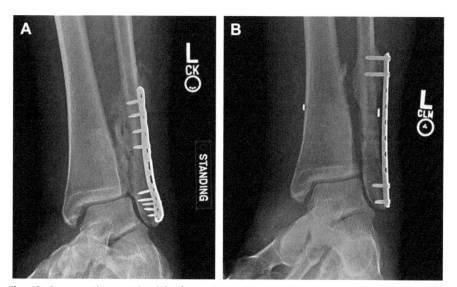

Fig. 13. Preoperative mortise (*A*) of a patient with an untreated syndesmotic injury who developed a significant synostosis. The 12-month postoperative radiograph (*B*) demonstrates excision of the synostosis with stable reduction of the syndesmosis and medial clear space.

Coetzee[192] who also recommended arthrodesis for patients with an injury older than 6 months, severe incongruity, or a recurrence of diastasis after removal of fixation. The authors thought this procedure should be reserved for low-demand patients (**Fig. 14**). Overcompression of the syndesmosis should be avoided, as this creates a nonanatomic mortise increasing the risk of tibiotalar arthritis.

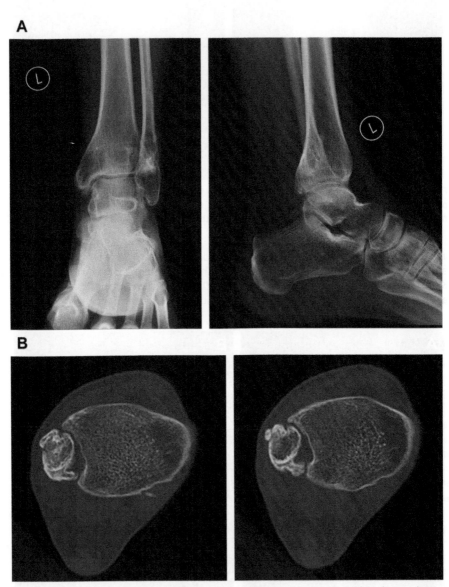

Fig. 14. Preoperative radiographs (*A*) of a patient with persistent pain within the syndesmosis without clear evidence of tibiotalar arthritis. CT scan (*B*) reveals clear evidence of tibiofibular degenerative changes that precludes reconstruction. Postoperative radiographs (*C*) after syndesmotic fusion with allograft to maintain the appropriate relationship of the tibia and fibula.

C

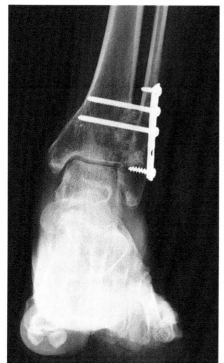 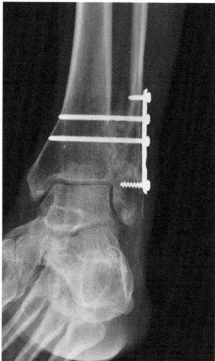

Fig. 14. (*continued*)

SUMMARY

Injuries to the syndesmosis are a diagnostic and therapeutic challenge to the orthopedic surgeon. The lack of clear radiographic parameters on which to make surgical decisions places greater importance on the physical examination and advanced imaging. Lack of injury to the deltoid ligament and PITFL based on MRI imaging is a reliable determinant to consider nonoperative treatment. Injury to the deltoid ligament or disruption of the relationship of the tibia and fibula typically is treated with surgical reduction and fixation. Use of the contralateral lower extremity is the most reliable in determining the normal relationship of the tibia and fibula for the patient both preoperatively and intraoperatively. Sagittal instability is more critical than coronal instability and must be taken into account when considering reduction of fixation of the syndesmosis. Further studies will determine the need for primary repair of the deltoid ligament and fixation of the posterior malleolus in the setting of ankle fracture and syndesmotic injuries. As the understanding of the longer-term outcomes following injury to the syndesmosis advances, a logical algorithm to the treatment of these injuries should emerge.

REFERENCES

1. Bartonicek J. Anatomy of the tibiofibular syndesmosis and its clinical relevance. Surg Radiol Anat 2003;25:379–86.

2. Lepojarvi S, Pakarinen H, Savola O, et al. Posterior translation of the fibula may indicate malreduction: CT study of normal variation in uninjured ankles. J Orthop Trauma 2014;28:205–9.

3. Mendelsohn ES, Hoshino CM, Harris TG, et al. CT characterizing the anatomy of uninjured ankle syndesmosis. Orthopedics 2014;37:e157–60.

4. Dikos GD, Heisler J, Choplin RH, et al. Normal tibiofibular relationships at the syndesmosis on axial CT imaging. J Orthop Trauma 2012;26:433–8.

5. Kelikian AS, Sarrafian SK, Sarrafian SK. Sarrafian's anatomy of the foot and ankle: descriptive, topographical, functional. 3rd edition. Philadelphia: Wolters Kluwer Health/Lippincott Williams & Wilkins; 2011.

6. Hermans JJ, Beumer A, de Jong TA, et al. Anatomy of the distal tibiofibular syndesmosis in adults: a pictorial essay with a multimodality approach. J Anat 2010;217:633–45.

7. Williams BT, Ahrberg AB, Goldsmith MT, et al. Ankle syndesmosis: a qualitative and quantitative anatomic analysis. Am J Sports Med 2015;43:88–97.

8. McKeon KE, Wright RW, Johnson JE, et al. Vascular anatomy of the tibiofibular syndesmosis. J Bone Joint Surg Am 2012;94:931–8.

9. Michelson JD, Helgemo SL Jr. Kinematics of the axially loaded ankle. Foot Ankle Int 1995;16:577–82.

10. Beumer A, Valstar ER, Garling EH, et al. Kinematics of the distal tibiofibular syndesmosis: radiostereometry in 11 normal ankles. Acta Orthop Scand 2003;74:337–43.

11. Espinosa N, Smerek JP, Myerson MS. Acute and chronic syndesmosis injuries: pathomechanisms, diagnosis and management. Foot Ankle Clin 2006;11:639–57.

12. Ogilvie-Harris DJ, Reed SC, Hedman TP. Disruption of the ankle syndesmosis: biomechanical study of the ligamentous restraints. Arthroscopy 1994;10:558–60.

13. Xenos JS, Hopkinson WJ, Mulligan ME, et al. The tibiofibular syndesmosis. Evaluation of the ligamentous structures, methods of fixation, and radiographic assessment. J Bone Joint Surg Am 1995;77:847–56.

14. Ramsey PL, Hamilton W. Changes in tibiotalar area of contact caused by lateral talar shift. J Bone Joint Surg Am 1976;58:356–7.

15. Lloyd J, Elsayed S, Hariharan K, et al. Revisiting the concept of talar shift in ankle fractures. Foot Ankle Int 2006;27:793–6.

16. Norkus SA, Floyd RT. The anatomy and mechanisms of syndesmotic ankle sprains. J Athl Train 2001;36:68–73.

17. Lauge-Hansen N. Fractures of the ankle. II. Combined experimental-surgical and experimental-roentgenologic investigations. Arch Surg 1950;60:957–85.

18. Pankovich AM. Maisonneuve fracture of the fibula. J Bone Joint Surg Am 1976;58:337–42.

19. Haraguchi N, Armiger RS. A new interpretation of the mechanism of ankle fracture. J Bone Joint Surg Am 2009;91:821–9.

20. Dubin JC, Comeau D, McClelland RI, et al. Lateral and syndesmotic ankle sprain injuries: a narrative literature review. J Chiropr Med 2011;10:204–19.

21. Kellett JJ. The clinical features of ankle syndesmosis injuries: a general review. Clin J Sport Med 2011;21:524–9.

22. Roemer FW, Jomaah N, Niu J, et al. Ligamentous injuries and the risk of associated tissue damage in acute ankle sprains in athletes: a cross-sectional MRI study. Am J Sports Med 2014;42:1549–57.

23. Vosseller JT, Karl JW, Greisberg JK. Incidence of syndesmotic injury. Orthopedics 2014;37:e226–9.

24. Hunt KJ, George E, Harris AH, et al. Epidemiology of syndesmosis injuries in intercollegiate football: incidence and risk factors from National Collegiate Athletic Association injury surveillance system data from 2004-2005 to 2008-2009. Clin J Sport Med 2013;23:278–82.

25. Wright RW, Barile RJ, Surprenant DA, et al. Ankle syndesmosis sprains in National Hockey League players. Am J Sports Med 2004;32:1941–5.

26. Clanton TO, Paul P. Syndesmosis injuries in athletes. Foot Ankle Clin 2002;7: 529–49.

27. Fritschy D. An unusual ankle injury in top skiers. Am J Sports Med 1989;17: 282–5 [discussion: 285–6].

28. Flik K, Lyman S, Marx RG. American collegiate men's ice hockey: an analysis of injuries. Am J Sports Med 2005;33:183–7.

29. Hopkinson WJ, St Pierre P, Ryan JB, et al. Syndesmosis sprains of the ankle. Foot Ankle 1990;10:325–30.

30. Nussbaum ED, Hosea TM, Sieler SD, et al. Prospective evaluation of syndesmotic ankle sprains without diastasis. Am J Sports Med 2001;29:31–5.

31. Gerber JP, Williams GN, Scoville CR, et al. Persistent disability associated with ankle sprains: a prospective examination of an athletic population. Foot Ankle Int 1998;19:653–60.

32. Kaplan LD, Jost PW, Honkamp N, et al. Incidence and variance of foot and ankle injuries in elite college football players. Am J Orthop (Belle Mead NJ) 2011;40: 40–4.

33. Morris MW, Rice P, Schneider TE. Distal tibiofibular syndesmosis reconstruction using a free hamstring autograft. Foot Ankle Int 2009;30:506–11.

34. Grass R, Rammelt S, Biewener A, et al. Peroneus longus ligamentoplasty for chronic instability of the distal tibiofibular syndesmosis. Foot Ankle Int 2003; 24:392–7.

35. Harper MC. Delayed reduction and stabilization of the tibiofibular syndesmosis. Foot Ankle Int 2001;22:15–8.

36. Taylor DC, Englehardt DL, Bassett FH 3rd. Syndesmosis sprains of the ankle. The influence of heterotopic ossification. Am J Sports Med 1992; 20:146–50.

37. Ward DW. Syndesmotic ankle sprain in a recreational hockey player. J Manipulative Physiol Ther 1994;17:385–94.

38. van Dijk CN, Lim LS, Bossuyt PM, et al. Physical examination is sufficient for the diagnosis of sprained ankles. J Bone Joint Surg Br 1996;78:958–62.

39. van Dijk CN, Mol BW, Lim LS, et al. Diagnosis of ligament rupture of the ankle joint. Physical examination, arthrography, stress radiography and sonography compared in 160 patients after inversion trauma. Acta Orthop Scand 1996;67: 566–70.

40. Beumer A, van Hemert WL, Swierstra BA, et al. A biomechanical evaluation of clinical stress tests for syndesmotic ankle instability. Foot Ankle Int 2003;24: 358–63.

41. Boytim MJ, Fischer DA, Neumann L. Syndesmotic ankle sprains. Am J Sports Med 1991;19:294–8.

42. Ogilvie-Harris DJ, Reed SC. Disruption of the ankle syndesmosis: diagnosis and treatment by arthroscopic surgery. Arthroscopy 1994;10:561–8.

43. Teitz CC, Harrington RM. A biochemical analysis of the squeeze test for sprains of the syndesmotic ligaments of the ankle. Foot Ankle Int 1998;19:489–92.

44. Kiter E, Bozkurt M. The crossed-leg test for examination of ankle syndesmosis injuries. Foot Ankle Int 2005;26:187–8.

45. Williams GN, Jones MH, Amendola A. Syndesmotic ankle sprains in athletes. Am J Sports Med 2007;35:1197–207.

46. Beumer A, Swierstra BA, Mulder PG. Clinical diagnosis of syndesmotic ankle instability: evaluation of stress tests behind the curtains. Acta Orthop Scand 2002;73:667–9.

47. Sman AD, Hiller CE, Rae K, et al. Diagnostic accuracy of clinical tests for ankle syndesmosis injury. Br J Sports Med 2015;49:323–9.

48. de Cesar PC, Avila EM, de Abreu MR. Comparison of magnetic resonance imaging to physical examination for syndesmotic injury after lateral ankle sprain. Foot Ankle Int 2011;32:1110–4.

49. Ryan LP, Hills MC, Chang J, et al. The lambda sign: a new radiographic indicator of latent syndesmosis instability. Foot Ankle Int 2014;35:903–8.

50. Sman AD, Hiller CE, Refshauge KM. Diagnostic accuracy of clinical tests for diagnosis of ankle syndesmosis injury: a systematic review. Br J Sports Med 2013;47:620–8.

51. Alonso A, Khoury L, Adams R. Clinical tests for ankle syndesmosis injury: reliability and prediction of return to function. J Orthop Sports Phys Ther 1998; 27:276–84.

52. Harper MC, Keller TS. A radiographic evaluation of the tibiofibular syndesmosis. Foot Ankle 1989;10:156–60.

53. Croft S, Furey A, Stone C, et al. Radiographic evaluation of the ankle syndesmosis. Can J Surg 2015;58:58–62.

54. Beumer A, van Hemert WL, Niesing R, et al. Radiographic measurement of the distal tibiofibular syndesmosis has limited use. Clin Orthop Relat Res 2004;(423):227–34.

55. Pneumaticos SG, Noble PC, Chatziioannou SN, et al. The effects of rotation on radiographic evaluation of the tibiofibular syndesmosis. Foot Ankle Int 2002;23:107–11.

56. Shah AS, Kadakia AR, Tan GJ, et al. Radiographic evaluation of the normal distal tibiofibular syndesmosis. Foot Ankle Int 2012;33:870–6.

57. Hermans JJ, Wentink N, Beumer A, et al. Correlation between radiological assessment of acute ankle fractures and syndesmotic injury on MRI. Skeletal Radiol 2012;41:787–801.

58. Nielson JH, Gardner MJ, Peterson MG, et al. Radiographic measurements do not predict syndesmotic injury in ankle fractures: an MRI study. Clin Orthop Relat Res 2005;(436):216–21.

59. Edwards GS Jr, DeLee JC. Ankle diastasis without fracture. Foot Ankle 1984;4: 305–12.

60. Schock HJ, Pinzur M, Manion L, et al. The use of gravity or manual-stress radiographs in the assessment of supination-external rotation fractures of the ankle. J Bone Joint Surg Br 2007;89:1055–9.

61. Ebraheim NA, Lu J, Yang H, et al. Radiographic and CT evaluation of tibiofibular syndesmotic diastasis: a cadaver study. Foot Ankle Int 1997;18:693–8.

62. Knops SP, Kohn MA, Hansen EN, et al. Rotational malreduction of the syndesmosis: reliability and accuracy of computed tomography measurement methods. Foot Ankle Int 2013;34:1403–10.

63. Gifford PB, Lutz M. The tibiofibular line: an anatomical feature to diagnose syndesmosis malposition. Foot Ankle Int 2014;35:1181–6.

64. Nault ML, Hebert-Davies J, Laflamme GY, et al. CT scan assessment of the syndesmosis: a new reproducible method. J Orthop Trauma 2013;27:638–41.

65. Ebraheim NA, Elgafy H, Padanilam T. Syndesmotic disruption in low fibular fractures associated with deltoid ligament injury. Clin Orthop Relat Res 2003;(409):260–7.

66. Mukhopadhyay S, Metcalfe A, Guha AR, et al. Malreduction of syndesmosis–are we considering the anatomical variation? Injury 2011;42:1073–6.
67. Vogl TJ, Hochmuth K, Diebold T, et al. Magnetic resonance imaging in the diagnosis of acute injured distal tibiofibular syndesmosis. Invest Radiol 1997;32:401–9.
68. Clanton TO, Ho CP, Williams BT, et al. Magnetic resonance imaging characterization of individual ankle syndesmosis structures in asymptomatic and surgically treated cohorts. Knee Surg Sports Traumatol Arthrosc 2014. [Epub ahead of print].
69. Han SH, Lee JW, Kim S, et al. Chronic tibiofibular syndesmosis injury: the diagnostic efficiency of magnetic resonance imaging and comparative analysis of operative treatment. Foot Ankle Int 2007;28:336–42.
70. Oae K, Takao M, Naito K, et al. Injury of the tibiofibular syndesmosis: value of MR imaging for diagnosis. Radiology 2003;227:155–61.
71. Sikka RS, Fetzer GB, Sugarman E, et al. Correlating MRI findings with disability in syndesmotic sprains of NFL players. Foot Ankle Int 2012;33:371–8.
72. Brown KW, Morrison WB, Schweitzer ME, et al. MRI findings associated with distal tibiofibular syndesmosis injury. AJR Am J Roentgenol 2004;182:131–6.
73. Campbell SE, Warner M. MR imaging of ankle inversion injuries. Magn Reson Imaging Clin N Am 2008;16:1–18, v.
74. Hunt KJ. Syndesmosis injuries. Curr Rev Musculoskelet Med 2013;6:304–12.
75. Gardner MJ, Demetrakopoulos D, Briggs SM, et al. Malreduction of the tibiofibular syndesmosis in ankle fractures. Foot Ankle Int 2006;27:788–92.
76. Schottel PC, Berkes MB, Little MT, et al. Comparison of clinical outcome of pronation external rotation versus supination external rotation ankle fractures. Foot Ankle Int 2014;35:353–9.
77. Pakarinen HJ, Flinkkila TE, Ohtonen PP, et al. Syndesmotic fixation in supination-external rotation ankle fractures: a prospective randomized study. Foot Ankle Int 2011;32:1103–9.
78. Weening B, Bhandari M. Predictors of functional outcome following trans-syndesmotic screw fixation of ankle fractures. J Orthop Trauma 2005;19:102–8.
79. Jenkinson RJ, Sanders DW, Macleod MD, et al. Intraoperative diagnosis of syndesmosis injuries in external rotation ankle fractures. J Orthop Trauma 2005;19:604–9.
80. Stark E, Tornetta P 3rd, Creevy WR. Syndesmotic instability in Weber B ankle fractures: a clinical evaluation. J Orthop Trauma 2007;21:643–6.
81. Tornetta P 3rd, Axelrad TW, Sibai TA, et al. Treatment of the stress positive ligamentous SE4 ankle fracture: incidence of syndesmotic injury and clinical decision making. J Orthop Trauma 2012;26:659–61.
82. Ebraheim NA, Weston JT, Ludwig T, et al. The association between medial malleolar fracture geometry, injury mechanism, and syndesmotic disruption. Foot Ankle Surg 2014;20:276–80.
83. Choi Y, Kwon SS, Chung CY, et al. Preoperative radiographic and CT findings predicting syndesmotic injuries in supination-external rotation-type ankle fractures. J Bone Joint Surg Am 2014;96:1161–7.
84. Pakarinen H, Flinkkila T, Ohtonen P, et al. Intraoperative assessment of the stability of the distal tibiofibular joint in supination-external rotation injuries of the ankle: sensitivity, specificity, and reliability of two clinical tests. J Bone Joint Surg Am 2011;93:2057–61.
85. Cotton FJ. Dislocations and joint-fractures. 2nd edition. Philadelphia; London: W.B. Saunders Company; 1924.

86. Candal-Couto JJ, Burrow D, Bromage S, et al. Instability of the tibio-fibular syndesmosis: have we been pulling in the wrong direction? Injury 2004;35: 814–8.
87. Matuszewski PE, Dombroski D, Lawrence JT, et al. Prospective intraoperative syndesmotic evaluation during ankle fracture fixation: stress external rotation versus lateral fibular stress. J Orthop Trauma 2015;29(4):e157–60.
88. Stoffel K, Wysocki D, Baddour E, et al. Comparison of two intraoperative assessment methods for injuries to the ankle syndesmosis. A cadaveric study. J Bone Joint Surg Am 2009;91:2646–52.
89. Jiang KN, Schulz BM, Tsui YL, et al. Comparison of radiographic stress tests for syndesmotic instability of supination-external rotation ankle fractures: a cadaveric study. J Orthop Trauma 2014;28:e123–7.
90. Sri-Ram K, Robinson AH. Arthroscopic assessment of the syndesmosis following ankle fracture. Injury 2005;36:675–8.
91. Takao M, Ochi M, Naito K, et al. Arthroscopic diagnosis of tibiofibular syndesmosis disruption. Arthroscopy 2001;17:836–43.
92. Takao M, Ochi M, Oae K, et al. Diagnosis of a tear of the tibiofibular syndesmosis. The role of arthroscopy of the ankle. J Bone Joint Surg Br 2003;85:324–9.
93. de Souza LJ, Gustilo RB, Meyer TJ. Results of operative treatment of displaced external rotation-abduction fractures of the ankle. J Bone Joint Surg Am 1985; 67:1066–74.
94. Jones MH, Amendola A. Syndesmosis sprains of the ankle: a systematic review. Clin Orthop Relat Res 2007;(455):173–5.
95. Mak MF, Gartner L, Pearce CJ. Management of syndesmosis injuries in the elite athlete. Foot Ankle Clin 2013;18:195–214.
96. Kortekangas TH, Pakarinen HJ, Savola O, et al. Syndesmotic fixation in supination-external rotation ankle fractures: a prospective randomized study. Foot Ankle Int 2014;35:988–95.
97. Jones CR, Nunley JA 2nd. Deltoid ligament repair vs. syndesmotic fixation in bi-malleolar equivalent ankle fractures. J Orthop Trauma 2015;29:245–9.
98. Thordarson DB, Motamed S, Hedman T, et al. The effect of fibular malreduction on contact pressures in an ankle fracture malunion model. J Bone Joint Surg Am 1997;79:1809–15.
99. Mohammed R, Syed S, Metikala S, et al. Evaluation of the syndesmotic-only fixation for Weber-C ankle fractures with syndesmotic injury. Indian J Orthop 2011; 45:454–8.
100. Miller AN, Barei DP, Iaquinto JM, et al. Iatrogenic syndesmosis malreduction via clamp and screw placement. J Orthop Trauma 2013;27:100–6.
101. Phisitkul P, Ebinger T, Goetz J, et al. Forceps reduction of the syndesmosis in rotational ankle fractures: a cadaveric study. J Bone Joint Surg Am 2012;94: 2256–61.
102. Marmor M, Hansen E, Han HK, et al. Limitations of standard fluoroscopy in detecting rotational malreduction of the syndesmosis in an ankle fracture model. Foot Ankle Int 2011;32:616–22.
103. Schreiber JJ, McLawhorn AS, Dy CJ, et al. Intraoperative contralateral view for assessing accurate syndesmosis reduction. Orthopedics 2013;36:360–1.
104. Koenig SJ, Tornetta P 3rd, Merlin G, et al. Can we tell if the syndesmosis is reduced using fluoroscopy? J Orthop Trauma 2015. [Epub ahead of print].
105. Summers HD, Sinclair MK, Stover MD. A reliable method for intraoperative evaluation of syndesmotic reduction. J Orthop Trauma 2013;27:196–200.

106. Ruan Z, Luo C, Shi Z, et al. Intraoperative reduction of distal tibiofibular joint aided by three-dimensional fluoroscopy. Technol Health Care 2011;19: 161–6.

107. Davidovitch RI, Weil Y, Karia R, et al. Intraoperative syndesmotic reduction: three-dimensional versus standard fluoroscopic imaging. J Bone Joint Surg Am 2013;95:1838–43.

108. Franke J, von Recum J, Suda AJ, et al. Intraoperative three-dimensional imaging in the treatment of acute unstable syndesmotic injuries. J Bone Joint Surg Am 2012;94:1386–90.

109. Sagi HC, Shah AR, Sanders RW. The functional consequence of syndesmotic joint malreduction at a minimum 2-year follow-up. J Orthop Trauma 2012;26: 439–43.

110. Miller AN, Carroll EA, Parker RJ, et al. Direct visualization for syndesmotic stabilization of ankle fractures. Foot Ankle Int 2009;30:419–26.

111. Bava E, Charlton T, Thordarson D. Ankle fracture syndesmosis fixation and management: the current practice of orthopedic surgeons. Am J Orthop (Belle Mead NJ) 2010;39:242–6.

112. Ahmad J, Raikin SM, Pour AE, et al. Bioabsorbable screw fixation of the syndesmosis in unstable ankle injuries. Foot Ankle Int 2009;30:99–105.

113. Hovis WD, Kaiser BW, Watson JT, et al. Treatment of syndesmotic disruptions of the ankle with bioabsorbable screw fixation. J Bone Joint Surg Am 2002;84-A: 26–31.

114. Thordarson DB, Samuelson M, Shepherd LE, et al. Bioabsorbable versus stainless steel screw fixation of the syndesmosis in pronation-lateral rotation ankle fractures: a prospective randomized trial. Foot Ankle Int 2001;22: 335–8.

115. Kaukonen JP, Lamberg T, Korkala O, et al. Fixation of syndesmotic ruptures in 38 patients with a malleolar fracture: a randomized study comparing a metallic and a bioabsorbable screw. J Orthop Trauma 2005;19:392–5.

116. Sinisaari IP, Luthje PM, Mikkonen RH. Ruptured tibio-fibular syndesmosis: comparison study of metallic to bioabsorbable fixation. Foot Ankle Int 2002;23: 744–8.

117. Beumer A, Campo MM, Niesing R, et al. Screw fixation of the syndesmosis: a cadaver model comparing stainless steel and titanium screws and three and four cortical fixation. Injury 2005;36:60–4.

118. Sun H, Luo CF, Zhong B, et al. A prospective, randomised trial comparing the use of absorbable and metallic screws in the fixation of distal tibiofibular syndesmosis injuries: mid-term follow-up. Bone Joint J 2014;96-B:548–54.

119. Hansen M, Le L, Wertheimer S, et al. Syndesmosis fixation: analysis of shear stress via axial load on 3.5-mm and 4.5-mm quadricortical syndesmotic screws. J Foot Ankle Surg 2006;45:65–9.

120. Thompson MC, Gesink DS. Biomechanical comparison of syndesmosis fixation with 3.5- and 4.5-millimeter stainless steel screws. Foot Ankle Int 2000;21: 736–41.

121. Markolf KL, Jackson SR, McAllister DR. Syndesmosis fixation using dual 3.5 mm and 4.5 mm screws with tricortical and quadricortical purchase: a biomechanical study. Foot Ankle Int 2013;34:734–9.

122. Hoiness P, Stromsoe K. Tricortical versus quadricortical syndesmosis fixation in ankle fractures: a prospective, randomized study comparing two methods of syndesmosis fixation. J Orthop Trauma 2004;18:331–7.

123. Wikeroy AK, Hoiness PR, Andreassen GS, et al. No difference in functional and radiographic results 8.4 years after quadricortical compared with tricortical syndesmosis fixation in ankle fractures. J Orthop Trauma 2010;24:17–23.

124. Moore JA Jr, Shank JR, Morgan SJ, et al. Syndesmosis fixation: a comparison of three and four cortices of screw fixation without hardware removal. Foot Ankle Int 2006;27:567–72.

125. Nousiainen MT, McConnell AJ, Zdero R, et al. The influence of the number of cortices of screw purchase and ankle position in Weber C ankle fracture fixation. J Orthop Trauma 2008;22:473–8.

126. Gardner R, Yousri T, Holmes F, et al. Stabilization of the syndesmosis in the Maisonneuve fracture–a biomechanical study comparing 2-hole locking plate and quadricortical screw fixation. J Orthop Trauma 2013;27:212–6.

127. Babis GC, Papagelopoulos PJ, Tsarouchas J, et al. Operative treatment for Maisonneuve fracture of the proximal fibula. Orthopedics 2000;23:687–90.

128. Stufkens SA, van den Bekerom MP, Doornberg JN, et al. Evidence-based treatment of Maisonneuve fractures. J Foot Ankle Surg 2011;50:62–7.

129. Dunn WR, Easley ME, Parks BG, et al. An augmented fixation method for distal fibular fractures in elderly patients: a biomechanical evaluation. Foot Ankle Int 2004;25:128–31.

130. Degroot H, Al-Omari AA, El Ghazaly SA. Outcomes of suture button repair of the distal tibiofibular syndesmosis. Foot Ankle Int 2011;32:250–6.

131. Laflamme M, Belzile EL, Bedard L, et al. A prospective randomized multicenter trial comparing clinical outcomes of patients treated surgically with a static or dynamic implant for acute ankle syndesmosis rupture. J Orthop Trauma 2015; 29:216–23.

132. Naqvi GA, Cunningham P, Lynch B, et al. Fixation of ankle syndesmotic injuries: comparison of tightrope fixation and syndesmotic screw fixation for accuracy of syndesmotic reduction. Am J Sports Med 2012;40:2828–35.

133. Naqvi GA, Shafqat A, Awan N. Tightrope fixation of ankle syndesmosis injuries: clinical outcome, complications and technique modification. Injury 2012;43: 838–42.

134. Rigby RB, Cottom JM. Does the Arthrex TightRope(R) provide maintenance of the distal tibiofibular syndesmosis? A 2-year follow-up of 64 TightRopes(R) in 37 patients. J Foot Ankle Surg 2013;52:563–7.

135. Schepers T. Acute distal tibiofibular syndesmosis injury: a systematic review of suture-button versus syndesmotic screw repair. Int Orthop 2012;36:1199–206.

136. Teramoto A, Suzuki D, Kamiya T, et al. Comparison of different fixation methods of the suture-button implant for tibiofibular syndesmosis injuries. Am J Sports Med 2011;39:2226–32.

137. Thornes B, Shannon F, Guiney AM, et al. Suture-button syndesmosis fixation: accelerated rehabilitation and improved outcomes. Clin Orthop Relat Res 2005;(431):207–12.

138. Willmott HJ, Singh B, David LA. Outcome and complications of treatment of ankle diastasis with tightrope fixation. Injury 2009;40:1204–6.

139. Cottom JM, Hyer CF, Philbin TM, et al. Transosseous fixation of the distal tibiofibular syndesmosis: comparison of an interosseous suture and endobutton to traditional screw fixation in 50 cases. J Foot Ankle Surg 2009; 48:620–30.

140. Ebramzadeh E, Knutsen AR, Sangiorgio SN, et al. Biomechanical comparison of syndesmotic injury fixation methods using a cadaveric model. Foot Ankle Int 2013;34:1710–7.

141. Forsythe K, Freedman KB, Stover MD, et al. Comparison of a novel FiberWire-button construct versus metallic screw fixation in a syndesmotic injury model. Foot Ankle Int 2008;29:49–54.
142. Qamar F, Kadakia A, Venkateswaran B. An anatomical way of treating ankle syndesmotic injuries. J Foot Ankle Surg 2011;50:762–5.
143. Storey P, Gadd RJ, Blundell C, et al. Complications of suture button ankle syndesmosis stabilization with modifications of surgical technique. Foot Ankle Int 2012;33:717–21.
144. Westermann RW, Rungprai C, Goetz JE, et al. The effect of suture-button fixation on simulated syndesmotic malreduction: a cadaveric study. J Bone Joint Surg Am 2014;96:1732–8.
145. McBryde A, Chiasson B, Wilhelm A, et al. Syndesmotic screw placement: a biomechanical analysis. Foot Ankle Int 1997;18:262–6.
146. Verim O, Er MS, Altinel L, et al. Biomechanical evaluation of syndesmotic screw position: a finite-element analysis. J Orthop Trauma 2014;28:210–5.
147. Kukreti S, Faraj A, Miles JN. Does position of syndesmotic screw affect functional and radiological outcome in ankle fractures? Injury 2005;36:1121–4.
148. Schepers T, van der Linden H, van Lieshout EM, et al. Technical aspects of the syndesmotic screw and their effect on functional outcome following acute distal tibiofibular syndesmosis injury. Injury 2014;45:775–9.
149. van den Bekerom MP, Hogervorst M, Bolhuis HW, et al. Operative aspects of the syndesmotic screw: review of current concepts. Injury 2008;39:491–8.
150. Kennedy MT, Carmody O, Leong S, et al. A computed tomography evaluation of two hundred normal ankles, to ascertain what anatomical landmarks to use when compressing or placing an ankle syndesmosis screw. Foot (Edinb) 2014;24:157–60.
151. Olerud C. The effect of the syndesmotic screw on the extension capacity of the ankle joint. Arch Orthop Trauma Surg 1985;104:299–302.
152. Tornetta P 3rd, Spoo JE, Reynolds FA, et al. Overtightening of the ankle syndesmosis: is it really possible? J Bone Joint Surg Am 2001;83-A:489–92.
153. Bragonzoni L, Russo A, Girolami M, et al. The distal tibiofibular syndesmosis during passive foot flexion. RSA-based study on intact, ligament injured and screw fixed cadaver specimens. Arch Orthop Trauma Surg 2006;126:304–8.
154. Gardner MJ, Brodsky A, Briggs SM, et al. Fixation of posterior malleolar fractures provides greater syndesmotic stability. Clin Orthop Relat Res 2006;447:165–71.
155. Miller AN, Carroll EA, Parker RJ, et al. Posterior malleolar stabilization of syndesmotic injuries is equivalent to screw fixation. Clin Orthop Relat Res 2010;468:1129–35.
156. Nelson OA. Examination and repair of the AITFL in transmalleolar fractures. J Orthop Trauma 2006;20:637–43.
157. Jelinek JA, Porter DA. Management of unstable ankle fractures and syndesmosis injuries in athletes. Foot Ankle Clin 2009;14:277–98.
158. Hsu YT, Wu CC, Lee WC, et al. Surgical treatment of syndesmotic diastasis: emphasis on effect of syndesmotic screw on ankle function. Int Orthop 2011;35:359–64.
159. Symeonidis PD, Iselin LD, Chehade M, et al. Common pitfalls in syndesmotic rupture management: a clinical audit. Foot Ankle Int 2013;34:345–50.

160. Egol KA, Tejwani NC, Walsh MG, et al. Predictors of short-term functional outcome following ankle fracture surgery. J Bone Joint Surg Am 2006;88: 974–9.
161. Egol KA, Pahk B, Walsh M, et al. Outcome after unstable ankle fracture: effect of syndesmotic stabilization. J Orthop Trauma 2010;24:7–11.
162. Litrenta J, Saper D, Tornetta P 3rd, et al. Does syndesmotic injury have a negative effect on functional outcome? A multicenter prospective evaluation. J Orthop Trauma 2015. [Epub ahead of print].
163. Kortekangas T, Flinkkila T, Niinimaki J, et al. Effect of syndesmosis injury in SER IV (Weber B)-type ankle fractures on function and incidence of osteoarthritis. Foot Ankle Int 2015;36:180–7.
164. Kennedy JG, Soffe KE, Dalla Vedova P, et al. Evaluation of the syndesmotic screw in low Weber C ankle fractures. J Orthop Trauma 2000;14:359–66.
165. Chissell HR, Jones J. The influence of a diastasis screw on the outcome of Weber type-C ankle fractures. J Bone Joint Surg Br 1995;77:435–8.
166. Mendelsohn ES, Hoshino CM, Harris TG, et al. The effect of obesity on early failure after operative syndesmosis injuries. J Orthop Trauma 2013;27:201–6.
167. Wukich DK, Kline AJ. The management of ankle fractures in patients with diabetes. J Bone Joint Surg Am 2008;90:1570–8.
168. Franke J, von Recum J, Suda AJ, et al. Predictors of a persistent dislocation after reduction of syndesmotic injuries detected with intraoperative three-dimensional imaging. Foot Ankle Int 2014;35:1323–8.
169. Pelton K, Thordarson DB, Barnwell J. Open versus closed treatment of the fibula in Maissoneuve injuries. Foot Ankle Int 2010;31:604–8.
170. Needleman RL, Skrade DA, Stiehl JB. Effect of the syndesmotic screw on ankle motion. Foot Ankle 1989;10:17–24.
171. Miller AN, Paul O, Boraiah S, et al. Functional outcomes after syndesmotic screw fixation and removal. J Orthop Trauma 2010;24:12–6.
172. Dattani R, Patnaik S, Kantak A, et al. Injuries to the tibiofibular syndesmosis. J Bone Joint Surg Br 2008;90:405–10.
173. Schepers T. To retain or remove the syndesmotic screw: a review of literature. Arch Orthop Trauma Surg 2011;131:879–83.
174. Schepers T, Van Lieshout EM, de Vries MR, et al. Complications of syndesmotic screw removal. Foot Ankle Int 2011;32:1040–4.
175. Jordan TH, Talarico RH, Schuberth JM. The radiographic fate of the syndesmosis after trans-syndesmotic screw removal in displaced ankle fractures. J Foot Ankle Surg 2011;50:407–12.
176. Stuart K, Panchbhavi VK. The fate of syndesmotic screws. Foot Ankle Int 2011; 32:S519–25.
177. Bell DP, Wong MK. Syndesmotic screw fixation in Weber C ankle injuries–should the screw be removed before weight bearing? Injury 2006;37:891–8.
178. Hamid N, Loeffler BJ, Braddy W, et al. Outcome after fixation of ankle fractures with an injury to the syndesmosis: the effect of the syndesmosis screw. J Bone Joint Surg Br 2009;91:1069–73.
179. Boyle MJ, Gao R, Frampton CM, et al. Removal of the syndesmotic screw after the surgical treatment of a fracture of the ankle in adult patients does not affect one-year outcomes: a randomised controlled trial. Bone Joint J 2014;96-B: 1699–705.
180. Tucker A, Street J, Kealey D, et al. Functional outcomes following syndesmotic fixation: a comparison of screws retained in situ versus routine removal - is it really necessary? Injury 2013;44:1880–4.

181. Manjoo A, Sanders DW, Tieszer C, et al. Functional and radiographic results of patients with syndesmotic screw fixation: implications for screw removal. J Orthop Trauma 2010;24:2–6.

182. Song DJ, Lanzi JT, Groth AT, et al. The effect of syndesmosis screw removal on the reduction of the distal tibiofibular joint: a prospective radiographic study. Foot Ankle Int 2014;35:543–8.

183. Pettrone FA, Gail M, Pee D, et al. Quantitative criteria for prediction of the results after displaced fracture of the ankle. J Bone Joint Surg Am 1983;65:667–77.

184. Roberts RS. Surgical treatment of displaced ankle fractures. Clin Orthop Relat Res 1983;(172):164–70.

185. Stiehl JB, Schwartz HS. Long-term results of pronation-external rotation ankle fracture-dislocations treated with anatomical open reduction, internal fixation. J Orthop Trauma 1990;4:339–45.

186. Veltri DM, Pagnani MJ, O'Brien SJ, et al. Symptomatic ossification of the tibiofibular syndesmosis in professional football players: a sequela of the syndesmotic ankle sprain. Foot Ankle Int 1995;16:285–90.

187. Leeds HC, Ehrlich MG. Instability of the distal tibiofibular syndesmosis after bi-malleolar and trimalleolar ankle fractures. J Bone Joint Surg Am 1984;66:490–503.

188. Moravek JE, Kadakia AR. Surgical strategies: doubled allograft reconstruction for chronic syndesmotic injuries. Foot Ankle Int 2010;31:834–44.

189. Malhotra G, Cameron J, Toolan BC. Diagnosing chronic diastasis of the syndesmosis: a novel measurement using computed tomography. Foot Ankle Int 2014;35:483–8.

190. Wagener ML, Beumer A, Swierstra BA. Chronic instability of the anterior tibiofibular syndesmosis of the ankle. Arthroscopic findings and results of anatomical reconstruction. BMC Musculoskelet Disord 2011;12:212.

191. Lui TH. Tri-ligamentous reconstruction of the distal tibiofibular syndesmosis: a minimally invasive approach. J Foot Ankle Surg 2010;49:495–500.

192. Pena FA, Coetzee JC. Ankle syndesmosis injuries. Foot Ankle Clin 2006;11:35–50, viii.

193. Olson KM, Dairyko GH Jr, Toolan BC. Salvage of chronic instability of the syndesmosis with distal tibiofibular arthrodesis: functional and radiographic results. J Bone Joint Surg Am 2011;93:66–72.

Chronic Ankle Instability (Medial and Lateral)

Markus Knupp, MD*, Tamara Horn Lang, PhD, Lukas Zwicky, MSc, Patrick Lötscher, MD, Beat Hintermann, MD

KEYWORDS

- Ankle instability • Ankle sprain • Medial ankle ligaments • Lateral ankle ligaments

KEY POINTS

- Up to 40% of patients with ankle sprains develop symptomatic instability.
- Arthroscopy as a diagnostic adjunct allows functional testing and assessment of the instability pattern (distinction of isolated medial/lateral or combined pathologies).
- Treatment of acute medial injuries and the postoperative protocol of the deltoid ligaments should be more restrictive than for the lateral ankle ligaments.
- The aim of surgical treatment is to restore the anatomy. Tenodesis procedures should be avoided.
- In severely altered conditions of the ligaments, tendon grafts can be used to restore joint stability.

INTRODUCTION

Ankle sprains are among the most common injuries, comprising up to one-third of all sport injuries.[1] A recent study, analyzing the ankle sprains presenting to emergency departments in the United States has shown an incidence of 2.15 per 1000 person-years.[2] Independent of the initial treatment strategy and the number of ligaments involved, up to 40% of the patients suffering from lateral ligament injuries end up having chronic ankle instability (CAI).[3]

Factors that may contribute to the development of CAI are functional and/or anatomic deficiencies. Functional deficiencies may be owing to impaired proprioception,[4] muscular imbalance,[5] or an impaired neuromuscular control, such as a delayed muscular reaction of the joint bridging muscles.[6] Suggested predisposing anatomic factors include hindfoot varus,[7] pathologic ligament laxity,[8] and an osseous configuration of the ankle joint, where the talus is less restrained in the ankle mortise.[9]

The authors have nothing to disclose.
Department of Orthopaedic Surgery, Kantonsspital Baselland, Rheinstrasse 26, Liestal CH-4410, Switzerland
* Corresponding author.
E-mail address: markus.knupp@ksbl.ch

The aim of this article is to summarize the different entities and various therapy approaches in CAI.

DIAGNOSIS OF CHRONIC ANKLE INSTABILITY
History and Clinical Findings

The diagnosis of CAI is based on the patients' medical history and clinical findings. Patients often complain of experiencing insecurity, instability, and "giving way" on uneven ground, leading to limitations in daily activities and difficulties in sports. Recurrent sprains, pain, tenderness, and at times bruising over the lateral or medial aspect or both of the ankle are common symptoms. Approximately 30% of patients suffering from CAI may be asymptomatic between the events, whereas others may present with chronic lateral and/or medial pain, tenderness, swelling, or "giving way."[10] Clinical tests such as the talar tilt test or anterior drawer test are positive in patients with structural ligament insufficiency, whereas these tests may be negative when only functional ankle instability is present.[11]

Imaging

Plain, weight-bearing, anteroposterior and lateral radiographs of the ankle joint are recommended to exclude fractures and malalignment. If a deformity is present, additional radiographs—dorsoplantar and lateral views of the foot and a hindfoot alignment view—are recommended. Particularly in chronic and recurrent instability, the physician must exclude osseous contributing factors such as frontal plane deformity of the hindfoot (varus/valgus) or forefoot-driven hindfoot deformities (such as the plantar flexed first metatarsal in a cavus foot leading to a hindfoot varus). Further imaging such as MRI may exclude osteochondral lesions and concomitant pathologies of the tendons. Particularly in CAI, comorbidities of the peroneal tendons are frequent. These comorbidities can be detected by MRI with a sensitivity of 84% and a specificity of 75%.[12] However, MRI has been shown to be clearly less reliable in detecting ligamentous deficits than arthroscopic assessment.[13]

Intraoperative Diagnostic Measures

Operative treatment is initiated with the completion of diagnosis using intraoperative fluoroscopy and arthroscopy, with the patient under anesthesia. Clinical tests include the talar tilt in the mortise and the anterior drawer test (**Fig. 1**). Stress views may additionally allow assessing syndesmotic stability.

In the United States, nearly one-half of the patients undergo arthroscopic evaluation before ligament reconstruction.[14] Arthroscopy has been found to be helpful to detect intraarticular damage, such as injuries to the syndesmosis, cartilage, and distal tibiofibular joint.[15–19] Therefore, a majority of the authors recommend arthroscopic evaluation to define the extent and origin of instability (medial/lateral) and to exclude intraarticular damage.[15,20,21]

In a large majority of patients, injury to the ligament is observed at the proximal insertion site. Intraoperatively, a bare area of periosteum on the lateral/medial malleolus, around the region of the detached ligament (the insertion site), is characteristically found. Functional arthroscopic testing includes:

- Axial traction to quantify the opening of the tibiotalar space
- Anterior drawer test to assess the medial and anteromedial instability
- Tilt test (valgus stress) to detect laxity or instability of the medial ligaments
- Tilt test (varus stress) to detect laxity or instability of the lateral ligaments

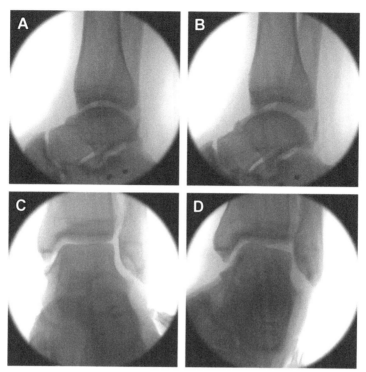

Fig. 1. Intraoperative testing of the drawer test (*A, B*) and the talar tilt test (*C, D*) in a 34-year-old male patient with combined, recurrent medial instability, 5 years after lateral ligament reconstruction. (*A, B*) Positive anterior drawer. (*C, D*) Positive talar tilt test. The drawer is positive owing to the injured left anterior talofibular ligament, calcaneofibular ligament, and the superficial deltoid. Valgus tilt is only partially negative owing to the remaining deep deltoid.

Finally, endoscopy of the peroneal and tibialis posterior tendon completes the intraoperative diagnostics.

CHRONIC LATERAL INSTABILITY
Anatomy of the Anterior Talofibular and the Calcaneofibular Ligament

In chronic lateral ankle instability the anterior talofibular ligament (ATFL) and/or the calcaneofibular ligament (CFL) are often altered, leading to joint hypermobility. Depending on the position of the foot, each of these lateral ligaments takes over a stabilizing role of the ankle or subtalar joint. In dorsiflexion, the posterior talofibular ligament is maximally stressed and the CFL is taut, whereas the ATFL is loose. Conversely, in plantarflexion, the ATFL is taut and the CFL and posterior talofibular ligaments are loose.[22]

The ATFL blends with the anterior capsule of the ankle, and spans the anterolateral aspect of the ankle joint (**Fig. 2**). The ligament originates at the anterior edge of the fibula, just lateral to the articular cartilage of the lateral malleolus. The center of attachment lies 10 mm proximal to the tip of the fibula. The insertion on the talus begins directly distal to the articular surface, and the center is 18 mm proximal to the subtalar joint.[23] Precisely owing to the ATFL's insertion and origin, it is the first ligament restricting supination of the foot, and is most frequently injured in ankle sprains.

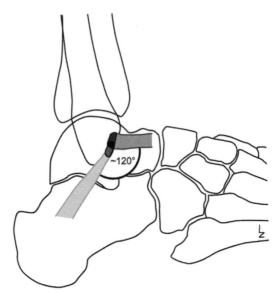

Fig. 2. Anatomy of the right anterior talofibular ligament and the calcaneofibular ligament. The 2 ligaments have overlapping insertion sites at the anterior margin of the distal fibula.

In contrast with popular belief, the CFL does not originate from the apex of the tip of the lateral malleolus (see **Fig. 2**). Its attachment is on the anterior edge of distal fibula, centered 8.5 mm from the distal tip just below the origin of the ATFL. The ligament courses medially, posteriorly, and inferiorly from its fibular origin to the calcaneal insertion. The calcaneal insertion begins 13 mm distal to the subtalar joint with its proximal edge on a line nearly perpendicular to the subtalar joint.[23] The CFL effectively spans the ankle and subtalar joints, which have markedly different axes of rotation.[24–26] Thus, this ligament must be attached so that it does not restrict motion of either joint, whether they move independently or simultaneously. The CFL resists ankle and subtalar joint supination, restricting inversion and internal rotation of the subtalar joint. Strain in the CFL increases with dorsiflexion; when it becomes more vertically orientated, and takes over the role of the lateral collateral ligament of the ankle. Chronic insufficiency of the CFL is combined typically with a pathologic talar tilt test in neutral ankle position.

Operative Treatment

Indications
Patients who fail to become asymptomatic with conservative measures (see also chronic medial instability) are considered for operative treatment. In particular, patients with ongoing instability, recurrent ankle sprains, pain, and limitations in their professional and recreational activities, as well as patients suffering from CAI owing to a nonunited osseous detachment of the lateral ligaments generally benefit from reconstructive surgery. The aims of surgery are to reestablish joint stability and reduce the risk for future ankle sprains, and thereby reduce damage to the cartilage.

Operative stabilization
The operative procedure chosen depends on the extent and the pattern of instability and is usually initiated by diagnostic arthroscopy.

Simple suture technique (Broström) The Broström procedure[10] is the gold standard when anatomic reconstruction of the lateral ankle ligaments is attempted. The goal of anatomic reconstruction is to restore the physiologic anatomy by suturing the ligament itself. If necessary, reconstruction can be reinforced by the extensor retinaculum of the foot[27] or by a periosteal flap of the fibula. Exposure of the lateral ankle ligaments can be achieved through a curved incision from the fibula directed anteriorly or posteriorly. The incision directed posteriorly allows a good exposure of the lateral ligaments; however, it has the disadvantage of not being extendable distally. Therefore, many surgeons prefer the curved incision directed anteriorly toward the base of the fourth metatarsal.

If the preoperative examination of the peroneal tendons resulted in unclear diagnostic findings, it is recommended that the tendons be exposed through the same access to possibly identify and repair existing lesions. Painful accessory ossicles in the area of the lateral ligaments are removed. Unfortunately, this can sometimes lead to considerable soft tissue damage that may greatly complicate ligament reconstruction.[28] Hence, screw fixation of the fragments to the distal fibula should be considered for very large accessory ossicles.

After reconstruction of the ligament, the ATFL and/or the CFL are reattached to the distal fibula using suture anchors or transosseous sutures.[29] If required, the reconstruction can be reinforced using the extensor retinaculum.

Reconstruction with a graft Reinforcement of the lateral ligaments using tendon grafts is done in the absence of sufficient local tissue (or by poor quality/quantity of local tissue) or by revision surgery. When using tendon grafts one distinguishes between anatomic reconstruction and tenodesis (Watson–Jones [1940], Chrisman–Snook [1969],[30] Elmslie [1934][31]). Tenodesis, a nonanatomic reconstruction, leads to nonphysiologic intraarticular pressure peaks, sacrifices a dynamic stabilizer, and causes movement restrictions and should therefore only be used when all other treatment options have failed.[32] When anatomic reconstruction using tendon autograft is aimed for, many surgeons prefer to use the plantaris longus tendon (**Fig. 3**).[33] The tendon is harvested through a separate medial incision and used for reconstruction of the ATFL and the CFL. For this purpose, drill holes are made in the distal fibula, the talar neck, and the lateral wall of the calcaneus; the tendon is weaved subsequently into the lateral aspect of the ankle joint (see **Fig. 3**). Alternatively, the use of the hamstrings[34,35] or bone–tendon–bone grafts[36] have been described in the literature.

Postoperative Treatment

Postoperative treatment is similar to the treatment advised after an acute ankle sprain. **Table 1** provides an overview of the recommendations according to a Cochrane review.[37]

CHRONIC MEDIAL INSTABILITY
Anatomy of the Deltoid Ligament

The deltoid ligament spreads in a fan-shaped manner over the medial part of the ankle joint, and is an important structure with regard to stability against valgus and rotatory forces. It consists of 6 distinct components: 4 superficial and 2 deep ligaments (**Fig. 4**). The superficial ligaments (tibiospring ligament, tibionavicular ligament, superficial posterior tibiotalar ligament, and tibiocalcaneal ligament) cross the ankle and the subtalar joint, whereas the deep components (deep posterior tibiotalar ligament and anterior tibiotalar ligament) only cross the ankle joint.[38] Owing to the broad insertion of the

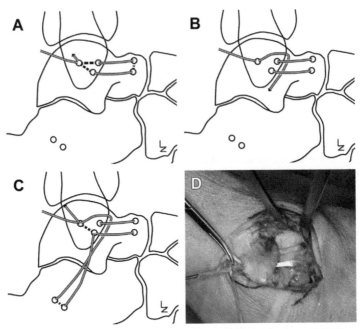

Fig. 3. Anatomic reconstruction of the right anterior talofibular ligament (LFTA) and the calcaneofibular ligament (CFL) using a plantaris tendon graft. (*A*) Reconstruction of the LFTA. (*B*, *C*) Reconstruction of the CFL. (*D*) Intraoperative image of a reconstructed LFTA with a plantaris tendon graft.

superficial deltoid ligament on the spring ligament, this complex also plays an important role in the stabilizing function of the medial ligaments. The superficial layers of the deltoid ligament particularly limit talar abduction, whereas the deep layers limit external rotation. Both deep and superficial layers are equally effective in limiting pronation of the talus.[24]

In contrast with the lateral ligaments, the deltoid ligament is involved significantly in the coupling mechanism between the leg and the foot. This is especially well-illustrated when sectioning the ligaments: sectioning the lateral ligaments does not affect tibial rotation and foot inversion–eversion while sectioning the medial ligaments

Table 1 Treatment after an acute ankle sprain		
Weeks	**Patient Mobilization**	**Physiotherapy**
1–2	Rest, Ice, Compression and Elevation (RICE) Orthosis Walker	Lymphatic drainage
3–6	Walker Weight bearing as tolerated	ROM max PF/DF 20°/0°/10 No inversion/eversion Proprioceptive training
7–12	Orthosis if needed	Unrestricted ROM, proprioceptive training, coordination training and force

Abbreviations: DF, dorsiflexion; PF, plantarflexion; ROM, range of motion.

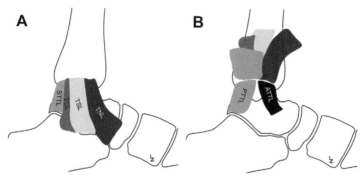

Fig. 4. Medial ligaments. Note that a majority of the ligaments are located posterior to the longitudinal axis of the tibia. (*A*) Shows the superficial part and the superficial posterior tibiotalar ligament of the deltoid and (*B*) Depicts the deep part without the posterior tibiotalar ligament. ATTL, anterior tibiotalar ligament; PTTL, posterior tibiotalar ligament; STTL, superficial posterior tibiotalar ligament; TCL, tibiocalcaneal ligament; TNL, tibionavicular ligament; TSL, tibiospring ligament.

greatly alters the physiologic force transmission pattern of the leg to the foot.[39,40] Therefore, the physiologic gait pattern depends highly on deltoid integrity.

Conservative Treatment

Conservative treatment may include physical therapy, such as muscular strengthening, proprioceptive training, and coordination training. Orthotics with a medial support, bracing, or taping may be used additionally to provide mechanical support and enhance proprioception through skin pressure. If conservative treatment has failed, operative treatment is necessary.

Operative Treatment

A slightly curved incision, 4 to 8 cm in length, is made, starting 1 to 2 cm proximal to the medial malleolar tip and toward the medial aspect of the navicular bone. After the dissection of the fascia, the deltoid ligament and the posterior tibial tendon are exposed. The extent and location of ligament injuries determine the lesion type: (a) injuries at the proximal part of the deltoid (type I lesions), (b) injuries at the intermediate part of the deltoid (type II lesions), and (c) injuries at the distal part of the deltoid and spring ligaments (type III lesions).[41] In type I lesions, the insertion area at the anterior aspect of the medial malleolus is exposed. The insertion area at the anterior border of the medial malleolus is roughened and an anchor is placed 4 to 6 mm above the tip (eg, anterior colliculus) of the medial malleolus. The detached ligament is taken with the suture and the open interval is closed firmly. In type II lesions, the incompetent and typically hypertrophic ligament is divided into 2 flaps. The deep part, which has its origin at the navicular tuberosity, is fixed to the medial malleolus using a bony anchor, as is done when treating a proximal lesion. The superficial part, which has its origin at the medial malleolus, is fixed distally to the superior edge of the navicular tuberosity using another bony anchor. In type III lesions, a bony anchor is used to fix the detached deltoid and spring ligaments to the navicular tuberosity. If the remaining tissue of the spring ligament is of bad quality, the distal part of the posterior tibial tendon is used to augment the ligament reconstruction.[42]

In patients where ankle instability persists and ligament quality is insufficient, direct reconstruction with anchors may not be possible. In these cases, autologous reconstruction using a free tendon graft is the surgical treatment of choice.[43] The graft is passed through 2 drill holes of 3.2 mm at 2 to 8 mm above the medial malleolar tip and through another dorsoplantar drill hole in the navicular bone. Holding the foot in a neutral position, the graft is fixed with resorbable sutures under slight tension. Attention needs to be paid to reconstruct the tendon in a strict anatomic position and to not overtighten the ligament construct.

Postoperative Treatment

Because the medial ligaments are involved significantly in force transmission from the leg to the foot, the authors tend to be more restrictive in the postoperative rehabilitation. The ankle is usually protected in a weight bearing lower leg cast for 6 weeks. Thereafter physiotherapy is initiated with gradual return to activities. Running is allowed 4 to 6 months after surgery and high-impact sports after 6 to 9 months.

SUMMARY

Up to one-third of the all sport injuries involve a sprained ankle. A large majority of these injuries are successfully treated conservatively. However, up to 40% of these patients report symptoms of CAI, which restrict their daily activities and the ability to return to sports. Once conservative treatment has failed, surgical reconstruction may restore ankle joint stability. Surgery is usually initiated by arthroscopy to assess the instability pattern. The ligaments are reconstructed anatomically and tenodesis procedures should be avoided. If the local soft tissues do not allow direct reconstruction, tendon grafts are used to augment the ligaments. The preferred grafts are the plantaris and the hamstring tendons.

REFERENCES

1. Garrick JG, Requa RK. The epidemiology of foot and ankle injuries in sports. Clin Sports Med 1988;7(1):29–36.
2. Waterman BR, Owens BD, Davey S, et al. The epidemiology of ankle sprains in the United States. J Bone Joint Surg Am 2010;92(13):2279–84.
3. van Rijn RM, van Os AG, Bernsen RM, et al. What is the clinical course of acute ankle sprains? A systematic literature review. Am J Med 2008;121(4):324–31.e6.
4. Hoch MC, Staton GS, Medina McKeon JM, et al. Dorsiflexion and dynamic postural control deficits are present in those with chronic ankle instability. J Sci Med Sport 2012;15(6):574–9.
5. Hubbard TJ, Kramer LC, Denegar CR, et al. Contributing factors to chronic ankle instability. Foot Ankle Int 2007;28(3):343–54.
6. Kavanagh JJ, Bisset LM, Tsao H. Deficits in reaction time due to increased motor time of peroneus longus in people with chronic ankle instability. J Biomech 2012; 45(3):605–8.
7. Morrison KE, Hudson DJ, Davis IS, et al. Plantar pressure during running in subjects with chronic ankle instability. Foot Ankle Int 2010;31(11):994–1000.
8. Crim JR, Beals TC, Nickisch F, et al. Deltoid ligament abnormalities in chronic lateral ankle instability. Foot Ankle Int 2011;32(9):873–8.
9. Frigg A, Magerkurth O, Valderrabano V, et al. The effect of osseous ankle configuration on chronic ankle instability. Br J Sports Med 2007;41(7):420–4.
10. Brostrom L. Sprained ankles. VI. Surgical treatment of "chronic" ligament ruptures. Acta Chir Scand 1966;132(5):551–65.
11. Peters JW, Trevino SG, Renstrom PA. Chronic lateral ankle instability. Foot Ankle 1991;12(3):182–91.

12. Park HJ, Cha SD, Kim SS, et al. Accuracy of MRI findings in chronic lateral ankle ligament injury: comparison with surgical findings. Clin Radiol 2012;67(4):313–8.

13. Hermans JJ, Wentink N, Beumer A, et al. Correlation between radiological assessment of acute ankle fractures and syndesmotic injury on MRI. Skeletal Radiol 2012;41(7):787–801.

14. Werner BC, Burrus MT, Park JS, et al. Trends in ankle arthroscopy and its use in the management of pathologic conditions of the lateral ankle in the United States: a national database study. Arthroscopy 2015;31(7):1330–7.

15. Takao M, Ochi M, Oae K, et al. Diagnosis of a tear of the tibiofibular syndesmosis. The role of arthroscopy of the ankle. J Bone Joint Surg Br 2003;85(3):324–9.

16. Komenda GA, Ferkel RD. Arthroscopic findings associated with the unstable ankle. Foot Ankle Int 1999;20(11):708–13.

17. Di Giovanni B, Fraga CJ, Cohen BE, et al. Associated injuries found in chronic lateral ankle instability. Foot Ankle Int 2000;21(10):809–15.

18. Choi WJ, Lee JW, Han SH, et al. Chronic lateral ankle instability: the effect of intra-articular lesions on clinical outcome. Am J Sports Med 2008;36(11):2167–72.

19. Hintermann B, Boss A, Schafer D. Arthroscopic findings in patients with chronic ankle instability. Am J Sports Med 2002;30(3):402–9.

20. Kerr HL, Bayley E, Jackson R, et al. The role of arthroscopy in the treatment of functional instability of the ankle. Foot Ankle Surg 2013;19(4):273–5.

21. Guillo S, Bauer T, Lee JW, et al. Consensus in chronic ankle instability: aetiology, assessment, surgical indications and place for arthroscopy. Orthop Traumatol Surg Res 2013;99(8 Suppl):S411–9.

22. Colville MR, Marder RA, Boyle JJ, et al. Strain measurement in lateral ankle ligaments. Am J Sports Med 1990;18(2):196–200.

23. Burks RT, Morgan J. Anatomy of the lateral ankle ligaments. Am J Sports Med 1994;22(1):72–7.

24. Close JR. Some applications of the functional anatomy of the ankle joint. J Bone Joint Surg Am 1956;38-A(4):761–81.

25. Larsen E. Experimental instability of the ankle. A radiographic investigation. Clin Orthop Relat Res 1986;(204):193–200.

26. Michelson JD, Clarke HJ, Jinnah RH. The effect of loading on tibiotalar alignment in cadaver ankles. Foot Ankle 1990;10(5):280–4.

27. Gould N, Seligson D, Gassman J. Early and late repair of lateral ligament of the ankle. Foot Ankle 1980;1(2):84–9.

28. Kim BS, Choi WJ, Kim YS, et al. The effect of an ossicle of the lateral malleolus on ligament reconstruction of chronic lateral ankle instability. Foot Ankle Int 2010; 31(3):191–6.

29. Cho BK, Kim YM, Kim DS, et al. Comparison between suture anchor and trans-osseous suture for the modified-Brostrom procedure. Foot Ankle Int 2012;33(6): 462–8.

30. Chrisman OD, Snook GA. Reconstruction of lateral ligament tears of the ankle. An experimental study and clinical evaluation of seven patients treated by a new modification of the Elmslie procedure. J Bone Joint Surg Am 1969;51(5):904–12.

31. Elmslie RC. Recurrent subluxation of the ankle-joint. Ann Surg 1934;100(2): 364–7.

32. Hennrikus WL, Mapes RC, Lyons PM, et al. Outcomes of the Chrisman-Snook and modified-Brostrom procedures for chronic lateral ankle instability. A prospective, randomized comparison. Am J Sports Med 1996;24(4):400–4.

33. Hintermann B, Renggli P. Anatomische Rekonstruktion der lateralen Sprungge-lenkbänder mit der Plantarissehne zur Behandlung der chronischen Instabilität.

[Anatomic reconstruction of the lateral ligaments of the ankle using a plantaris tendon graft in the treatment of chronic ankle joint instability]. Orthopade 1999; 28(9):778–84.

34. Richter J, Volz R, Immendorfer M, et al. Reconstruction of the lateral ankle ligaments with hamstring tendon autograft in patients with chronic ankle instability. Oper Orthop Traumatol 2012;24(1):50–60 [in German].

35. Coughlin MJ, Matt V, Schenck RC Jr. Augmented lateral ankle reconstruction using a free gracilis graft. Orthopedics 2002;25(1):31–5.

36. Sugimoto K, Takakura Y, Kumai T, et al. Reconstruction of the lateral ankle ligaments with bone-patellar tendon graft in patients with chronic ankle instability: a preliminary report. Am J Sports Med 2002;30(3):340–6.

37. de Vries JS, Krips R, Sierevelt IN, et al. Interventions for treating chronic ankle instability. Cochrane Database Syst Rev 2011;(8):CD004124.

38. Hintermann B. Medial ankle instability. Foot Ankle Clin 2003;8(4):723–38.

39. Hintermann B, Nigg BM, Sommer C, et al. Transfer of movement between calcaneus and tibia in vitro. Clin Biomech 1994;9(6):349–55.

40. Hintermann B, Sommer C, Nigg BM. Influence of ligament transection on tibial and calcaneal rotation with loading and dorsi-plantarflexion. Foot Ankle Int 1995;16(9):567–71.

41. Hintermann B, Knupp M, Pagenstert GI. Deltoid ligament injuries: diagnosis and management. Foot Ankle Clin 2006;11(3):625–37.

42. Lötscher P, Hintermann B. Medial ankle ligament injuries in athletes. Oper Tech Sports Med 2014;22(4):290–5.

43. Deland JT, de Asla RJ, Segal A. Reconstruction of the chronically failed deltoid ligament: a new technique. Foot Ankle Int 2004;25(11):795–9.

Arthroscopic Approach to Osteochondral Defects, Impingement, and Instability

Roger Walker, DO, William Aaron Kunkle, DO,
Dominic S. Carreira, MD*

KEYWORDS

- Osteochondral defects • Impingement • Instability • Sports injuries • Foot • Ankle

KEY POINTS

- Arthroscopic treatment of talar dome osteochondral defect lesions is a common and highly effective technique.
- Ankle impingement treated arthroscopically allows quicker return to sport.
- Arthroscopic ankle stabilization is an evolving field with limited clinical evidence.

INTRODUCTION
Osteochondral Defects

Osteochondral injury involves damage to the articular cartilage and its corresponding bone. In the ankle, it is widely believed that the etiology of osteochondral lesions is traumatic, leading to partial or complete detachment of the osteochondral fragment of the talus, although several other proposed etiologies exist.[1,2] Osteochondral injuries are estimated to occur in one-half of all acute ankle sprains and up to 73% of ankle fractures.[3–5] Loren and Ferkel reported a 60% incidence of traumatic articular surface lesions in unstable ankle fractures undergoing arthroscopic evaluation.[6] Traumatic etiologies are associated with 70% of medial and 98% of lateral lesions of the talus.[7] Seventy percent of osteochondral defects (OCD) of the talus occur in men, especially athletes, with an average age range of 20 to 35 years.[2] Patients with an acute inversion injury, chronic ankle pain, and a history of ankle trauma with instability are more likely to experience an osteochondral lesion of the talus.

Disclosures: Dr W.A. Kunkle and Dr R. Walker have identified no professional or financial affiliations for themselves or their spouse/partner. Dr D. Carreira is the paid consultant for Biomet.
Sports Medicine and Orthopedics, Broward Health Medical Center, 1601 South Andrews Avenue, 2nd Floor, Fort Lauderdale, FL 33316, USA
* Corresponding author.
E-mail address: dcarreira@gmail.com

Raikin and colleagues developed a 3 × 3 grid system in which they stratified OCD location and morphology in 428 lesions based on MRI findings. Medial central talar lesions were the most common (53%) and were also the largest in surface dimension and depth. Lateral lesions were the second most commonly observed (26%).

Nonrecognition or misidentification of OCD symptoms is problematic in effective diagnosis and treatment.[1,8] Symptoms of OCD may include pain, catching, grinding, feelings of instability, giving way, and effusion.[1,2] Ankle stability should also be assessed and surgically corrected if present when treating OCDs.

Zengerink and colleagues[1] and McCollum and colleagues[9] differentiate between the clinical presentation of acute and chronic symptoms. Acute OCDs often present similar to other acute ankle injuries, with lateral or medial ankle pain, swelling, and limited range of motion being most common. If these symptoms do not resolve within 4 to 6 weeks after an isolated ligamentous ankle injury, an OCD should be suspected.[9] Deep lateral or medial ankle pain, associated with weight bearing, can be associated with chronic OCDs.[1,9] Based on patient history and physical examination, MRI and CT images are often obtained when an OCD is suspected.[1,2,8,9] Plain film radiographs have low sensitivity (50%) in detecting OCDs.[10] CT may help to define the exact anatomy of the osseous defect.[1,9] Specific cartilage-sensitive pulse sequences have been developed allowing for differentiation of native articular cartilage, reparative fibrocartilage, and synovial fluid.[11]

The staging of osteochondral lesions may be relevant in determining treatment outcomes, particularly when identifying cystic lesions, which may be more appropriately managed with bone grafting.[12]

Surgical Management

Surgical management is considered in patients with OCDs that remain symptomatic after failed nonoperative modalities and that consist of displaced fragments. Given the variety of options available, the surgical treatment of OCDs is a challenging and controversial problem in orthopedics. The goal of creating a homogenous and durable articular chondral surface is well-understood. However, the reconstructive technique that best produces such a result, along with pain relief, remains an area of debate, especially in light of the fact that no large studies with long-term outcomes have been performed to compare the various options. There is considerable evidence with short- to medium-term results for using bone marrow stimulation techniques in smaller defects and transplant techniques in larger cystic lesions. Surgical options include those listed in **Box 1**.[12,13]

Box 1
Surgical options for osteochondral defect lesions

1. Bone marrow stimulation (BMS)[a]

2. Autologous chondrocyte implantation (ACI)

3. Matrix-associated autologous chondrocyte implantation (MACI)

4. Particulated juvenile cartilage allograft

5. Debridement

   [a] Investigational augments-concentrated bone marrow aspirates, platelet-rich plasma, extracellular matrix scaffolds.

Improvements in instrumentation have helped to gain access and treat OCDs, including small curved shavers and burrs, and ankle specific instrumentation for bone marrow stimulation (Ankle Arthroscopy Tray, Smith and Nephew, Andover, MA).

Indications for arthroscopy depend on a number of variables, including lesion size, location (accessibility of lesion on the tibial or talar articular surface), and the bony component of the OCD. Strict guidelines related to these factors differ across studies. The advantages of arthroscopy include faster recovery, less pain, and lower infection rates, and must be weighed against the limitations of arthroscopic techniques. Cystic defects, larger lesions, and uncontained lesions have been demonstrated to have less success with debridement and/or bone marrow stimulation techniques.[14]

OCD lesion sizes less than 150 mm^2 treated with bone marrow stimulation techniques have been shown to produce clinical outcomes with good to excellent results in 87% of patients.[14,15]

The location of the OCD should be considered preoperatively. Anterior arthroscopy can be used to access OCD lesions on the anterior one-half of the talus and posterior arthroscopy should be considered for those lesions outside these limits.[16] Ankle positioning, for example, full plantar flexion for anterior lesions, may improve access to OCDs,[13] but malleolar osteotomies must be considered, particularly in lesions that are more central and posterior. Accessory portals may also serve to gain access. Flick and Gould[7] described a "grooving" technique of the anteromedial tibia surface for exposure of medial lesions. An alternative combined anteromedial and posteromedial approach described by Thompson and Loomer[17] was also found effective for the medial lesion exposure. Other portals described include portals at the Achilles (immediately medial or lateral, or less commonly, trans-Achilles) and adjacent to the peroneal tendons. The neurovascular anatomy relative to these portals should be understood to prevent iatrogenic injury. Lesions within the posterior third of the plafond may be accessed with posterior ankle arthroscopy in the prone position.[18]

OCDs that are larger, cystic, uncontained, and those having failed prior bone marrow stimulation may be managed with osteochondral transplants, autologous chondrocyte transplantation, or juvenile particulated cartilage. These procedures can be assisted arthroscopically for surface preparation, but are performed more commonly with an open approach, with or without malleolar osteotomy (**Fig. 1**).

Surgical Techniques

Arthroscopic bone marrow stimulation techniques include microfracture or drilling. Noninvasive distraction, either with a metal distractor or with waist distraction, opens the tibiotalar space to improve access. In the microfracture technique, the OCD is prepared with complete debridement of loose unstable cartilage and the creation of stable shoulders to the lesion. Multiple holes are punctured with a microfracture awl and with a mallet to penetrate into the subchondral plate at 3 to 4 mm of spacing to maintain a stable bone bridge.[13,19] The depth of penetration of the microfracture should be assessed intraoperatively by reducing pump pressure and by visualizing bleeding bone or fat droplet extravasation.[13] Growth factors and an initial fibrin clot form to create fibrocartilage, primarily over the first 6 weeks. Fibrocartilage from microfracture, composed primarily of type 1 collagen, has inferior biological and biomechanical properties when compared with native tissue.[20,21] However, it has remained a standard to which other cartilage repair techniques are compared. Augmentation of microfracture with bone marrow aspirate and/or platelet-rich plasma has been proposed to promote differentiation of the fibrocartilage to a more hyaline cartilage structure with greater quantities of type 2 collagen and chondroitin sulfate.[20,22,23]

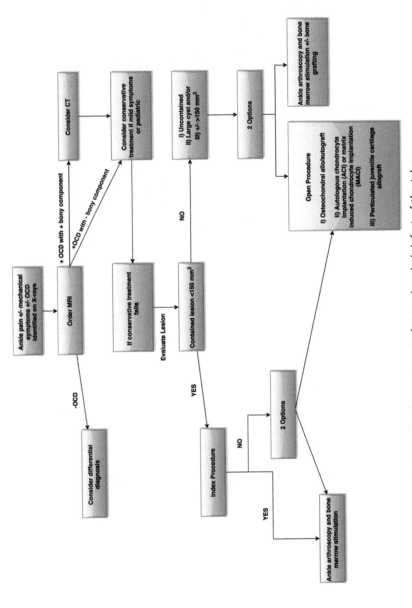

Fig. 1. An evidence-based treatment algorithm for the treatment of osteochondral defect of the talus.

Tissue transplantation with particulated juvenile cartilage, typically performed as an open procedure, contains viable chondrocytes. In the setting of bone defects greater than 5 mm, such as in the case of a cystic lesion, bone grafting may be performed before the delivery of chondrocytes.[24] Fibrin glue is delivered to secure the chondrocytes in place.

Postoperative Management and Rehabilitation

Patients treated arthroscopically initiate range of motion within 2 weeks to promote nutrient flow to the cartilage surface and to decrease scarring and stiffness. For bone marrow stimulation techniques, a period of non–weight-bearing, 6 weeks, has been the norm, although 2 recent reports challenge this practice. Zengerink and colleagues[1] recently published excellent results with progression to full weight-bearing in smaller lesions. Lee and colleagues[25] reported on a randomized control trial comparing early weight-bearing at 2 weeks (N = 40) and delayed weight-bearing (DWB) at 6 weeks (N = 41) in 81 patients treated with arthroscopic microfracture of a single osteochondral talus lesion with mean size of 1.0 cm^2. Comparison of the 2 study groups found equivocal American Orthopedic Foot and Ankle Society score, visual analog scale score and Ankle Activity Score. The authors recommended early weight-bearing regiments for small OCD lesions treated with microfracture.

Clinical Outcomes

The literature on microfracture of OCD shows good to excellent results in 65% to 90% of patients in the short term, but poorer outcomes beyond 5 years. Recent studies have focused on the confounding factors that may affect clinical outcome, such as lesion size, patient age, body mass index, lesion classification, containment, duration of symptoms, and traumatic etiology.

Choi and colleagues[15] demonstrated lesions with an area greater than 150 mm^2 showed clinical failure in 80% of the treated patients. There was no association with outcome and patient age, duration of symptoms, trauma, and location of lesion. A more recent retrospective review of 130 patients treated with marrow stimulation techniques found statistically significant higher incidence of poor outcomes with OCD larger than 150 mm^2.[14]

Saxena and Eakin[4] reported on a prospective case series of athletes treated with microfracture and bone graft of OCD lesions. The treatment plan was based on the MRI Hepple classification with stages 2 through 4 lesions treated with microfracture and stage 5 lesions with bone graft. The microfracture group had faster return to athletics at 15.1 weeks than the bone graft group, at 19.6 weeks (P = .006). Patients treated for anterior lesions with arthroscopic microfracture had faster return to athletics at 15.8 weeks than those with central posterior lesions treated with arthrotomy, whose return to athletics was 17.5 weeks (P = .30). Postoperative American Orthopedic Foot and Ankle Society scores were also similar between the microfracture and bone graft groups (94.4 and 93.4). The authors also noted that anterolateral lesions had significantly faster return to athletics with higher postoperative scores.

There is limited evidence on particulated juvenile cartilage transplants. Coetzee and colleagues[24] reported on a case series of 24 ankles with a minimum of 12 month follow-up. Mean lesion size was 125 mm^2 with a depth of 7 mm. Outcomes proportioned to lesion size found 92% good to excellent results in lesions 10 to 15 mm in size. The authors proposed this technique as a possible bridge between microfracture and osteochondral autograft transfer procedures for lesions within this range.

Clanton and colleagues reported on 7 patients in which microfracture with extracellular matrix augmentation prepared with concentrated bone marrow aspirate was used for treatment of talus OCD. The mean follow-up was 8.4 months with overall improvement in Foot and Ankle Disability Index activities of daily living subscale, Foot and Ankle Disability Index sports subscale, and Foot and Ankle Disability Index total score.

ANKLE IMPINGEMENT

The symptoms associated with ankle impingement (AI) include anterior or posterior ankle pain with decreased range of motion.[26,27] Palpation of the joint line is typically painful, with palpable osteophytes and swelling.[28] AI may be caused by osseous impingement and/or soft tissue impingement. The pathogenesis of impingement is thought to originate from an inciting traumatic event, such as a sprain, chronic instability, or repetitive trauma at the extremes of motion.

Soft tissue impingement has been cited as the most common cause of chronic pain after an ankle sprain.[27,29,30] Anterior soft tissue impingent can occur as a result of synovial meniscoid scar tissue formed as a result of an injury to the surrounding capsule, anterior talofibular ligament or calcaneofibular ligaments. The distal fascicle of the anterior inferior tibiofibular ligament or Bassett's ligament may also cause anterior impingement.[28]

Anterior bony impingement occurs anteromedially or anterolaterally. It is common in high-level athletes, as noted in 60% of elite soccer players.[31] The end stage of chronic anteromedial AI may result in medial malleolar stress fracture in elite running and jumping athletes.[32]

Posterior impingement is most commonly caused by an elongated posterior lateral talar tubercle (Stieda process) or by an os trigonum. Other causes include a prominent posterior calcaneal tuberosity, downward slopping tibia, malunion, or loose body. Soft tissue etiologies include the flexor hallucis longus, deltoid ligament, peroneal tendons, posterior inferior tibiofibular ligament, posterior talofibular ligament, posterior tibiotalar ligament, intermaleollar ligament, and fibular ligaments as sources of impingement.[33,34]

Radiographic evaluation of impingement includes standard 3-view ankle radiographs and may be supplemented with an oblique anteromedial impingement view. This impingement view is obtained by angling the beam 45° craniocaudal with the leg in 30° of external rotation.[35] Advanced imaging with MRI is recommended to evaluate the extent of swelling and impingement in addition to evaluating ankle ligaments and joint cartilage.[36] A diagnostic injection of local anesthetic may be used confirm the diagnosis.[36]

Surgical Management

Nonsurgical management with rest, activity modification, heel lifts, and intraarticular injections are recommended but infrequently successful.[27,37,38] Surgical management of AI is the treatment of choice in athletes.[36] The operative procedure is guided by the source of impingement and should address all sources of impingement.

Assessing the severity of tibiotalar arthritic change has been correlated with patient results. In a case series by van Dijk (N = 57), patient outcomes were stratified based on preexisting osteoarthritic changes in the ankle joint. They reported 82% good to excellent results in patients with osteophytes without joint space narrowing and 50% good to excellent results in patients with joint space narrowing.[29]

Operative Techniques

Patient positioning for anterior impingement is supine and for posterior impingement is prone. For the anterior approach, standard arthroscopic portals are used. The use of traction decreases the anterior working space,[29] and therefore the senior author recommends traction intermittently using waist distraction. Placing the foot on the operator's abdomen and into passive dorsiflexion, can reveal engaging lesions while protecting the talar dome from iatrogenic damage.[29] Dynamic impingement can be accessed with passive dorsiflexion under direct visualization.[29] During this maneuver, the interaction of the anterior tibia and talus can be inspected for kissing lesions or impinging soft tissue.[37]

The 2 portal para-Achilles hindfoot endoscopy technique, as described by van Dijk and colleagues,[39] is a commonly used approach for the management of posterior impingement.[40] A working area is created first before visualizing the impinging lesion. The flexor hallucis longus tendon serves as the landmark for the neurovascular bundle (**Fig. 2**).[41]

Postoperative Management and Rehabilitation

Postoperatively, the patient is placed in a controlled ankle motion (CAM) boot with partial weight-bearing restrictions for 1 week. Range of motion can be started immediately postoperatively.

Beginning at 2 weeks postoperatively, sport-specific physical therapy can be instituted for range of motion, strengthening, and proprioception.[42,43] Field training and return to sports may begin as early as 4 weeks.[43] In many cases, impingement is treated concomitantly with instability and OCD lesions, which alter rehabilitation timing and protocols.

Clinical Outcomes

The results of arthroscopic management of AI are good to excellent in more than 77% of patients.[20,44–47] More than 95% of athletes return to the same level of sport.[19,45,48,49] Open procedures have shown similar return to sport outcomes, but with longer recovery times.[50–52] Patients obtain pain-free range of motion and small increases in dorsiflexion postoperatively.[52] Factors associated with poor results of arthroscopic management of AI were older patients, longer delay between inciting

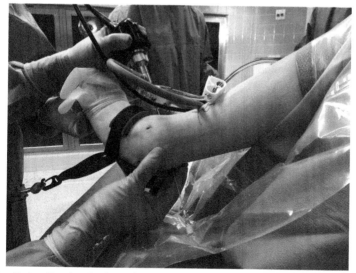

Fig. 2. Needle localization for lateral portal placement adjacent to Achilles tendon.

trauma and surgical treatment, ankle laxity, and osteoarthritic joint space narrowing changes.[50]

Support for early operative intervention was reported by Murawski and Kennedy, who noted a 7-week average return to sport after operative intervention versus a 6-week trial of nonoperative management.[20]

Long-term studies with 5 to 7 years of follow-up in patients with grade 1 to 3 lesions have demonstrated a high recurrence rate of spurs in 66% to 100% of cases. However, these patients remained asymptomatic.[44,51,52] Coull and colleagues[48] found no correlation between recurrence of osteophytes and with recurrence of symptoms.

The outcome of posterior ankle arthroscopy is (approximately 95%) experiencing improvement in symptoms and return to sport.[34,43,49,53] Most of the literature on athletes involves elite soccer players and dancers. Arthroscopically treated, athletes return sport faster than those who undergo open procedures.[35,54] Longer times for return to sport are reported for dancers and when bony procedures are performed. Calder and colleagues[48] reported on a case series of 28 elite soccer players finding return to sport was faster and significant after flexor halluces longus debridement (mean, 28 days) than with bony surgery (mean, 40 days). Guo and colleagues compared return to sport in dancers and soccer players treated arthroscopically versus open procedures for posterior impingement. Soccer players treated arthroscopically returned to sport in 4 to 6 weeks compared with 6 to 12 weeks with open procedures. Dancers returned to sport faster with arthroscopic management as well at 6 to 8 weeks versus 8 to 24 weeks with open techniques.[54]

The largest and most comprehensive study looking at complications after posterior arthroscopy was reported by Nickisch and colleagues[55] and demonstrated a complication rate of 8.5%. Open surgery complication rates have been reported between 10% and 24% (**Fig. 3**).[56]

ANKLE INSTABILITY

Ankle sprains are the most commonly sustained injuries in all sports,[57] and the most frequently encountered injury seen by general practitioners and emergency departments.[58] They account for 25% of musculoskeletal injuries, and more than 20,000 cases of ankle sprains are seen in the United States every day.[59,60] A history of ankle sprains is the main predisposing factor leading to chronic ankle instability (CAI).[61,62] Up to 55% of people sustaining ankle sprains choose not to seek professional analysis and treatment[63]; lack of treatment has been shown to increase the chances of residual symptoms and the development of secondary conditions, including CAI.[64]

The ligaments surrounding the ankle are the main contributors to ankle stability. These include the tibiofibular syndesmosis, deltoid ligament, anterior tibial fibular ligament, calcaneal fibular, and posterior talofibular ligaments.[65] The anterior talofibular ligament is in a plane parallel to the axis of movement (flexion–extension) when the ankle is in a neutral position, and is both the main stabilizer of the ankle and the ligament most susceptible to injuries.[66] However, the etiology of ankle sprains and CAI are far from homogenous. All of the following have been implicated as contributing factors to the development of ankle sprains and/or CAI:

- Lower limb varus malalignment[67];
- Anatomic variations of the tibiotalar joint, for example, axis of rotation, talar dome radius, or retroposition of the lateral malleolus[56,68–70];
- Limited dorsiflexion, chondral problems, and bimalleolar diastasis of the tibiotalar joint[70];
- Subtalar joint anatomic variations and pathologies[57];

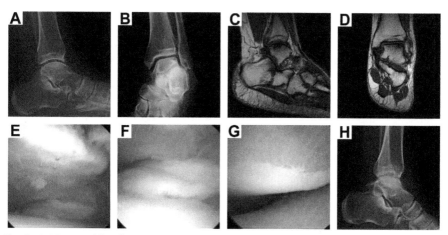

Fig. 3. A 28-year-old male presented with anterior ankle pain with swelling and a history of multiple ankle sprains diagnosed with concomitant osteochondral defect (OCD) lesion and anterior impingement. The patient underwent arthroscopy for debridement, removal of anterior osteophyte and microfracture of OCD lesion. (A) Lateral radiograph demonstrating anterior tibial plafond osteophyte. (B) Anteroposterior (AP) radiograph with subtle lateral talar dome lucency. (C) Sagittal T1 MRI with central talar signal loss in region of OCD and anterior tibial plafond osteophyte. (D) Coronal T1 MRI with lateral talar OCD. (E) Anterior medial portal view of anterior tibial osteophyte and chondral loose body in background. (F) Anterior medial portal view of chondral loose body. (G) Anterior tibial plafond after debridement and osteophyte shaving. (H) Postoperative lateral radiograph.

- Anatomic or histologic variations of the collateral lateral ligament[64,70–72];
- Peroneal tendons pathologies[73]; and
- Pathologies with a proprioceptive deficit or imbalance in neuromuscular control.[67,74]

Common symptoms of CAI include frequent inversion injuries, pain and swelling, and repeated instances of the ankle "giving way."[57,58] One or more ankle inversion injuries always precede the symptoms of CAI. Nonradiographic examinations for quantifying ankle instability include the talar tilt and the anterior drawer tests.[59,75,76] Krips and colleagues[58] describe both tests, and recommend the anterior drawer test as the "most important test for detection of acute and chronic ankle instability." Owing to inconsistent and unreliable results, the talar tilt test was found to be less advantageous.[58] MRI is useful for determining the extent of damage to ankle ligaments and other coexisting pathologies.[57,58]

Therapeutic Options and Surgical Technique

CAI encompasses both mechanical and functional instability. Mechanical instability is defined as chronic laxity in the medial or lateral ligamentous structures.[49] Operative intervention should be considered in patients with continued complaints of pain or instability despite appropriate conservative treatment including physical therapy (proprioceptive and strength training) and bracing or taping. Fewer than 10% of patients who sustain acute ankle ligament injuries will require stabilization surgery.[76] The historical modes of treatment for CAI involved tenodesis such as the Evans, Watson–Jones, and Chrismann–Snook procedures. These nonanatomic reconstructions have had varying levels of success but have been associated with recurrent laxity, limitations in subtalar motion, and the development of arthritis.[34,42,57,77,78] Other open anatomic reconstructions of the lateral ankle ligaments have been published that have included reinforcement with local tissues, namely, inferior extensor retinaculum (Gould modification), autograft or allograft tendon, or a periosteal sleeve. The open modified Brostrom Gould procedure remains the gold standard of ankle ligament stabilization for the majority of patients. It has demonstrated 85% to 100% good to excellent short- and long-term clinical outcomes using various outcome scoring systems.[39] However, arthroscopic approaches have been developed in hopes of decreasing the morbidity of open procedures.

Arthroscopic Techniques

Ankle arthroscopy, in the setting of CAI, has advantages when compared with open surgery, including direct intraarticular evaluation of chondral surfaces, defects, ligaments, scarring, and potential loose bodies. Thermal shrinkage, adapted from the shoulder, has been abandoned because of concerns of capsular necrosis. Other early arthroscopic-assisted treatments of CAI included the use of a percutaneous staple for lateral ligament repair.[79,80]

More recently, treatment has progressed from arthroscopically assisted to all inside anatomic repair of the lateral ankle ligaments, in hopes of minimizing complications such as suture anchor prominence and neuritis.[50] Similar to open repair of ligaments, arthroscopic lateral ankle repair requires that the lateral ankle ligaments have sufficient remnants available for repair. Concern for whether sufficient tissue exists to regain stability of the native ligaments, particularly in the arthroscopic setting, has been raised.

For the arthroscopic technique, utilization of an accessory anterolateral portal is often required for anatomic suture anchor placement and subsequent repair.[50] By using this portal, in conjunction with an understanding of the anatomy of the anterior tibular fibular ligament and calcaneal fibular ligament, suture anchors can be placed.[50]

Clinical Outcomes

Studies are limited related to arthroscopic ankle stabilization. In cadaveric studies, Giza and colleagues[48] found no difference between the strength or stiffness in open versus arthroscopic lateral ankle ligament repair. However, the study did show a high incidence of failure at the suture anchor sites.[48] Drakos and colleagues[43] again demonstrated nearly equivalent results between open versus arthroscopic stabilization of CAI, except in the position of 15° of inversion and plantarflexion, where stability was decreased.

In clinical studies, Kim and colleagues[49] used arthroscopy for anterior tibial fibular ligament reconstruction with inferior extensor retinaculum augmentation and showed that all patients in their cohort were able to return to preinjury activity level. Nery and colleagues[32] also showed promising early functional results using an arthroscopic Broström–Gould technique for stabilization of CAI.

Postoperative Management and Rehabilitation

Rehabilitation protocols are limited for arthroscopic lateral ankle ligament repair. Vega and colleagues[81] proposed the following rehab protocol for arthroscopic lateral ankle ligament repair: a sterile postoperative splint placed for 2 to 3 days, at which time the patient is placed in a CAM boot and progressed to partial weight-bearing. At postoperative week 3, the CAM boot is exchanged for an ankle brace, which is worn for another 3 weeks. Physical therapy is initiated between postoperative weeks 3 and 4 with no inversion or eversion for 6 weeks. The patient returns to noncontact sports in approximately 6 to 8 weeks, and to full participation at approximately 3 months.[50]

SUMMARY

The role of arthroscopy in the management of OCD talar lesions depends on lesion size, character, and location. It is recommended to treat lesions less than 150 mm^2 arthroscopically with bone marrow stimulation. Arthroscopic treatment of larger osteochondral lesions, particularly with a cystic component, remains controversial.

Arthroscopic management of AI in athletes provides a faster return to play with high success rates in both the short and long term. Surgically addressing the extent of both the bony and soft tissue component of impingement is critical. Long-term studies demonstrate recurrence of asymptomatic osteophytic changes.

The gold standard for ankle instability remains open anatomic reconstruction using the Brostrom Gould procedure. Biomechanically, arthroscopy has shown promising results for the treatment of CAI but clinical outcome studies are lacking.

REFERENCES

1. Zengerink M, Szerb I, Hangody L, et al. Current concepts: treatment of osteochondral ankle defects. Foot Ankle Clin 2006;11(2):331–59, vi.
2. Marchant MH Jr, Anderson S, Easley M, et al. Osteochondral lesions of the talus. 2013. Available at: http://www.wheelessonline.com/ortho/osteochondral_lesions_of_the_talus_dup_of_5051. Accessed January 30, 2015.
3. Soboroff SH, Pappius EM, Komaroff AL. Benefits, risks, and costs of alternative approaches to the evaluation and treatment of severe ankle sprain. Clin Orthop Relat Res 1984;183:160–8.
4. Saxena A, Eakin C. Articular talar injuries in athletes: results of microfracture and autogenous bone graft. Am J Sports Med 2007;35(10):1680–7.
5. Savage-Elliott I, Ross KA, Smyth NA, et al. Osteochondral lesions of the talus: a current concepts review and evidence-based treatment paradigm. Foot Ankle Spec 2014;7(5):414–22.
6. Loren GJ, Ferkel RD. Arthroscopic assessment of occult intra-articular injury in acute ankle fractures. Arthroscopy 2002;18(4):412–21.
7. Flick AB, Gould N. Osteochondritis dissecans of the talus (transchondral fractures of the talus): review of the literature and new surgical approach for medial dome lesions. Foot Ankle 1985;5(4):165–85.
8. Dunlap BJ, Ferkel RD, Applegate GR. The "LIFT" lesion: lateral inverted osteochondral fracture of the talus. Arthroscopy 2013;29(11):1826–33.
9. McCollum GA, Calder JD, Longo UG, et al. Talus osteochondral bruises and defects: diagnosis and differentiation. Foot Ankle Clin 2013;18(1):35–47.
10. Golano P, Vega J, de Leeuw PA, et al. Anatomy of the ankle ligaments: a pictorial essay. Knee Surg Sports Traumatol Arthrosc 2010;18(5):557–69.
11. Mintz DN, Tashjian GS, Connell DA, et al. Osteochondral lesions of the talus: a new magnetic resonance grading system with arthroscopic correlation. Arthroscopy 2003;19(4):353–9.
12. Canale ST, Belding RH. Osteochondral lesions of the talus. J Bone Joint Surg Am 1980;62(1):97–102.
13. Clanton T, Nicholas J, Matheny L. Use of cartilage extracellular matrix and bone marrow aspirate concentrate in treatment of osteochondral lesions of the talus. Techniques in Foot and Ankle Surgery 2014;13:212–20.
14. Cuttica DJ, Smith WB, Hyer CF, et al. Osteochondral lesions of the talus: predictors of clinical outcome. Foot Ankle Int 2011;32(11):1045–51.
15. Choi WJ, Park KK, Kim BS, et al. Osteochondral lesion of the talus: is there a critical defect size for poor outcome? Am J Sports Med 2009;37(10):1974–80.

16. van Bergen CJ, Tuijthof GJ, Maas M, et al. Arthroscopic accessibility of the talus quantified by computed tomography simulation. Am J Sports Med 2012;40(10): 2318–24.

17. Thompson JP, Loomer RL. Osteochondral lesions of the talus in a sports medicine clinic. A new radiographic technique and surgical approach. Am J Sports Med 1984;12(6):460–3.

18. Elias I, Zoga AC, Morrison WB, et al. Osteochondral lesions of the talus: localization and morphologic data from 424 patients using a novel anatomical grid scheme. Foot Ankle Int 2007;28(2):154–61.

19. Hannon CP, Smyth NA, Murawski CD, et al. Osteochondral lesions of the talus: aspects of current management. Bone Joint J 2014;96-B(2):164–71.

20. Murawski CD, Foo LF, Kennedy JG. A review of arthroscopic bone marrow stimulation techniques of the talus: the good, the bad, and the causes for concern. Cartilage 2010;1(2):137–44.

21. Nehrer S, Spector M, Minas T. Histologic analysis of tissue after failed cartilage repair procedures. Clin Orthop Relat Res 1999;(365):149–62.

22. Potier E, Ferreira E, Dennler S, et al. Desferrioxamine-driven upregulation of angiogenic factor expression by human bone marrow stromal cells. J Tissue Eng Regen Med 2008;2(5):272–8.

23. Mehta S, Watson JT. Platelet rich concentrate: basic science and current clinical applications. J Orthop Trauma 2008;22(6):432–8.

24. Coetzee JC, Giza E, Schon LC, et al. Treatment of osteochondral lesions of the talus with particulated juvenile cartilage. Foot Ankle Int 2013;34(9):1205–11.

25. Lee DH, Lee KB, Jung ST, et al. Comparison of early versus delayed weightbearing outcomes after microfracture for small to midsized osteochondral lesions of the talus. Am J Sports Med 2012;40(9):2023–8.

26. Bassett FH 3rd, Gates HS 3rd, Billys JB, et al. Talar impingement by the anteroinferior tibiofibular ligament. A cause of chronic pain in the ankle after inversion sprain. J Bone Joint Surg Am 1990;72(1):55–9.

27. Cutsuries AM, Saltrick KR, Wagner J, et al. Arthroscopic arthroplasty of the ankle joint. Clin Podiatr Med Surg 1994;11(3):449–67.

28. van den Bekerom MP, Raven EE. The distal fascicle of the anterior inferior tibiofibular ligament as a cause of tibiotalar impingement syndrome: a current concepts review. Knee Surg Sports Traumatol Arthrosc 2007;15(4):465–71.

29. Tol JL, Verheyen CP, van Dijk CN. Arthroscopic treatment of anterior impingement in the ankle. J Bone Joint Surg Br 2001;83(1):9–13.

30. Ferkel R. Soft-tissue lesions of the ankle. In: Whipple T, editor. Arthroscopic surgery: the foot and ankle. Philadelphia: Lippincott-Raven; 1996. p. 121–43.

31. Massada JL. Ankle overuse injuries in soccer players. Morphological adaptation of the talus in the anterior impingement. J Sports Med Phys Fitness 1991;31(3):447–51.

32. Jowett AJ, Birks CL, Blackney MC. Medial malleolar stress fracture secondary to chronic ankle impingement. Foot Ankle Int 2008;29(7):716–21.

33. Hess GW. Ankle impingement syndromes: a review of etiology and related implications. Foot Ankle Spec 2011;4(5):290–7.

34. Solakoglu C, Kiral A, Pehlivan O, et al. Late-term reconstruction of lateral ankle ligaments using a split peroneus brevis tendon graft (Colville's technique) in patients with chronic lateral instability of the ankle. Int Orthop 2003;27(4):223–7.

35. van Dijk CN, Wessel RN, Tol JL, et al. Oblique radiograph for the detection of bone spurs in anterior ankle impingement. Skeletal Radiol 2002;31(4):214–21.

36. Murawski CD, Kennedy JG. Anteromedial impingement in the ankle joint: outcomes following arthroscopy. Am J Sports Med 2010;38(10):2017–24.

37. Ferkel RD, Scranton PE Jr. Arthroscopy of the ankle and foot. J Bone Joint Surg Am 1993;75(8):1233–42.
38. Liu SH, Baker CL. Comparison of lateral ankle ligamentous reconstruction procedures. Am J Sports Med 1994;22(3):313–7.
39. van Dijk CN, de Leeuw PA, Scholten PE. Hindfoot endoscopy for posterior ankle impingement. Surgical technique. J Bone Joint Surg Am 2009;91(Suppl 2): 287–98.
40. Rosenbaum D, Becker HP, Sterk J, et al. Long-term results of the modified Evans repair for chronic ankle instability. Orthopedics 1996;19(5):451–5.
41. Trevino SG, Davis P, Hecht PJ. Management of acute and chronic lateral ligament injuries of the ankle. Orthop Clin North Am 1994;25(1):1–16.
42. Messer TM, Cummins CA, Ahn J, et al. Outcome of the modified Brostrom procedure for chronic lateral ankle instability using suture anchors. Foot Ankle Int 2000; 21(12):996–1003.
43. Pierrard G, Acquitter Y, Vandamme G, et al. Arthroscopic treatment of anterior ankle impingement: results of a 70 patient multicenter prospective study. Arthroscopy 2012;28(9):370.
44. Coull R, Raffiq T, James LE, et al. Open treatment of anterior impingement of the ankle. J Bone Joint Surg Br 2003;85(4):550–3.
45. Gulish HA, Sullivan RJ, Aronow M. Arthroscopic treatment of soft-tissue impingement lesions of the ankle in adolescents. Foot Ankle Int 2005;26(3):204–7.
46. Kim SH, Ha KI. Arthroscopic treatment for impingement of the anterolateral soft tissues of the ankle. J Bone Joint Surg Br 2000;82(7):1019–21.
47. Smyth NA, Murawski CD, Levine DS, et al. Hindfoot arthroscopic surgery for posterior ankle impingement: a systematic surgical approach and case series. Am J Sports Med 2013;41(8):1869–76.
48. Calder JD, Sexton SA, Pearce CJ. Return to training and playing after posterior ankle arthroscopy for posterior impingement in elite professional soccer. Am J Sports Med 2010;38(1):120–4.
49. Noguchi H, Ishii Y, Takeda M, et al. Arthroscopic excision of posterior ankle bony impingement for early return to the field: short-term results. Foot Ankle Int 2010; 31(5):398–403.
50. Bell SJ, Mologne TS, Sitler DF, et al. Twenty-six-year results after Brostrom procedure for chronic lateral ankle instability. Am J Sports Med 2006;34(6): 975–8.
51. Walsh SJ, Twaddle BC, Rosenfeldt MP, et al. Arthroscopic treatment of anterior ankle impingement: a prospective study of 46 patients with 5-year follow-up. Am J Sports Med 2014;42(11):2722–6.
52. Tol JL, van Dijk CN. Anterior ankle impingement. Foot Ankle Clin 2006;11(2): 297–310, vi.
53. Rosenbaum D, Becker HP, Sterk J, et al. Functional evaluation of the 10-year outcome after modified Evans repair for chronic ankle instability. Foot Ankle Int 1997;18(12):765–71.
54. Kim ES, Lee KT, Park JS, et al. Arthroscopic anterior talofibular ligament repair for chronic ankle instability with a suture anchor technique. Orthopedics 2011;34(4). http://dx.doi.org/10.3928/01477447-20110228-03.
55. Nickisch F, Barg A, Saltzman CL, et al. Postoperative complications of posterior ankle and hindfoot arthroscopy. J Bone Joint Surg Am 2012;94(5):439–46.
56. Guillo S, Bauer T, Lee JW, et al. Consensus in chronic ankle instability: aetiology, assessment, surgical indications and place for arthroscopy. Orthop Traumatol Surg Res 2013;99(8 Suppl):S411–9.

57. Krips R, de Vries J, van Dijk CN. Ankle instability. Foot Ankle Clin 2006;11(2): 311–29, vi.
58. van Dijk CN. On diagnostic strategies in patients with severe ankle sprain [master's]. Amsterdam: Universiteit van Amsterdam; 1994.
59. Klenerman L. The management of sprained ankle. J Bone Joint Surg Br 1998; 80(1):11–2.
60. Garrick JG. The frequency of injury, mechanism of injury, and epidemiology of ankle sprains. Am J Sports Med 1977;5(6):241–2.
61. Konradsen L, Bech L, Ehrenbjerg M, et al. Seven years follow-up after ankle inversion trauma. Scand J Med Sci Sports 2002;12(3):129–35.
62. McKay GD, Goldie PA, Payne WR, et al. Ankle injuries in basketball: injury rate and risk factors. Br J Sports Med 2001;35(2):103–8.
63. Pijnenburg AC, Van Dijk CN, Bossuyt PM, et al. Treatment of ruptures of the lateral ankle ligaments: a meta-analysis. J Bone Joint Surg Am 2000;82(6):761–73.
64. Wiersman P, Grifioen F. Variations of three lateral ligaments of the ankle: a descriptive anatomical study. Foot 1992;2:218–22.
65. Bronstroem L. Sprained ankles: a pathologic, arthrographic and clinical study [doctoral]. Stockholm (Sweden): Karolinska Institute; 1996.
66. Bonnel F, Toullec E, Mabit C, et al. Chronic ankle instability: biomechanics and pathomechanics of ligaments injury and associated lesions. Orthop Traumatol Surg Res 2010;96(4):424–32.
67. Coughlin M, Mann R, Saltzman C. Surgery of the foot and ankle. Philadelphia: Mosby Elsevier; 2007.
68. Sammarco GJ, Burstein AH, Frankel VH. Biomechanics of the ankle: a kinematic study. Orthop Clin North Am 1973;4(1):75–96.
69. Scranton PE Jr, McDermott JE, Rogers JV. The relationship between chronic ankle instability and variations in mortise anatomy and impingement spurs. Foot Ankle Int 2000;21(8):657–64.
70. Choi WJ, Lee JW, Han SH, et al. Chronic lateral ankle instability: the effect of intra-articular lesions on clinical outcome. Am J Sports Med 2008;36(11):2167–72.
71. Hubbard-Turner T. Relationship between mechanical ankle joint laxity and subjective function. Foot Ankle Int 2012;33(10):852–6.
72. Hatch GF, Labib SA, Rolf RH, et al. J Surg Orthop Adv 2007;16(4):187–91.
73. Hiller CE, Nightingale EJ, Lin CW, et al. Characteristics of people with recurrent ankle sprains: a systematic review with meta-analysis. Br J Sports Med 2011; 45(8):660–72.
74. van Dijk CN. CBO-guideline for diagnosis and treatment of the acute ankle injury. National organization for quality assurance in hospitals. Ned Tijdschr Geneeskd 1999;143(42):2097–101.
75. van Dijk CN, Lim LS, Bossuyt PM, et al. Physical examination is sufficient for the diagnosis of sprained ankles. J Bone Joint Surg Br 1996;78(6):958–62.
76. Snook GA, Chrisman OD, Wilson TC. Long-term results of the Chrisman-Snook operation for reconstruction of the lateral ligaments of the ankle. J Bone Joint Surg Am 1985;67(1):1–7.
77. van der Rijt AJ, Evans GA. The long-term results of Watson-Jones tenodesis. J Bone Joint Surg Br 1984;66(3):371–5.
78. Hawkins RB. Arthroscopic stapling repair for chronic lateral instability. Clin Podiatr Med Surg 1987;4(4):875–83.
79. Baums MH, Kahl E, Schultz W, et al. Clinical outcome of the arthroscopic management of sports-related "anterior ankle pain": a prospective study. Knee Surg Sports Traumatol Arthrosc 2006;14(5):482–6.

80. Lopez Valerio V, Seijas R, Alvarez P, et al. Endoscopic repair of posterior ankle impingement syndrome due to os trigonum in soccer players. Foot Ankle Int 2015;36(1):70–4.
81. Vega J, Golano P, Pellegrino A, et al. All-inside arthroscopic lateral collateral ligament repair for ankle instability with a knotless suture anchor technique. Foot Ankle Int 2013;34(12):1701–9.

Lisfranc Injuries
When to Observe, Fix, or Fuse

Jeffrey D. Seybold, MD*, J. Chris Coetzee, MD

KEYWORDS

- Lisfranc • Tarsometatarsal joint • Instability • Arthrodesis • Athlete

KEY POINTS

- A high index of suspicion is critical to adequately recognize subtle Lisfranc complex injuries. Weight-bearing radiographs of the injured foot, contralateral comparison radiographs, and stress views are all essential in the diagnosis of a subtle Lisfranc injury.
- Stable Lisfranc sprains, with no evidence of instability, may be treated with nonoperative management, with reliable return to competitive activity.
- Unstable Lisfranc complex injuries mandate operative stabilization. Anatomic reduction of the Lisfranc joint complex is critical and correlates with improved results, regardless of whether percutaneous or open methods are used.
- Arthrodesis is advised for purely ligamentous injuries that involve the medial and middle columns or for significantly comminuted fracture-dislocations. Failure to remove transarticular hardware essentially consigns patients to a pseudoarthrodesis.
- Athletes should be advised that Lisfranc complex injuries are serious; although the literature supports most athletes can return to competitive play after operative intervention, recovery may take up to 6 months to a year.

Injuries to the foot are common in the athletic population, accounting for approximately 16% of all sporting injuries.[1] Trauma to the tarsometatarsal (TMT) joints is the second most common injury pattern, second only to metatarsophalangeal (MTP) joint injuries, and occurs in up to 4% of professional American football players on an annual basis. Offensive linemen are responsible for 29.2% of these injuries.[2] The bony and ligamentous structures around the first and second TMT joints, or Lisfranc joint complex, are the most commonly involved in injuries to the midfoot because of the limited static and dynamic stability of this region. Rapid diagnosis of Lisfranc injuries is critical to allow for appropriate treatment and a more speedy return to play. Misdiagnosis or maltreatment of these potentially career-ending injuries may not

All authors certify that there are no relevant disclosures regarding funding or conflicts of interest pertaining to the following article.
Twin Cities Orthopedics, 4010 West, 65th Street, Edina, MN 55435, USA
* Corresponding author.
E-mail address: jseybold@tcomn.com

only prolong return to competitive play but can also lead to posttraumatic degenerative changes and pain that limit activity and quality of life in the future.

High-energy injuries that involve multiple fractures and/or dislocations of the TMT joints are relatively easy to recognize and are fortunately less common in the setting of athletic competition. Discussion of these more severe injuries is beyond the scope of this review. The appropriate management of Lisfranc or TMT joint injuries in the athlete is controversial, with multiple classification schemes and treatment methods and little evidence-based guidelines to help deliver appropriate care. This article reviews the current diagnosis and management principles for TMT injuries in the athletic population.

ANATOMY

The Lisfranc complex of the midfoot consists of an intricate interaction between the wedge-shaped bases of the first and second metatarsals, the corresponding articular surfaces of the medial and middle cuneiforms, and the ligamentous supports that traverse these joints. The base of the second metatarsal is recessed approximately 8 mm relative to the distal articular surface of the medial cuneiform and 4 mm relative to the lateral cuneiform and is recognized as a keystone that helps lock in stability to the midfoot and Lisfranc complex.[3] Although strong interosseous ligamentous structures support most of the midfoot joints, there is no intermetatarsal ligament between the bases of the first and second metatarsals. Therefore, stability of the Lisfranc complex depends on the weaker dorsal and interosseous Lisfranc ligaments and the stronger plantar Lisfranc ligament, which run between the base of the second metatarsal and the lateral and distal aspect of the medial cuneiform.[4] Cadaveric studies have demonstrated that the plantar Lisfranc ligament is 3 times stronger than the dorsal Lisfranc ligament and is the critical structure in differentiating a stable midfoot sprain from an unstable Lisfranc injury.[4,5] Any fracture or avulsion of bone at this complex confers inherent instability of the Lisfranc complex. Because the plane of the TMT joints is relatively perpendicular to the ground, there is little inherent bony stability of the TMT joints during stance, and the ligamentous support is critical to maintain appropriate alignment and articular contact. The arc of motion at the TMT joints is minimal because of both osseous and ligamentous constraints, with approximately 4° of dorsiflexion and 1° plantar flexion noted at the first TMT joint and even less arc of motion at the second and third TMT joints.[6] The lateral column of the midfoot, which includes the fourth and fifth TMT joints, has much more mobility than the remainder of the midfoot (nearly 10° of dorsiflexion and plantar flexion) and as a result is able to better tolerate subtle instability associated with athletic midfoot injuries.

MECHANISM OF INJURY

Injuries to the Lisfranc joint complex typically occur by one of 2 classically described mechanisms. Direct injury to the Lisfranc complex is seen most commonly in high-energy trauma, in which a crush or significant impact to the midfoot leads to fractures and dislocations of the TMT joints. Although this mechanism of injury is more commonly reported than low-energy scenarios, indirect or low-energy injuries are much more common in athletic competition.[7] Athletic Lisfranc complex injuries fall broadly into 2 categories: plantar flexion injuries and abduction injuries. Plantar flexion injuries occur when an axial load is applied to a plantar flexed foot and ankle while the toes are dorsiflexed at the MTP joints. The ligamentous complex at the TMT joints fails dorsally; as the body falls over the foot, rotational forces are applied to the midfoot with resulting joint subluxation or dislocations.[8-10] This injury is the traditional football lineman injury in which a tackled player falls onto the lineman's heel while the foot is planted on the ground during a block. Abduction injuries occur as the forefoot is suddenly abducted relative to a fixed hindfoot. This pattern typically occurs in sports in which the hindfoot remains secured within a stirrup or brace, such as surfing or equestrian sports.[8,9,11] In reality, a combination of forces often contributes to the athletic Lisfranc complex injury, and many cannot be simplified into one of these 2 categories.

CLINICAL PRESENTATION

A high clinical suspicion for injury is critical to identify patients with subtle Lisfranc complex injuries. Patients with subtle Lisfranc complex injuries may present with varied degrees of swelling throughout the midfoot, though reliably report pain with attempted weight-bearing activity.[10] Midfoot pain while walking down stairs is a valuable clue in diagnosing a subtle Lisfranc complex injury. Plantar ecchymosis is considered pathognomonic for a Lisfranc injury and should trigger a thorough clinical and radiographic evaluation, even if initial radiographs do not demonstrate an obvious fracture or instability.[12] Pain is commonly elicited with palpation directly over the dorsal aspect of the involved TMT joints. The piano-key test, in which the metatarsal is grasped and dorsiflexion and plantar flexion are performed at the TMT joint, may elicit pain at the involved joints. Shapiro and colleagues[10] illustrated 2 provocative tests that identify athletes with an injury to the Lisfranc complex: midfoot compression and dorsal and plantar manipulation of the first metatarsal head relative to the second metatarsal head. Myerson and Cerrato[9] cautioned that diagnosing a Lisfranc complex injury based on pain with manipulation of the first metatarsal in the sagittal plane might produce false-negative results, as the medial column may not be involved in the injury pattern. They described another clinical test that is more specific for Lisfranc complex injuries, which consists of compression between the first and second metatarsals in the coronal plane to place stress across the bases of the medial and middle columns. Pain or a palpable click indicates an injury to the Lisfranc complex.[9] Care must be taken to examine the entire foot and ankle for associated fractures or ligamentous injuries, which may require additional treatment.

RADIOGRAPHIC STUDIES

Weight-bearing anteroposterior (AP), 30° oblique, and lateral radiographs are the first, and typically most valuable, imaging studies obtained for patients with a suspected Lisfranc complex injury. If it is too painful for patients to cooperate with an adequate standing radiograph, allowing the foot to rest for a week and obtaining radiographs when patients are more comfortable placing weight down on the foot may be helpful. An ankle block or administration of intra-articular local anesthetic can be performed in order to obtain adequate weight-bearing radiographs or to perform abduction stress radiographs in a timely fashion. A small avulsion fracture at the medial base of the second metatarsal or the distal lateral corner of the medial cuneiform, the so-called fleck sign, indicates an unstable injury.[13] Non–weight-bearing radiographs may identify more severe or high-energy fracture-dislocations but are essentially useless in the evaluation of a subtle injury (**Fig. 1**). A comparison weight-bearing AP radiograph of the contralateral foot should be obtained to identify subtle subluxation or translation at the Lisfranc joint complex, which appears asymmetric in the injured foot (**Fig. 2**). This radiograph is particularly useful for cases with less than 2 mm of instability as this amount of displacement is often difficult to assess on a plain radiograph.[14]

One must always take care to complete a thorough radiographic review as associated fractures occur in 39% of patients with Lisfranc injuries.[15] These fractures include

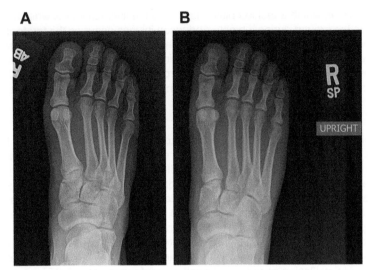

Fig. 1. (*A, B*) This patient demonstrated a nondisplaced medial cuneiform fracture on initial non–weight-bearing radiographs in the emergency department without obvious TMT joint subluxation (*A*). Subsequent weight-bearing radiographs obtained at the patient's initial clinic visit demonstrate definitive widening at the Lisfranc joint (*B*).

the nutcracker fracture, whereby the cuboid is crushed between the fourth and fifth metatarsal bases and the anterior calcaneus. Although more common in higher-energy injuries, this injury pattern has also been described in equestrian injuries[16,17] and is critical to recognize as operative fixation is required and best performed for the lateral column first to restore length and aid in reduction of the middle and medial

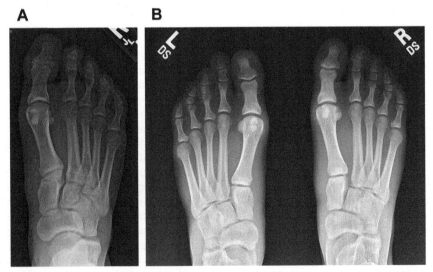

Fig. 2. (*A, B*) When an initial radiograph is inconclusive (*A*), a comparison weight-bearing radiograph of the contralateral foot (*B*) is frequently helpful to identify subtle widening at the Lisfranc joint in the injured foot.

columns.[9] Another variant of the Lisfranc complex injury is the longitudinal instability pattern, in which diastasis is present between the medial and middle cuneiforms and the second TMT joint may remain stable. A gap sign may be present on examination, with an asymmetric space appearing between the hallux and second toe.[18] This pattern also mandates operative stabilization of the intercuneiform joint.

More frequently, advanced imaging studies are used to identify or confirm a subtle injury, especially as up to 20% of Lisfranc complex injuries are missed on initial radiographs.[19] Thin-cut computed tomography (CT) imaging with reconstruction views will identify small fractures or possibly subluxation at the TMT joints[14] and may be particularly helpful if the foot can be loaded with a simulated weight-bearing study. MRI is both sensitive and specific in identifying partial and complete ligamentous injuries at the Lisfranc joint complex but is unnecessary for evaluation of injuries with obvious subluxation or dislocation.[9,20] A normal appearance of the plantar Lisfranc ligament on MRI is highly suggestive of a stable midfoot, whereas the best predictor for instability is a rupture or a grade-2 sprain of this ligament. MRI has demonstrated a sensitivity, specificity, and positive predictive value for detecting injury to the plantar Lisfranc ligament of 95%, 75%, and 94%, respectively.[21] Nunley and Vertullo[22] have supported the use of bone scans to identify occult injuries at the Lisfranc joint complex with excellent reported sensitivity,[2] though this modality may be difficult to access and is not typically used in the authors' evaluation of patients with midfoot injuries.

Abduction stress radiographs of the injured foot may identify dynamic instability at the Lisfranc joint complex in cases where plain weight-bearing radiographs are negative or equivocal but clinical suspicion remains high (**Fig. 3**). Traditionally, pronation

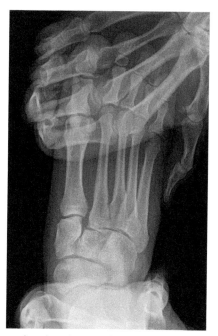

Fig. 3. Abduction stress can be placed across the midfoot to identify dynamic instability or confirm adequate fixation intraoperatively. This patient demonstrated dynamic instability at the Lisfranc joint with lateral translation of the second metatarsal base but no gapping at the first TMT joint.

and abduction stress at the midfoot has been used to reveal instability,[23] but a squeeze test between the medial and middle columns has also been advocated as a supplemental stress examination to identify unstable injuries.[24] The utility of stress radiographs has been called into question because of the variable forces applied by the examiner and lack of standardization to declare a positive test.[22] Other investigators have reported more reliable use of stress radiographs with patients placed under sedation or anesthesia as patients may not be able to comply with these radiographs in the clinic setting.[9] Although these concerns are valid, the authors' experience has supported the use of stress radiographs in the clinic setting as patients are often able to tolerate gentle, progressive stress across the midfoot with minimal complaint, limiting the expense and risk of evaluation under a nerve block or anesthesia. Stress radiographs are also of use when assessing the adequacy of reduction or fixation of the Lisfranc joint intraoperatively. Radiographic parameters typically used to identify instability at the Lisfranc and TMT joints are noted in **Table 1**.

CLASSIFICATION

Quenu and Kuss[25] first provided a classification system for TMT and Lisfranc injuries in 1909, dividing injuries into isolated, homolateral, and divergent groups. This system has since been revised by both Hardcastle and colleagues[26] and Myerson and colleagues[13]: Type A injuries demonstrate total incongruity of all of the TMT joints in either a medial or lateral direction; type B injuries demonstrate partial incongruity with injuries limited to a particular column; and type C injuries result in a divergent fracture pattern in which the medial column displaces medially and the middle column (and in type C2 cases the lateral column as well) displaces laterally. This classification system is most helpful to describe high-energy injuries but does not truly address the subtle or low-energy Lisfranc complex injuries.

More recently, Nunley and Vertullo[22] proposed a classification system that addresses the subtle Lisfranc complex injury that typically occurs with a low-energy mechanism (**Fig. 4**). Stage I injuries include those patients who demonstrate pain at the Lisfranc complex on examination and are unable to participate in athletic activity but do not demonstrate any evidence of instability on weight-bearing radiographs. In these cases, MRI is often positive for a sprain of the Lisfranc ligament and edema at the involved bones. Stage II injuries demonstrate 1 to 5 mm of diastasis at the Lisfranc joint on a weight-bearing AP radiograph without loss of arch height on the lateral radiograph. Stage III injuries demonstrate greater than 5 mm of diastasis at the Lisfranc joint

Table 1	
Radiographic parameters to identify Lisfranc or TMT injuries	
XR View	**Radiographic Finding**
AP	• Loss of contour along the medial border of the second MT base and the medial border of the middle cuneiform • Greater than 2 mm of diastasis between the base of the first and second MT • Greater than 1 mm of difference when measuring the diastasis between the first and second MT bases compared with the normal foot • Avulsion of the Lisfranc ligament (fleck sign)
Oblique	• Loss of contour along the medial border of the fourth MT and the medial border of the cuboid
Lateral	• Reduced distance between the plantar fifth metatarsal and medial cuneiform • Dorsal subluxation of the metatarsals at the TMT joints

Abbreviations: MT, metatarsal; TMT, tarsometatarsal; XR, X-ray.

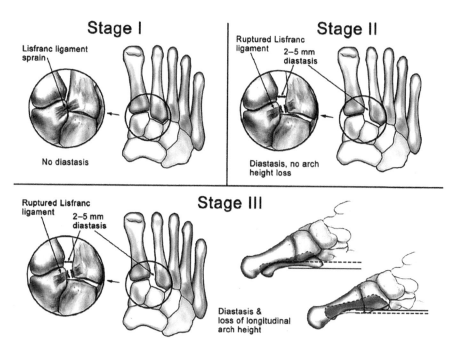

Fig. 4. The classification system proposed by Nunley and Vertullo.[22] Stage I injuries include patients with pain at the Lisfranc complex but no evidence of instability on weight-bearing radiographs. Stage II injuries demonstrate less than 5 mm of diastasis at the Lisfranc joint without loss of arch height. It should be noted that although the diagram from the article denotes 2 to 5 mm of diastasis, the text description by Nunley and Vertullo includes diastasis of 1 to 5 mm in stage II. Stage III injuries demonstrate greater than 5 mm of diastasis at the Lisfranc joint and loss of distance between the plantar aspect of the fifth metatarsal and medial cuneiform on the lateral radiograph. (*From* Nunley JA, Vertullo CJ. Classification, investigation, and management of midfoot sprains: Lisfranc injuries in the athlete. Am J Sports Med 2002;30(6):872; with permission.)

on the weight-bearing AP radiograph and loss of distance between the plantar aspect of the fifth metatarsal and medial cuneiform on the lateral radiograph. Nonoperative treatment was advised for stage I injuries, and operative reduction and internal fixation were recommended for stage II and III injuries.

A modification of this classification was proposed in a recent article by Eleftheriou and Rosenfeld.[27] Grade 1 injuries remain the same, with tenderness localized to the Lisfranc joint complex on examination but no evidence of instability on weight-bearing radiographs. Grade 2 injuries demonstrate 2 mm or less of displacement on weight-bearing radiographs and/or diastasis on CT or intraoperative fluoroscopy. Grade 3 injuries included any diastasis greater than 2 mm on weight-bearing radiographs or an injury that meets any of the Myerson classification parameters. Grade 1 injuries were managed nonoperatively with careful follow-up, and open reduction and internal fixation (ORIF) or arthrodesis were advised for grade 2 and 3 injuries.

MANAGEMENT

There are few foot and ankle traumatic injuries that elicit as much debate regarding appropriate management than Lisfranc fractures or dislocations. Few level 1 studies exist that define the best treatment course for these injuries, though there is little debate that a higher risk of posttraumatic degenerative changes and poor outcomes are present in unrecognized unstable injuries, inadequately stabilized injuries, and purely ligamentous injuries.[2,8,9,13,23,26,28–33]

Any patients with evidence of dynamic instability or clear diastasis at the Lisfranc joint complex require operative management. Controversy exists as to the most appropriate treatment of these injuries, even in high-energy mechanism injuries that have been well studied. Ultimately, each patient's age, extent of injury, activity level, and desired return to sport should be considered when selecting the most appropriate treatment.

In a 2008 Instructional Course Lecture, Myerson and Cerrato[9] presented several pertinent questions that remain critical to address in deciding the most appropriate management for each patient and are summarized here. When is surgery necessary? When should surgery be performed? Is the injury amenable to percutaneous fixation or is an open reduction required? What hardware should be used for fixation? How should patients be managed postoperatively? When should hardware be removed? When should a primary arthrodesis be performed? And lastly, when can an athlete expect to return to play? Each of these questions are addressed in the following paragraphs.

Nonoperative Management

Nonoperative treatment is reserved solely for patients with a Nunley and Vertullo[22] stage 1, completely stable injury (no diastasis noted at the Lisfranc complex). Excellent results have been reported whether immobilizing patients in a short-leg cast for 6 weeks[22] or allowing early weight bearing with a protective orthotic.[2] The authors recommend a protective but progressive approach to stable injuries, similar to those proposed by multiple other investigators.[9,27,34] Patients are initially immobilized in a short walker boot with protected weight bearing for 2 weeks, after which patients are reexamined. If tenderness over the Lisfranc complex resolves and there is no evidence of diastasis at the Lisfranc joint on repeat weight-bearing imaging, patients are allowed to progress weight-bearing activity as tolerated in the boot, often with the addition of a well-molded arch support orthotic. Weight bearing out of the boot is initiated once patients are pain free with abduction stress, typically by 6 to 8 weeks after injury. A stiff-soled shoe with rigid orthotic support is used for 6 months. Sport-specific rehabilitation can begin once the athlete can walk down several flights of stairs without inducing pain. Although patients are able to progress into in-line impact activity as tolerated after discontinuing boot immobilization, running on uneven surfaces and any cutting or twisting activities are not permitted for the first 3 to 4 months following injury to limit recurrent injury or continued pain. Patients should be able to do a single leg hop test pain free before these activities are permitted. Even with the variation noted in the management of stage I injuries, excellent results are noted throughout the literature with successful return to competitive play.[2,10,22,23] Curtis and colleagues[23] reviewed the cases of 9 patients who sustained a TMT joint injury without evidence of diastasis and noted good to excellent results in 7. Shapiro and colleagues[10] reported on a series of 9 athletes with isolated TMT ligament ruptures. All but one were treated with a removable splint for 4 to 6 weeks, and all returned to competitive activity.

Timing of Intervention

Low-energy mechanism injuries as seen in the athletic population are not typically associated with a severe degree of swelling that would limit the ability to proceed with surgery as soon as feasible. Nonetheless, a delay of 1 to 2 weeks from injury to definitive fixation has not been shown to negatively affect outcomes after ORIF.[29,35,36] Although some investigators advocate for definitive fixation to be performed within 6 weeks of the initial injury,[9,37,38] satisfactory outcomes have been noted with fixation performed 1 year after injury.[9] The authors generally support an attempt at internal fixation without an arthrodesis up to 4 months after injury, after which time arthrodesis will typically provide the best results. In cases whereby the initial diagnosis was missed or treatment is delayed for more than 6 weeks, open reduction of the involved joints is required to remove the thickened scar tissue between the joints that will prevent a stable closed reduction.[9]

Percutaneous Fixation Versus Open Reduction

Although some investigators propose that accurate, anatomic reduction is best achieved with open methods,[28,39] patients with a statically reduced Lisfranc joint but dynamic instability on abduction stress are excellent candidates for percutaneous reduction and internal fixation. It is critical to assess the reduction of the Lisfranc complex on AP and lateral fluoroscopic views in the operating room to ensure an anatomic reduction is achieved, as the quality of the reduction is correlated with patient outcomes.[13,26,28,29,31] Any persistent subluxation or inadequate reduction requires conversion to an open procedure.

Two small incisions are made medially at the base of the medial cuneiform and dorsally over the lateral base of the second metatarsal. A large pointed reduction forceps is secured across the Lisfranc complex, and the reduction is assessed under fluoroscopic imaging. At this point, multiple fixation options are available. A fully threaded 4.0-mm cannulated screw is frequently used, traveling from the base of the medial cuneiform across the Lisfranc joint and securing the second metatarsal base in bicortical fashion. It is the authors' experience that after securing the Lisfranc joint with a single screw, the first and second TMT joints will often stabilize and remain in a reduced position with abduction stress, limiting the need for further fixation (Fig. 5). If the medial column remains unstable, a closed reduction of the first TMT joint is achieved by manipulating the hallux MTP joint into slight varus and dorsiflexion while applying lateral pressure to the base of the first metatarsal. A guidewire can be advanced while maintaining the first TMT joint in a reduced position, and once again a fully threaded 4.0-mm cannulated screw is advanced across the first TMT joint from dorsal and distal to proximal and plantar.

If open reduction is required, the authors prefer to make a single incision centered over the Lisfranc joint, using an interval between the extensor hallucis longus and extensor digitorum longus tendons to the second toe. Soft tissue dissection is carefully carried down keeping in mind that the deep peroneal nerve and dorsalis pedis artery will often appear in this interval and require protection. If the third TMT joint is involved and requires fixation or arthrodesis, or concomitant injuries need to be addressed, then multiple incisions may be used; but a wide skin bridge is critical to limit skin and wound necrosis.

Surgical Hardware

Early reports of Lisfranc injury management described the so-called pin-and-plaster technique, relying on Kirschner wire fixation to maintain a stable reduction at the involved joints.[26,40] Although a few investigators still endorse this method, the authors do not advocate it for the athletic population. Numerous studies have demonstrated improved stability with screw and/or plate fixation, which also limits the risks of recurrent subluxation after early pin removal and pin site complications.[9,13,28,39,41] The

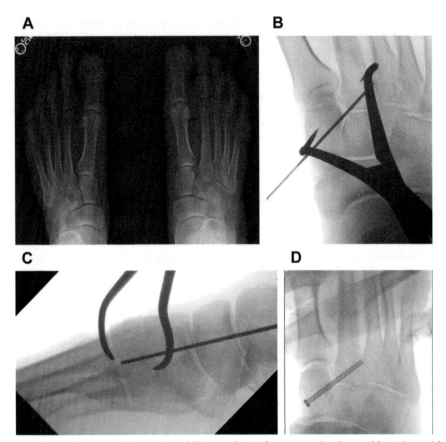

Fig. 5. (A–D) Patients with static stability at the Lisfranc complex but subluxation with weight bearing or abduction stress are excellent candidates for percutaneous reduction and internal fixation. Often, after stabilizing the Lisfranc joint, the first and second TMT joints remain stable with stress and do not require further fixation. This patient sustained a Lisfranc injury while playing ultimate Frisbee with an associated fleck fracture and coronal plane instability noted on weight-bearing radiographs (A). The midfoot stabilized with a single Lisfranc screw following percutaneous reduction (B–D).

authors do use Kirschner wires to stabilize injuries at the fourth and fifth TMT joints, advancing the wires from distal to proximal across the bases of the metatarsals into the cuboid. The wires are bent back or buried under the skin and typically removed in the clinic at 6 weeks after injury once adequate scar tissue formation has occurred.

The workhorse of Lisfranc joint complex fixation is a 4.0-mm fully threaded screw. Cannulated or noncannulated screws both provide adequate rigidity to the fixation construct, and the use of either is surgeon dependent. Partially threaded or lag screws are not recommended, as these increase pressure across the articular surfaces of the involved joints and may lead to cartilage death and posttraumatic degenerative changes.[29,42] Approximately 2.0% to 4.8% of the TMT joint articular surface is compromised with use of a transarticular screw (and the damage is likely more extensive because of thermal injury from drilling across the joint),[43] which has led to the more recent endorsement of dorsal transarticular or bridge plating and hybrid techniques. Alberta and colleagues[43] demonstrated equivalent results when comparing the degree of TMT joint displacement when stabilizing the joint with 3.5-mm transarticular screws or a dorsal one-third tubular plate. Advocates for bridge plating propose that avoiding further trauma to the articular surface of the injured joints further limits the risk of posttraumatic arthritis.[44–46] More extensive soft tissue dissection is required both at the time of implantation and hardware removal with use of dorsal plates, and more definitive studies are required before their use can be universally supported over screws. The authors typically reserve the use of dorsal locked bridge plating for grade 3 injuries with plantar instability and/or metatarsal base fractures that may limit the degree of stability achieved with transarticular screws (**Fig. 6**).

More recently, suture button devices have been used as the sole means of fixation or an augment to screw fixation of Lisfranc complex injuries and are an option when percutaneous methods are allowable (**Fig. 7**).[9,47,48] Recent studies have confirmed equivalent stability across the Lisfranc joint when using a suture button device as compared with screw fixation.[49,50] Even so, suture button devices should be used with extreme caution, as multi-plane instability cannot be adequately stabilized with flexible fixation. If any instability in the sagittal plane is noted on preoperative or intraoperative imaging, the authors recommend a screw for fixation after reduction of the Lisfranc complex. Hybrid techniques have also been advocated in which a suture device and screw are both secured across the Lisfranc joint. After the Lisfranc screw is removed, the suture device provides continued coronal plane stability. This construct has been used particularly in heavyweight athletes, such as football players; but any literature supporting this indication is lacking. When using a suture button device as

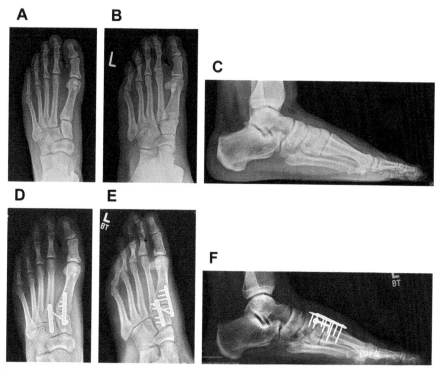

Fig. 6. (*A–F*) Dorsal plating has gained in popularity over recent years, and the authors typically use plates for patients with plantar instability or base fractures that limit stability achieved with transarticular screws.

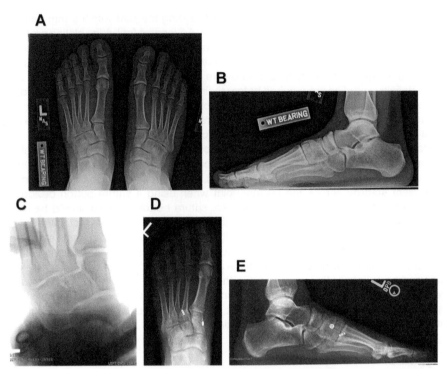

Fig. 7. (*A–E*) Suture button devices have an undefined role in Lisfranc complex injuries and should only be considered for patients with isolated coronal plane instability. This patient is a female collegiate athlete who demonstrated subtle coronal plane instability at the Lisfranc joint with dynamic stress (*A–C*) and underwent tightrope stabilization (*D–E*).

the sole means of fixation, similar restrictions are used for advancing weight-bearing activity postoperatively, though hardware removal is not required. Much more evidence is required before the use of suture button fixation can be universally advocated.

Postoperative Care

Patients remain non–weight bearing for 2 weeks following surgery and are immobilized in a short leg splint. Reliable patients who undergo percutaneous procedures may be immobilized in a short CAM walker boot. Sutures are typically removed at 2 weeks postoperatively when initial weight-bearing radiographs are obtained. Patients may begin partial weight bearing in a short CAM walker boot, placing weight down on their heel for balance; athletes can begin a program of water exercise and high-repetition, low-resistance exercise on a stationary bicycle. At 6 weeks postoperatively, progressive weight bearing is allowed in a short CAM walker boot and patients transition into a supportive shoe with a carbon fiber plate orthotic as comfort allows. Patients may participate in low-impact activity (eg, exercise bike, elliptical trainer, swimming) but refrain from impact activity until after the metalwork is removed. Following screw and/or plate removal, patients may bear weight as tolerated in a short CAM walker boot for 2 weeks and then transition into low-impact and eventually in-line impact activity as tolerated. Return to athletic activity is allowed as for nonoperative management. Sport-specific rehabilitation is initiated once the athlete can walk down several flights of stairs without inducing pain. Patients must be able to perform a single leg hop test pain free before running on uneven surfaces or twisting or cutting activities are permitted. A carbon fiber plate orthotic or stiff shoe is used as patients initiate running or jumping activity and is discontinued as the patients' comfort allows.

Patients who undergo suture button fixation alone may progress from low-impact to impact activity at 3 months following surgery, using a carbon fiber plate orthotic in their shoe until approximately 5 to 6 months after injury.

Wagner and colleagues[51] have proposed an early weight-bearing regimen starting 3 weeks after percutaneous fixation of Lisfranc complex injuries. Although the results from this study are promising, more data are needed to universally advocate early weight-bearing activity.

Hardware Removal

Regardless of the metalwork used, the authors universally recommend removal of hardware no earlier than 4 months after injury to allow restoration of more physiologic motion at the Lisfranc joint complex and limit the risk of hardware fatigue and failure. Failure to remove the hardware essentially consigns patients to a pseudoarthrodesis. If there is any question regarding adequate healing and stability at the Lisfranc joint complex, fixation is left in place as long as possible.

If persistent subluxation is noted with abduction stress under fluoroscopic imaging after extraction of hardware, a suture button device may be substituted in place of the screw or plate. Although this provides less rigid fixation across the Lisfranc joint, adequate stability may be conferred to allow return to athletic activity and prolong the need for eventual arthrodesis. This use of the suture button device has not been evaluated formally in the literature.

Primary Arthrodesis

Approximately 40% to 94% of patients develop posttraumatic arthritis even after ORIF of a Lisfranc complex injury, and often these patients will require conversion to a midfoot arthrodesis.[13,28–30,32,42] Although primary arthrodesis has been advocated for injuries that include significant intra-articular comminution at the involved TMT joints,[48] these are not typically encountered in the athlete population. More commonly, an athlete may present with a purely ligamentous TMT joint injury, a pattern that has demonstrated a tendency to insufficiently stabilize after ORIF and progress more rapidly to posttraumatic arthritis.[29,48] As a result, arthrodesis has gained support as a primary treatment option (**Fig. 8**). Ly and Coetzee[32] evaluated 41 patients with isolated ligamentous injuries and noted a more rapid recovery, better foot outcome scores, and improved return to function in patients who underwent primary arthrodesis as opposed to ORIF. Five patients who underwent ORIF eventually required arthrodesis in this study, though all were high-energy injuries and none were athletes. Multiple studies have noted a higher reoperation rate in patients after ORIF compared with arthrodesis.[32,52] Contrary to this study, Mulier and colleagues[42] noted a higher complication rate and increased complaints of stiffness in a cohort of patients treated with arthrodesis, as opposed to ORIF. Most patients with arthrodesis in this study, however, demonstrated preoperative deformity that required correction and were not the typical low-energy Lisfranc injury population. Although arthrodesis eliminates the risk of posttraumatic arthritis and associated pain, the stiffness and limited function of the foot following an arthrodesis procedure, especially if involving multiple TMT joints, may not be desirable for young athletic patients; careful discussion of the benefits and risks of ORIF versus arthrodesis must be undertaken. Multiple studies, however, have reported similar outcomes when comparing arthrodesis to

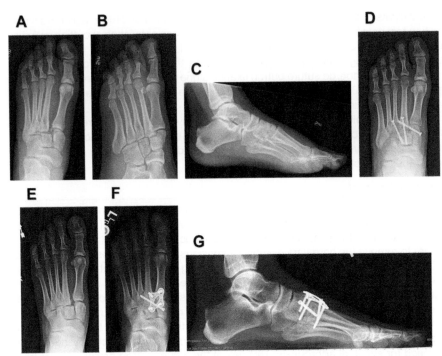

Fig. 8. (*A–G*) Patients with a purely ligamentous injury involving both the middle and medial columns or extensive articular comminution at the involved TMT joints are treated with primary arthrodesis. This 20-year-old athlete was initially treated elsewhere with ORIF (*A–D*) but demonstrated persistent instability and incongruity of the Lisfranc complex after hardware removal (*E*) and would have been better treated with an arthrodesis as the initial procedure (*F, G*).

ORIF cohorts,[32,52,53] and professional athletes have been able to return to competitive play even after a Lisfranc fusion.[54] In general, the authors recommend the use of arthrodesis for injuries with significant intra-articular comminution or purely ligamentous injuries that involve the entire medial and middle columns. Although there is no supporting literature to endorse the following as a rule, the authors have a lower threshold to fuse the first and second TMT joints in patients with a cavus foot. These patients have a very stiff midfoot at baseline, and sacrificing a minimal amount of TMT joint motion seldom makes a clinical difference for the sake of a definitive surgical treatment that eliminates the risk of posttraumatic arthritis and pain. In patients with a very flexible, mobile midfoot at baseline, ORIF and subsequent removal of hardware is likely the best first option.

Traditionally, screw constructs have been used for fusion at the TMT joints, though the advent of low-profile, locked dorsal plates have led to the widespread use of all-plate and hybrid arthrodesis constructs.[55] Nitinol staples may also be used for arthrodesis particularly of the second and third TMT joints, but their role has not yet been defined in the literature.

Patients who undergo arthrodesis remain non–weight bearing for at least 6 weeks in a cast or boot with gradual weight bearing allowed in a short CAM walker boot up to 3 months following surgery. Low-impact activity is permissible in the boot once patients are fully comfortable bearing weight; impact activity may be attempted at 3 to 4 months following surgery, typically with a carbon fiber plate orthotic in the athletic shoe.

Return to Play

Patients should expect at least a 6-month recovery period until return to competitive athletic activity. Earlier return to athletic activity has been reported by Nunley and Vertullo,[22] who observed an average of 14.4 weeks for return to play after surgery. This rapid return to sport has not been the authors' usual experience. Vertullo and Nunley[54] completed a survey of the American Orthopaedic Foot and Ankle Society members in 2002, with 103 surgeons responding to questions regarding participation in a variety of sports after different arthrodesis procedures of the foot and ankle and results of arthrodesis in professional athletes.[54] Ninety-seven percent of surgeons would allow patients to return to golf and skiing after a Lisfranc arthrodesis, and greater than 75% would allow tennis and jogging activity. Football, soccer, and basketball were permissible by 62% to 66% of the surveyed physicians. Return to running activity was allowed by only 54%. Interestingly, 12% of surgeons allowed the patients to return to all sports irrespective of their arthrodesis. Although the investigators did not comment on how many professional athletes were not able to return to competitive play after a Lisfranc arthrodesis, 5 athletes did return to their professional sport: 2 National Football League football players, 2 National Basketball Association basketball players, and 1 AAA baseball player. Although little literature exists to support the guidelines for return to athletic play after a Lisfranc arthrodesis, the authors supported the following discussion points, which help provide realistic expectations after a severe injury. Points specific to a midfoot or Lisfranc arthrodesis are summarized next.

1. Preoperatively, patients should be aware of the potential functional limitation after an arthrodesis.
2. The arthrodesis must be clinically and radiologically healed and pain free.
3. Patients should be aware of the possibility of accelerated periarticular arthrosis and stress fracture after arthrodesis, though the authors note that there is not a single report in the literature supporting this notion.
4. Patients with a lower extremity arthrodesis who suffer pain during sports participation should be counseled to seek medical attention.

COMPLICATIONS

Short-term complications after fixation or arthrodesis of a Lisfranc complex injury are similar to those experienced with any traumatic injury to the foot. Wound dehiscence, infection, and neurovascular injury are all relatively low risk with careful attention to soft tissue handling and allowing for adequate resolution of soft tissue swelling before operative intervention. Patients are placed on pharmacologic deep vein thrombosis prophylaxis for the period of time they remain non–weight bearing and immobilized. Long-term complications include stiffness, difficulty returning to athletic activity, periarticular degenerative disease, and flatfoot deformity. Hardware irritation is not uncommon, with up to 16% of patients requiring removal of metalwork.[56] Radiographic progression of degenerative disease is commonly seen in patients with Lisfranc complex injuries, but there is no clear association between the degree of radiographic arthritis and patient symptoms.[13,28–30,32,42]

FUTURE STUDIES/TECHNOLOGY

The increasing availability and use of suture button fixation has supplemented the authors' approach to Lisfranc complex injuries and adds another potential tool to help restore or preserve stability at the TMT joints while avoiding the potential risk of painful metalwork or the need for removal of hardware after fixation. As noted earlier, much more research is required before these devices can be wholeheartedly supported in the athletic population. Bioabsorbable screw technology has also been explored as an option for Lisfranc complex fixation,[36,57] again eliminating the need for future hardware removal or the risk of painful metalwork, but is not widely used and has fallen into disfavor. Future studies are also required to determine when is the best time to remove hardware in the athletic population and what activities or limitations should be expected for patients from the high school or amateur athlete to the professional. Given the diverse treatment options and algorithms presented for care of the subtle Lisfranc complex injury, multicenter, prospective, randomized trials will be required to determine the best treatment pathway for these injuries.

SUMMARY

Significant debate persists regarding the optimal treatment of subtle or low-energy TMT injuries, and decisions regarding treatment and return to activity can be particularly difficult when managing a high-level or professional athlete. There is little debate regarding the need for a high index of suspicion when evaluating patients with midfoot pain following an athletic injury. The use of comparison and weight-bearing radiographs is critical to identify patients with subtle instability at the Lisfranc joint complex. Most evidence supports fixation of injuries that demonstrate any signs of instability, and removal of hardware is recommended after at least 4 months postoperatively to allow for adequate healing at the TMT joints and restore more normal kinematics of the midfoot. Failure to remove hardware after ORIF essentially consigns patients to a pseudoarthrodesis. Although arthrodesis has been traditionally avoided for athletic injuries, there have been good reported results with satisfactory return to play in a select population. The role of suture button techniques or hybrid dorsal plate and screw technology continues to evolve. Ultimately, patients must all be consulted that unstable Lisfranc complex injuries are potentially career threatening and it may take up to a year to return to a previous level of competition.

REFERENCES

1. Garrick JG, Requa RK. The epidemiology of foot and ankle injuries in sports. Clin Sports Med 1988;7(1):29–36.
2. Meyer SA, Callaghan JJ, Albright JP, et al. Midfoot sprains in collegiate football players. Am J Sports Med 1994;22(3):392–401.
3. Sarrafian SK, Kelikian AS. Syndesmology. In: Kelikian AS, editor. Sarrafian's anatomy of the foot and ankle: descriptive, topographic, functional. Philadelphia: Lippincott; 2011. p. 208–12.
4. de Palma L, Santucci A, Sabetta SP, et al. Anatomy of the Lisfranc joint complex. Foot Ankle Int 1997;18(6):356–64.
5. Solan MC, Moorman CT 3rd, Miyamoto RG, et al. Ligamentous restraints of the second tarsometatarsal joint: a biomechanical evaluation. Foot Ankle Int 2001; 22(8):637–41.
6. Ouzounian TJ, Sheref MJ. In vitro determination of midfoot motion. Foot Ankle 1989;10(3):140–6.
7. Faciszewski T, Burks RT, Manaster BJ. Subtle injuries of the Lisfranc joint. J Bone Joint Surg Am 1990;72(10):1519–22.
8. Myerson M. The diagnosis and treatment of injuries to the Lisfranc joint complex. Orthop Clin North Am 1989;20(4):655–64.
9. Myerson MS, Cerrato RA. Current management of tarsometatarsal injuries in the athlete. J Bone Joint Surg Am 2008;90(11):2522–33.

10. Shapiro MS, Wascher DC, Finerman GA. Rupture of Lisfranc's ligament in athletes. Am J Sports Med 1994;22(5):687–91.

11. Ceroni D, De Rosa V, De Coulon G, et al. The importance of proper shoe gear and safety stirrups in the prevention of equestrian foot injuries. J Foot Ankle Surg 2007;46(1):32–9.

12. Ross G, Cronin R, Hauzenblas J, et al. Plantar ecchymosis sign: a clinical aid to diagnosis of occult Lisfranc tarsometatarsal injuries. J Orthop Trauma 1996;10(2): 119–22.

13. Myerson MS, Fisher RT, Burgess AR, et al. Fracture dislocations of the tarsometatarsal joints: end results correlated with pathology and treatment. Foot Ankle 1986;6(5):225–42.

14. Lu J, Ebraheim NA, Skie M, et al. Radiographic and computed tomographic evaluation of Lisfranc dislocation: a cadaver study. Foot Ankle Int 1997;18(6):351–5.

15. Vuori JP, Aro HT. Lisfranc joint injuries: trauma mechanisms and associated injuries. J Trauma 1993;35(1):40–5.

16. Hermel MB, Gershon-Cohen J. The nutcracker fracture of the cuboid by indirect violence. Radiology 1953;60(6):850–4.

17. Hsu JC, Chang JH, Wang SJ, et al. The nutcracker fracture of the cuboid in children: a case report. Foot Ankle Int 2004;25(6):423–5.

18. Davies MS, Saxby TS. Intercuneiform instability and the "gap" sign. Foot Ankle Int 1999;20(9):606–9.

19. Mantas JP, Burks RT. Lisfranc injuries in the athlete. Clin Sports Med 1994;13(4): 719–30.

20. Potter HG, Deland JT, Gusmer PB, et al. Magnetic resonance imaging of the Lisfranc ligament of the foot. Foot Ankle Int 1998;19(7):438–46.

21. Raikin SM, Elias I, Dheer S, et al. Prediction of midfoot instability in the subtle Lisfranc injury. Comparison of magnetic resonance imaging with intraoperative findings. J Bone Joint Surg Am 2009;91(4):892–9.

22. Nunley JA, Vertullo CJ. Classification, investigation, and management of midfoot sprains: Lisfranc injuries in the athlete. Am J Sports Med 2002;30(6):871–8.

23. Curtis MJ, Myerson M, Szura B. Tarsometatarsal joint injuries in the athlete. Am J Sports Med 1993;21(4):497–502.

24. Coss HS, Manos RE, Buoncristiani A, et al. Abduction stress and AP weight bearing radiography of purely ligamentous injury in the tarsometatarsal joint. Foot Ankle Int 1998;19(8):537–41.

25. Quénu EK, Kuss G. Etude sur les luxations du métatarse (Luxations métatarso-tarsiennes). Du diastasis entre le 1er et le 2e métatarsien. Rev Chir Paris 1909; 39:231–336, 720–91, 1093–134.

26. Hardcastle PH, Reschauer R, Kutscha-Lissberg E, et al. Injuries to the tarsometatarsal joint. Incidence, classification and treatment. J Bone Joint Surg Br 1982; 64(3):349–56.

27. Eleftheriou KI, Rosenfeld PF. Lisfranc injury in the athlete: evidence supporting management from sprain to fracture dislocation. Foot Ankle Clin 2013;18(2): 219–36.

28. Arntz CT, Veith RG, Hansen ST Jr. Fractures and fracture-dislocations of the tarsometatarsal joint. J Bone Joint Surg Am 1988;70(2):173–81.

29. Kuo RS, Tejwani NC, Digiovanni CW, et al. Outcome after open reduction and internal fixation of Lisfranc joint injuries. J Bone Joint Surg Am 2000;82-A(11): 1609–18.

30. Sangeorzan BJ, Veith RG, Hansen ST Jr. Salvage of Lisfranc's tarsometatarsal joint by arthrodesis. Foot Ankle 1990;10(4):193–200.

31. Teng AL, Pinzur MS, Lomasney L, et al. Functional outcome following anatomic restoration of tarsal-metatarsal fracture dislocation. Foot Ankle Int 2002;23(10): 922–6.

32. Ly TV, Coetzee JC. Treatment of primarily ligamentous Lisfranc joint injuries: primary arthrodesis compared with open reduction and internal fixation. A prospective, randomized study. J Bone Joint Surg Am 2006;88(3):514–20.

33. Richter M, Wippermann B, Krettek C, et al. Fractures and fracture dislocations of the midfoot: occurrence, causes and long-term results. Foot Ankle Int 2001;22(5): 392–8.

34. Lattermann C, Goldstein JL, Wukich DK, et al. Practical management of Lisfranc injuries in athletes. Clin J Sport Med 2007;17(4):311–5.

35. Buzzard BM, Briggs PJ. Surgical management of acute tarsometatarsal fracture dislocation in the adult. Clin Orthop Relat Res 1998;(353):125–33.

36. DeOrio M, Erickson M, Usuelli FG, et al. Lisfranc injuries in sport. Foot Ankle Clin 2009;14(2):169–86.

37. Trevino SG, Kodros S. Controversies in tarsometatarsal injuries. Orthop Clin North Am 1995;26(2):229–38.

38. Philbin T, Rosenberg G, Sferra JJ. Complications of missed or untreated Lisfranc injuries. Foot Ankle Clin 2003;8(1):61–71.

39. Schepers T, Oprel PP, Van Lieshout EM. Influence of approach and implant on reduction accuracy and stability in Lisfranc fracture-dislocation at the tarsometatarsal joint. Foot Ankle Int 2013;34(5):705–10.

40. Resch S, Stenstrom A. The treatment of tarsometatarsal injuries. Foot Ankle 1990; 11(3):117–23.

41. Lee CA, Birkedal JP, Dickerson EA, et al. Stabilization of Lisfranc joint injuries: a biomechanical study. Foot Ankle Int 2004;25(5):365–70.

42. Mulier T, Reynders P, Sioen W, et al. The treatment of Lisfranc injuries. Acta Orthop Belg 1997;63(2):82–90.

43. Alberta FG, Aronow MS, Barrero M, et al. Ligamentous Lisfranc joint injuries: a biomechanical comparison of dorsal plate and transarticular screw fixation. Foot Ankle Int 2005;26(6):462–73.

44. Hu SJ, Chang SM, Li XH, et al. Outcome comparison of Lisfranc injuries treated through dorsal plate fixation versus screw fixation. Acta Ortop Bras 2014;22(6): 315–20.

45. Purushothaman B, Robinson E, Lakshmanan P, et al. Extra-articular fixation for treatment of Lisfranc injury. Surg Technol Int 2010;19:199–202.

46. Stern RE, Assal M. Dorsal multiple plating without routine transarticular screws for fixation of Lisfranc injury. Orthopedics 2014;37(12):815–9.

47. Brin YS, Nyska M, Kish B. Lisfranc injury repair with the TightRope device: a short-term case series. Foot Ankle Int 2010;31(7):624–7.

48. Coetzee JC. Making sense of Lisfranc injuries. Foot Ankle Clin 2008;13(4): 695–704, ix.

49. Panchbhavi VK, Vallurupalli S, Yang J, et al. Screw fixation compared with suture-button fixation of isolated Lisfranc ligament injuries. J Bone Joint Surg Am 2009; 91(5):1143–8.

50. Pelt CE, Bachus KN, Vance RE, et al. A biomechanical analysis of a tensioned suture device in the fixation of the ligamentous Lisfranc injury. Foot Ankle Int 2011;32(4):422–31.

51. Wagner E, Ortiz C, Villalon IE, et al. Early weight-bearing after percutaneous reduction and screw fixation for low-energy Lisfranc injury. Foot Ankle Int 2013; 34(7):978–83.

52. Henning JA, Jones CB, Sietsema DL, et al. Open reduction internal fixation versus primary arthrodesis for Lisfranc injuries: a prospective randomized study. Foot Ankle Int 2009;30(10):913–22.
53. Reinhardt KR, Oh LS, Schottel P, et al. Treatment of Lisfranc fracture-dislocations with primary partial arthrodesis. Foot Ankle Int 2012;33(1):50–6.
54. Vertullo CJ, Nunley JA. Participation in sports after arthrodesis of the foot or ankle. Foot Ankle Int 2002;23(7):625–8.
55. Filippi J, Myerson MS, Scioli MW, et al. Midfoot arthrodesis following multi-joint stabilization with a novel hybrid plating system. Foot Ankle Int 2012;33(3):220–5.
56. Stavlas P, Roberts CS, Xypnitos FN, et al. The role of reduction and internal fixation of Lisfranc fracture-dislocations: a systematic review of the literature. Int Orthop 2010;34(8):1083–91.
57. Thordarson DB, Hurvitz G. PLA screw fixation of Lisfranc injuries. Foot Ankle Int 2002;23(11):1003–7.

Turf Toe and Disorders of the Sesamoid Complex

Lyndon W. Mason, MB BCh, MRCS (Eng), FRCS (Tr&Orth)*,
Andrew P. Molloy, MBChB, MRCS (Ed), FRCS (Tr&Orth)

KEYWORDS

- Turf toe • Sesamoid fracture • Osteochondral injury • Traumatic hallux valgus

KEY POINTS

- Turf toe injuries are common in athletes.
- The incidence of turf toe injuries has been decreasing since the 1970s because of an improvement in playing surfaces and shoe wear.
- Most turf toe injuries are mild; however, severe injuries can occur, resulting in sesamoid fractures, cartilage injury, and traumatic hallux valgus.
- Nonoperative treatment is generally sufficient in the treatment of mild and moderate turf toe injuries.

INTRODUCTION

A functional first metatarsophalangeal joint (MTPJ) is an important factor in the normal biomechanics of bipedal gait. In normal walking gait, it has the ability to transfer large forces over a small area, with McBride and colleagues[1] calculating that on barefoot walking, $0.8 \times$ body weight passes through the MTPJ on toe-off. This value increases to 200% to 300% of body weight with athletic activity and can increase to 800% of body weight with running and jumping.[2] Injury to the first MTPJ complex is common, although often underappreciated. Clanton and Ford[3] reported that foot injuries were the third leading cause of missed time in University athletes, with a significant proportion of these involving the first MTPJ. If undiagnosed and not appropriately managed, the injury can have severe detrimental effects on the foot function in athletes, such as persistent pain, weakness in push-off, stiffness, deformity, and development of joint

Disclosure: The authors have no affiliations with or involvement in any organization or entity with any financial interest or nonfinancial interest in the subject matter or materials discussed in this article.
Foot and Ankle Unit, University Hospital Aintree, Lower Lane, Liverpool L9 7AL, UK
* Corresponding author.
E-mail address: lyndon.mason@aintree.nhs.uk

Clin Sports Med 34 (2015) 725–739
http://dx.doi.org/10.1016/j.csm.2015.06.008
0278-5919/15/$ – see front matter © 2015 Elsevier Inc. All rights reserved.

arthritis. Significant delays in return to sporting activities have been reported in the literature following first MTPJ injury.[4]

BACKGROUND

Turf toe is an umbrella term applied to a variety of injuries of the plantar aspect of the first MTPJ. The term was coined by Bowers and Martin[5] in 1976, describing the injury in collegiate football players. Rodeo and colleagues[6] subsequently reported an incidence of 45% in professional football players, with 83% of cases occurring on artificial turf. Later studies have seen a reduction in the rate of reported turf toe injuries, with Kaplan and colleagues[7] reporting an incidence of 11% in the National Football League. This reduction in incidence has also been seen in soccer.[8] The perceived decline in the incidence of turf toe injuries in football has been hypothesized to be secondary to improved artificial surfaces and/or new shoe designs with increased forefoot stiffness.[9] An investigation of the National Collegiate Athletic Association Injury Surveillance System identified several risk factors associated with turf toe injury (**Table 1**).

Most turf toe injuries are sustained as a result of contact with the playing surface or contact with another player. A combination of hyperdorsiflexion and axial load with the foot fixed in equinus is the most commonly described mechanism.[10] Garcia and colleagues[11] found that extension of the MTPJ had a profound effect on increasing forefoot plantar soft-tissue stiffness and decreasing plantar soft-tissue thickness, which leaves the joint vulnerable to rapid increases in joint extension and thus injury. Others believe forced hyperextension of the first MTPJ to be the primary mechanism of injury.[3–6] Rodeo and colleagues[6] reported a 12% incidence of MTPJ injury due to plantarflexion, which Frey and colleagues[12] differentiated from turf toe by calling it sand toe. A valgus force can be associated with turf toe injuries causing disruption of the plantar medial capsuloligamentous structures or the tibial sesamoid, resulting in a traumatic hallux valgus deformity.

ANATOMY

The first MTPJ is a ginglymoarthrodial joint that works with a combined movement as a hinge and a sliding joint. Joseph[13] reported that normal active dorsiflexion of the first MTPJ approximates 80°. The joint has no inherent bony stability because of the shallow articulation between the convex metatarsal head and concave base of the proximal phalanx articular surface. It therefore relies on the complex attachments of

Table 1
Risk factors related to turf toe injury

Risk Factor	Description
Playing surface	85% higher risk of turf toe injury on artificial surfaces than on natural grass
Time of season	More common in regular season than in preseason or postseason More common in game time than in practice sessions
Team position	More common in running backs, quarter backs, and line receivers
Player activity	Most common in general play than in other set plays (ie, blocking drill, kick-off coverage)

Adapted from George E, Harris AH, Dragoo JL, et al. Incidence and risk factors for turf toe injuries in intercollegiate football: data from the National Collegiate Athletic Association injury surveillance system. Foot Ankle Int 2014;35(2):108–15.

the capsule and ligaments, further enhanced by musculotendinous structures that surround the joint. An intra-articular meniscus is common; this is a transverse band extending across the intra-articular surface of the planter plate from one sesamophalangeal ligament to the other.[14] The first MTPJ differs from that of the lesser MTPJs because of the sesamoids and the interplay of the medial and lateral intrinsic muscles (abductor and adductor hallucis), which work to stabilize the joint and provide motor strength to the first ray.[15]

The hallucal sesamoids are a consistent entity in humans, appearing within the seventh or eighth week of embryonic development as islands of undifferentiated connective tissue within the tendons of flexor hallucis brevis (FHB). They do not ossify until age 8 years in girls and age 10 years in boys, through multiple ossification centers.[16,17] Often, these centers of ossification do not coalesce and remain partite. Munuera and colleagues[18] reported on an analysis of 474 radiographs a rate of partition of at least 1 sesamoid in 14.6%. The function of the sesamoids is to increase the power of plantar flexion of the first ray by increasing the moment of the intrinsic flexors. They also operate by elevating the first metatarsal head and in doing so spread applied forces over the metatarsal head.[19]

The sesamoids are closely connected with the fibrous layer of the joint capsule as well as with the medial and lateral sesamoid ligaments that are blended with the capsule.[20] Sharpey fibers from the sesamoid ligaments penetrate the sesamoids on their capsular side. Anterior to the medial and lateral sesamoid ligaments are the collateral ligaments that fan out distally and plantarward connecting to the base of the proximal phalanx.[21] The dense fibrous plantar pad enshrouds the plantar aspect of the sesamoids and anchors the sesamoid complex to the base of the proximal phalanx. The tendons of FHB are attached to the plantar surface of the sesamoids. However, the tendons of adductor and abductor hallucis mainly bypass the sesamoids, with only some inner fibers of these tendons connecting to the sesamoids on their plantar side.[20] The intersesamoid ligament connects the sesamoids. The collagenous fibers of the intersesamoid ligament form an interwoven lattice consisting of transverse, longitudinal, and vertical bundles.[20] The flexor hallucis longus nestles on the plantar aspect between the sesamoids, with the intersesamoid ligament blending with its synovial tendon sheath.[20] The anatomy of the first MTPJ is illustrated in **Figs. 1** and **2**.

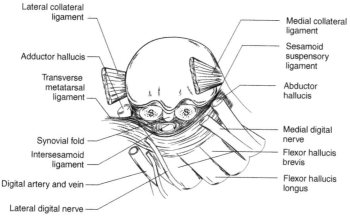

Fig. 1. An exploded view of the first MTPJ/sesamoid complex with the proximal phalanx removed and head-on view of the first metatarsal head.

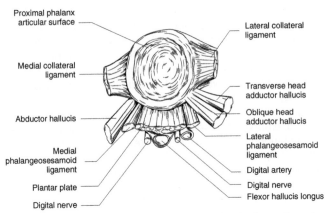

Fig. 2. Corresponding view of the proximal phalangeal articular surface showing the insertions of the ligaments of the MTPJ/sesamoid complex.

The blood supply to each sesamoid bone arrives via the sesamoid artery. The sesamoid arteries branch off from the digital plantar arteries of the hallux, which, in turn, are derived from the medial plantar artery and the plantar arch.[22] The arteries enter the sesamoids via the plantar nonarticular area, from the lateral aspect of the lateral sesamoid and medial aspect of the medial sesamoid. The number of sesamoid arteries varies from 1 to 3, the number increasing with increasing size of the sesamoid bones.[22] This information is important when considering the approach to the plantar aspect of the foot in cases of surgical repair. The hallucal nerves run in close proximity to the hallucal sesamoids, traversing the plantar medial and plantar lateral aspect of the medial and lateral sesamoids, respectively. They pass underneath the crural fascia, covered by vertical fibers investing the plantar fat pad at the level of the MTPJ.[23] The medial plantar nerve then comes into close proximity to the flexor hallucis longus sheath distal to the MTPJ and is at risk of iatrogenic nerve injury when surgical procedures are performed to the flexor hallucis longus sheath.[24]

CLASSIFICATION

Jahss[25] was the first to describe a classification system for turf toe. Several other investigators have described anatomic, pathologic, and clinical classification systems.[3,6,26–29] These systems have been summarized in **Table 2**. First MTPJ dislocations have been illustrated in **Fig. 3**.

CLINICAL PRESENTATION

Assessment at presentation is directed toward identifying the severity and location of the injury, as this ultimately guides treatment. As indicated in **Table 2**, the patient's presentation is dictated by the severity of injury. In low-grade injuries, the patient's clinical signs may be limited to just pain, and therefore, clinical suspicion is necessary. On examination, the patient generally displays an antalgic gait, with forefoot supination in an attempt to offload the painful area. A reluctance to progress through the third rocker of gait should be expected. Periarticular swelling and ecchymosis are typically present. All aspects of the joint should be palpated. Mild injuries present with plantar or plantar medial tenderness. Dorsal tenderness is

Table 2
Turf toe classifications

Grade	Pathology	Clinical	Radiographs	MRI
Jahss pathology classification (see Fig. 1)				
I	Dorsal dislocation of the proximal phalanx and sesamoids with intersesamoidal ligament intact	—	—	—
IIa	Dorsal dislocation of the proximal phalanx and the sesamoids with rupture of the intersesamoidal ligament	—	—	—
IIb	Type IIa with transverse fracture of one of the sesamoids	—	—	—
IIc	Type IIa with fracture of both sesamoids	—	—	—
Clanton clinical classification				
I	—	Plantar or medial tenderness, minimal swelling, no ecchymosis	—	—
II	—	Diffuse tenderness, mild to moderate swelling, ecchymosis, decreased range of motion	—	—
III	—	Severe diffuse tenderness, maximally dorsally, marked swelling and ecchymosis, marked decrease in range of motion	—	—
Rodeo clinical classification				
I	Acute sprain of plantar capsule. No bony pathology or joint instability	Localized tenderness, swelling, pain with dorsiflexion	Normal	—

(continued on next page)

Table 2
(continued)

Grade	Pathology	Clinical	Radiographs	MRI
II	Acute sprain of plantar capsule with significant capsular disruption	More extensive ecchymosis, loss of motion, painful dorsiflexion, possible diastasis of a partite sesamoid, and/or joint instability	Normal	—
III	Chronic symptoms involving the first MTPJ due to MTPJ injury	Loss of motion	Significant radiographic changes of either hallux rigidus or degenerative joint disease	—
Anderson clinical classification				
I	Strain of the capsule without a loss of continuity	Normal range of motion, no visible ecchymosis, and the patient can bear weight	Normal	Intact soft-tissue complex with surrounding edema
II	Partial tear of the plantar plate and capsule	Painful motion and difficulty bearing weight	Normal	Soft-tissue edema and high signal intensity that does not extend through the full thickness of the plantar plate
III	Complete tear with loss of continuity of the plantar plate and capsule	Associated injuries including sesamoid fracture, diastasis of bipartite sesamoids, dorsal metatarsal articular impaction, and proximal sesamoid migration	May show avulsion fracture of the proximal phalanx, sesamoid fracture, proximally migrated sesamoid, MTPJ dislocation	High signal intensity completely traversing the plantar capsuloligamentous complex and sesamoid and chondral injury
Anderson anatomic classification				
Hyperextension injury (turf toe)				
I	Stretching of plantar capsular ligamentous complex	Localized tenderness, minimal swelling, minimal ecchymosis	—	—
II	Partial tear of plantar capsular ligamentous complex	Diffuse tenderness, moderate swelling, ecchymosis, restricted movement with pain	—	—

III	Frank tear of plantar capsular ligamentous complex; Possible associated injuries: Medial/lateral injury, sesamoid fracture/bipartite diastasis, articular cartilage/subchondral bone bruise	Severe tenderness, marked swelling and ecchymosis, limited movement with pain, vertical Lachman test positive	—
Hyperflexion (sand toe)			
	Hyperflexion injury to hallux MTPJ or IPJ	May involve injury to lesser MTPJs as well	—
Dislocation			
I	Dislocation of the hallux with the sesamoids	No disruption of the intersesamoid ligament, frequently irreducible	—
IIA	Associated disruption of the intersesamoid ligament	Usually reducible	—
IIB	Associated transverse fracture of one or both sesamoids, partial disruption of the plantar plate with disruption of medial or lateral sesamoid	Usually reducible	—
III	Complete disruption of intersesamoid ligament with fracture of one of the sesamoids	Usually reducible	—
IIIA[a]	Dislocation with complete soft-tissue disruption of the plantar complex from the proximal phalanx	—	—
IIIB[a]	Dislocation with complete plantar plate disruption, including disruption of 1 sesamoid	—	—

Abbreviation: IPJ, interphalangeal joint.
[a] IIIA and IIIB are added by Maskill.
Data from Refs. [4,6,25–29]

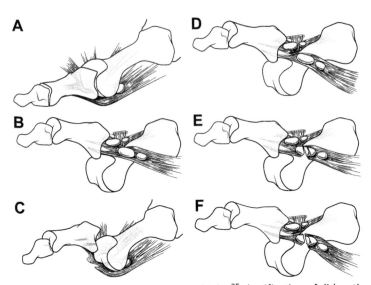

Fig. 3. (A) Normal anatomy of the first MTPJ and Jahss[25] classification of dislocations of the MTP joint. (B) Type IA dislocation. (C) Type IB dislocation. (D) Type IIA dislocation. (E) Type IIB dislocation. (F) Type IIC dislocation. (*Adapted from* Mittlmeier T, Haar P. Sesamoid and toe fractures. Injury 2004;35(Suppl 2):SB93; with permission.)

elicited in more severe capsular disruption. Dorsal or medial joint tenderness is also an indication of sand toe and traumatic hallux valgus. A palpable plantar defect may be noted, indicating a partial or complete disruption of the plantar plate-sesamoid mechanism.[30]

Limitation of joint movement depends on the severity of injury. Push-off is impaired with running, and it may be difficult to crouch with the MTPJ extended.[5] Range of motion and maneuvers to load the joint also elicit discomfort on physical examination.[5] The presence of an intrinsic-minus posture (metatarsophalangeal [MTP] extension, interphalangeal flexion) suggests disruption of the FHB tendon insertion.[31] Weak plantarflexion strength of the hallux can indicate an injury to the plantar plate, FHB, or flexor hallucis longus. Joint stability assessment with respect to dorsoplantar stress and varus/valgus stress is essential. Anderson and Shawen[28] described the use of a vertical Lachman test to assess joint excursion. Serial examinations are useful to identify resolution of the pain or presence of progressive deformity.[31] In the most severe injuries, fracture-dislocation of the joint can occur with obvious joint deformity (**Fig. 4**).

IMAGING

Anteroposterior, lateral, and axial sesamoid weight-bearing radiographs are important in the initial evaluation of the injury. In severe injuries, obtaining weight-bearing radiographs may not be possible (**Fig. 5**). Comparative anteroposterior views with the contralateral limb can be useful to assess for proximal migration of the sesamoids and sesamoid fracture diastasis. In addition, a lateral 40° oblique view helps visualize the lateral sesamoid, whereas a medial 40° oblique view visualizes the medial sesamoid.[31] In general, initial radiographs typically reveal only soft-tissue swelling, although subtle findings may be present.[4,5]

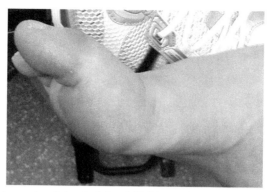

Fig. 4. Clinical picture of a dislocated first MTPJ in an international Rugby player before reduction.

Dorsiflexion stress test under fluoroscopy is an adjunctive test. A biomechanical study found that an injury producing a 3-mm change in movement of the sesamoids relative to the uninjured or intact side on a lateral radiograph is highly predictive of a severe turf toe injury involving at least 3 of the 4 plantar ligaments (medial collateral ligament, tibial phalangeal sesamoid ligament, fibular phalangeal sesamoid ligament, and lateral collateral ligament) of the plantar plate complex.[32]

MRI can be used to evaluate the presence and extent of capsular or plantar plate disruption, in addition to identifying injury to the flexor hallucis longus and the articular surface of the MTPJ (**Fig. 6**).[27,33] In addition, MRI reveals osseous or articular damage in the presence of normal findings on radiographs.[27] MRI is helpful in identifying avascularity in the metatarsal or sesamoid bones. It can, however, overestimate the injury. Dietrich and colleagues[34] performed a study in which healthy volunteers underwent MRI of the first MTPJ and found that cartilage defects, bone marrow edemalike signal changes, subchondral cysts, and plantar recesses were common occurrences. The collateral ligaments were often heterogeneous in structure and showed increased signal intensity.

NONOPERATIVE TREATMENTS

George and colleagues[9] found that of 147 turf toe injuries sustained in collegiate football players, only 2% required operative intervention. Several small retrospective case series recommend conservative management for the treatment of grade I and II injuries.[4,5,29,35] Kadakia and Molloy[31] thought this was sufficient evidence to make a grade B recommendation. There was, however, insufficient evidence to make a recommendation regarding grade III injuries. In the initial stages, ice, compression, and nonsteroidal anti-inflammatory drugs may be used.[2–5] Taping of the toe helps compress the joint and limit motion; this is useful for comfort and stabilization to aid healing.[36] Inserting a rigid forefoot insole, or a Morton extension, can reduce the third rocker motion of the first MTPJ to aid in both comfort and reduction of the rate of recurrent injury.[3–5] In the initial stages, the goals are to control swelling, reduce pain, and sustain a range of movement.[36] McCormick and Anderson[2] advised a walking boot in the more severe cases, which can use a hallucal relief (ie, an excavation under the hallux) to allow gentle range of motion exercises with addition of taping to limit movement.

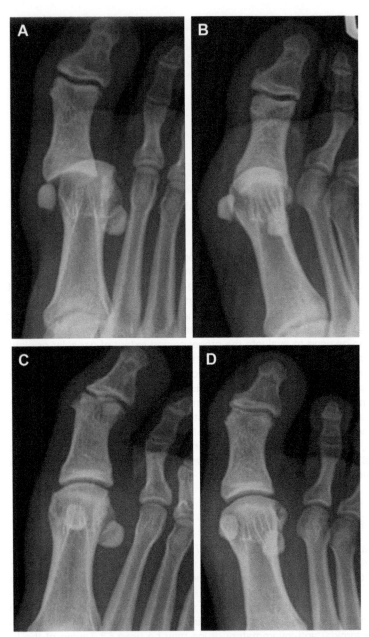

Fig. 5. Anteroposterior and oblique radiographs of a dislocated first MTPJ prereduction (*A*, *B*) and postreduction (*C*, *D*). The prereduction radiograph clearly shows that the head of the first metatarsal has separated the sesamoids illustrating an injury to the intersesamoid ligament and the retraction of the fibular hallucal sesamoid. Postreduction, the fibular hallucal sesamoidal retraction is more evident as the normal first ray length has been achieved.

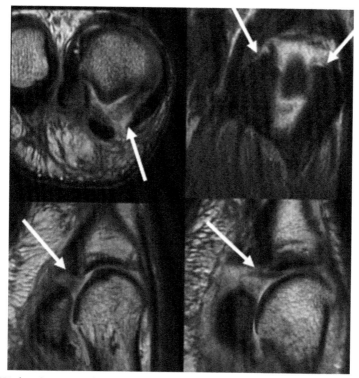

Fig. 6. MRI showing coronal, axial, and sagittal views of a plantar plate distal avulsion. Arrows illustrate the site of ligamentous disruption.

A gradual progression toward weight-bearing activities and normalized gait as symptoms allow is proposed. Time to return to play for mild to moderate injuries can vary from 2 to 6 weeks depending on rehabilitation progression and sport demands.[36] Ideally, the first MTPJ achieves a painless 50° to 60° dorsiflexion before running or explosive activities are attempted.[2] Intra-articular injections of steroids disguise symptoms or give temporary relief only and are not recommended.

OPERATIVE TREATMENT

Indications for operative treatment include a large capsular avulsion with unstable joint, diastasis or retraction of sesamoids, vertical instability, traumatic hallux valgus deformity, chondral injury, intra-articular loose body, sesamoid fracture, and failed conservative treatment.[2,9,37] An open repair of a capsular injury is occasionally performed, especially in the presence of a complete plantar plate injury.[35] The capsular disruption typically occurs distal to the sesamoid bones. If this is the only injury, McCormick and Anderson[38] advise a plantar soft-tissue direct repair end to end with nonabsorbable sutures. If there is no distal soft tissue attached to the proximal phalanx, then the plantar plate can be reattached to the plantar aspect of the proximal phalanx using bone anchors or bone tunnels.

In sesamoid fractures, there is a limited literature relevant to its surgical management. Kadakia and Molloy[31] thought there was not enough evidence to make a recommendation in regard to its operative management. When a sesamoid injury (fracture, osteonecrosis) occurred and did not heal successfully, Coughlin[30] thought that surgical excision may be warranted. However, because of the crucial role of the sesamoids, total sesamoidectomy without soft-tissue reconstruction is not recommended by others.[39] Partial (proximal) sesamoidectomy and reconstruction of the short flexor tendon is nevertheless a reasonable option to reduce pain and allow functional return.[40] After partial sesamoidectomy the soft tissues should be repaired to the remaining sesamoid by passing a suture through a drill hole in the sesamoid.[2] If excision of the sesamoid is completed, McCormick and Anderson[2] recommended detaching the abductor hallucis tendon from its distal insertion and transferring it plantarly into the soft-tissue defect left by the excised sesamoids. They thought that this acts as a plantar restraint to dorsiflexion forces and augments the flexion power of the hallux. Transfer of the abductor is most appropriate in the setting of a concomitant turf toe injury. Percutaneous procedures have been described for fixation of sesamoid fractures using small cannulated screws as an alternative to open procedures.[41] Acute fixation of sesamoid fractures is rarely indicated, and when doing so in the chronic setting, direct visualization is recommended given the narrow thickness of the sesamoid to minimize intra-articular hardware placement.

Several studies have reported favorably in the surgical treatment of first MTPJ osteochondral injuries.[42–44] Kadakia and Molloy[31] concluded that there was fair evidence to give a grade B recommendation on operative management of osteochondral injuries. Altman has reported open management of these injuries[45] with excellent results. There have been 4 reported case series of arthroscopic management of osteochondral lesions, again with excellent outcomes.[42–44,46] If surgical repair of the first MTPJ sesamoid ligament complex is also required, an open procedure is preferred. For cartilage defects larger than 50 mm^2 or in the presence of subchondral cysts, Kim and colleagues[47] recommended an osteochondral autograft.

McCormick and Anderson[2,37] advised an approach to the joint through a medial J incision or a combined medial and a lateral plantar longitudinal approach. However, the plantar medial hallucal nerve is at risk if a plantar medial approach is attempted rather than the midmedial approach to the first MTPJ.[23] A midmedial approach was also advocated by other researchers as the safest approach to prevent avascular necrosis of the sesamoids.[22,48] Owing to the avascular area of the intersesamoid ligament, Pretterklieber and Wanivenhaus[22] promoted an intersesamoid approach if a plantar approach was to be used, again to prevent avascular necrosis of the sesamoids. Chamberland and colleagues[48] state the importance of avoiding sesamoid proximal pole dissection because of a dominant single vessel blood supply and avoiding excessive soft-tissue stripping to prevent loss of capsular attachments.

Traumatic hallux valgus is an uncommon variant of turf toe. With a progressive hallux valgus deformity, it is likely that disruption of the medial or plantar medial capsule has occurred. With progression of pain and deformity, surgical repair is often necessary. However, the evidence of its surgical treatment in the literature is limited. In his series, Anderson[29] recommended acute surgical intervention for patients with traumatic hallux valgus with a slight modification of the repair required for grade III turf toe injuries.

CLINICAL OUTCOMES

Nihal and colleagues[49] and Anderson[29] described turf toe injury as potentially career ending. However, most injuries are mild and sensitive to nonoperative management as long as they are recognized early. George and colleagues[9] found an average time of 10 days lost to turf toe injury. In comparison to ankle injuries, turf toe injuries resulted in a greater average time loss from athletic activity.[35] Clanton and colleagues[4] reported on 20 athletes with turf toe injuries and noted a 50% incidence of persistent symptoms at least 5 years after the injury.[4] Nihal and colleagues described an incidence of 25% to 50% of residual pain and limited dorsiflexion despite 6 months of rehabilitation. Brophy and colleagues[50] assessed professional American football players with a history of turf toe injury and found decreased passive MTP dorsiflexion and increased hallucal plantar pressure.

ACKNOWLEDGMENTS

The authors thank K Hariharan (Royal Gwent Hospital, UK) and P Williams (Morriston Hospital, UK) for their image contributions.

REFERENCES

1. McBride ID, Wys UP, Cooke TD, et al. First metatarsophalangeal joint reaction forces during high-heel gait. Foot Ankle Int 1991;11(5):282–8.
2. McCormick JJ, Anderson RB. Rehabilitation following turf toe injury and plantar plate repair. Clin Sports Med 2010;29(2):313–23, ix.
3. Clanton TO, Ford JJ. Turf toe injury. Clin Sports Med 1994;13(4):731–41.
4. Clanton TO, Butler JE, Eggert A. Injuries to the metatarsophalangeal joints in athletes. Foot Ankle 1986;7(3):162–76.
5. Bowers KD Jr, Martin RB. Turf-toe: a shoe-surface related football injury. Med Sci Sports 1976;8(2):81–3.
6. Rodeo SA, O'Brien S, Warren RF, et al. Turf-toe: an analysis of metatarsophalangeal joint sprains in professional football players. Am J Sports Med 1990;18(3):280–5.
7. Kaplan LD, Jost PW, Honkamp N, et al. Incidence and variance of foot and ankle injuries in elite college football players. Am J Orthop (Belle Mead NJ) 2011;40(1):40–4.
8. Bjorneboe J, Bahr R, Andersen TE. Risk of injury on third-generation artificial turf in Norwegian professional football. Br J Sports Med 2010;44(11):794–8.
9. George E, Harris AH, Dragoo JL, et al. Incidence and risk factors for turf toe injuries in intercollegiate football: data from the National Collegiate Athletic Association injury surveillance system. Foot Ankle Int 2014;35(2):108–15.
10. Rodeo SA, Warren RF, O'Brien SJ, et al. Diastasis of bipartite sesamoids of the first metatarsophalangeal joint. Foot Ankle 1993;14(8):425–34.
11. Garcia CA, Hoffman SL, Hastings MK, et al. Effect of metatarsal phalangeal joint extension on plantar soft tissue stiffness and thickness. Foot (Edinb) 2008;18(2):61–7.
12. Frey C, Andersen GD, Feder KS. Plantarflexion injury to the metatarsophalangeal joint ("sand toe"). Foot Ankle Int 1996;17(9):576–81.
13. Joseph J. Range of movement of the great toe in men. J Bone Joint Surg Br 1954;36:450–7.
14. Dereymaeker G, Mulier T, Girisch P. The first metatarsophalangeal joint meniscus and its relation to hallux valgus deformity–an anatomical and clinical study. Foot Ankle Surg 2011;17(4):270–3.
15. Stein HC. Hallux valgus. Surg Gynecol Obstet 1938;66:889–98.
16. Leventen EO. Sesamoid disorders and their treatment. Clin Orthop 1991;269:236–40.
17. Sammarco GJ, Idusuyi OB. Complications after surgery of the hallux. Clin Orthop Relat Res 2001;(391):59–71.

18. Munuera PV, Dominguez G, Reina M, et al. Bipartite hallucal sesamoid bones: relationship with hallux valgus and metatarsal index. Skeletal Radiol 2007; 36(11):1043–50.

19. Aper RL, Saltzman CL, Brown T. The effect of hallux sesamoid excision on the flexor hallucis longus moment arm. Clin Orthop Relat Res 1996;325:209–17.

20. Brenner E, Gruber H, Fritsch H. Fetal development of the first metatarsophalangeal joint complex with special reference to the intersesamoidal ridge. Ann Anat 2002;184(5):481–7.

21. Alvarez R, Haddad RJ, Gould N, et al. The simple bunion: anatomy at the metatarsophalangeal joint of the great toe. Foot Ankle 1984;4(5):229–40.

22. Pretterklieber ML, Wanivenhaus A. The arterial supply of the sesamoid bones of the hallux: the course and source of the nutrient arteries as an anatomical basis for surgical approaches to the great toe. Foot Ankle 1992;13(1):27–31.

23. Phisitkul P, Sripongsai R, Chaichankul C, et al. Anatomy of the plantarmedial hallucal nerve in relation to the medial approach of the first metatarsophalangeal joint. Foot Ankle Int 2009;30(6):558–61.

24. Lui TH, Chan KB, Chan LK. Cadaveric study of zone 2 flexor hallucis longus tendon sheath. Arthroscopy 2010;26(6):808–12.

25. Jahss MH. Traumatic dislocations of the first metatarsophalangeal joint. Foot Ankle 1980;1(1):15–21.

26. Maskill JD, Bohay DR, Anderson JG. First ray injuries. Foot Ankle Clin 2006;11(1): 143–63. ix-x.

27. Tewes DP, Fischer DA, Fritts HM, et al. MRI findings of acute turf toe. A case report and review of anatomy. Clin Orthop Relat Res 1994;(304):200–3.

28. Anderson RB, Shawen SB. Great toe disorders. In: Porter DA, Schon LC, editors. Baxter's foot and ankle in sport. 2nd edition. Philadelphia: Elsevier Health Sciences; 2007. p. 423.

29. Anderson RB. Turf toe injuries of the hallux metatarsophalangeal joint. Tech Foot Ankle Surg 2002;1(2):102–11.

30. Coughlin MJ. Sesamoid pain: causes and surgical treatment. Instr Course Lect 1990;39:23–35.

31. Kadakia AR, Molloy A. Current concepts review: traumatic disorders of the first metatarsophalangeal joint and sesamoid complex. Foot Ankle Int 2011;32(8): 834–9.

32. Waldrop NE 3rd, Zirker CA, Wijdicks CA, et al. Radiographic evaluation of plantar plate injury: an in vitro biomechanical study. Foot Ankle Int 2013; 34(3):403–8.

33. Crain JM, Phancao JP, Stidham K. MR imaging of turf toe. Magn Reson Imaging Clin N Am 2008;16(1):93–103, vi.

34. Dietrich TJ, da Silva FL, de Abreu MR, et al. First metatarsophalangeal joint - MRI findings in asymptomatic volunteers. Eur Radiol 2015;25:970–9.

35. Coker TP, Arnold JA, Weber DL. Traumatic lesions of the metatarsophalangeal joint of the great toe in athletes. Am J Sports Med 1978;6(6):326–34.

36. Faltus J, Mullenix K, Moorman CT 3rd, et al. Case series of first metatarsophalangeal joint injuries in division 1 college athletes. Sports Health 2014;6(6):519–26.

37. McCormick JJ, Anderson RB. The great toe: failed turf toe, chronic turf toe, and complicated sesamoid injuries. Foot Ankle Clin 2009;14(2):135–50.

38. McCormick JJ, Anderson RB. Turf toe: anatomy, diagnosis, and treatment. Sports Health 2010;2(6):487–94.

39. Mittlmeier T, Haar P. Sesamoid and toe fractures. Injury 2004;35(Suppl 2): SB87–97.

40. Biedert R, Hintermann B. Stress fractures of the medial great toe sesamoids in athletes. Foot Ankle Int 2003;24(2):137–41.
41. Blundell CM, Nicholson P, Blackney MW. Percutaneous screw fixation for fractures of the sesamoid bones of the hallux. J Bone Joint Surg Br 2002;84(8): 1138–41.
42. Davies MS, Saxby TS. Arthroscopy of the first metatarsophalangeal joint. J Bone Joint Surg Br 1999;81(2):203–6.
43. Debnath UK, Hemmady MV, Hariharan K. Indications for and technique of first metatarsophalangeal joint arthroscopy. Foot Ankle Int 2006;27(12):1049–54.
44. van Dijk CN, Veenstra KM, Nuesch BC. Arthroscopic surgery of the metatarsophalangeal first joint. Arthroscopy 1998;14(8):851–5.
45. Altman A, Nery C, Sanhudo A, et al. Osteochondral injury of the hallux in beach soccer players. Foot Ankle Int 2008;29(9):919–21.
46. Ahn JH, Choy WS, Lee KW. Arthroscopy of the first metatarsophalangeal joint in 59 consecutive cases. J Foot Ankle Surg 2012;51(2):161–7.
47. Kim YS, Park EH, Lee HJ, et al. Clinical comparison of the osteochondral autograft transfer system and subchondral drilling in osteochondral defects of the first metatarsal head. Am J Sports Med 2012;40:1824–33.
48. Chamberland PD, Smith JW, Fleming LL. The blood supply to the great toe sesamoids. Foot Ankle 1993;14(8):435–42.
49. Nihal A, Trepman E, Nag D. First ray disorders in athletes. Sports Med Arthrosc 2009;17(3):160–6.
50. Brophy RH, Gamradt SC, Ellis SJ, et al. Effect of turf toe on foot contact pressures in professional American football players. Foot Ankle Int 2009;30(5):405–9.

Disorders of the Flexor Hallucis Longus and Os Trigonum

 CrossMark

Chamnanni Rungprai, MD[a,b], Joshua N. Tennant, MD, MPH[c],
Phinit Phisitkul, MD[a],*

KEYWORDS

- Os trigonum • Flexor hallucis longus • Stenosing tenosynovitis
- Posterior ankle impingement syndrome

KEY POINTS

- Os trigonum syndrome and flexor hallucis longus (FHL) tenosynovitis is a common cause of posterior ankle pain. Acute or repetitive forced plantarflexion causes injury or impingement of the os trigonum or trigonal process on the FHL.
- Diagnostic injection can confirm the diagnosis if the history, physical examination, and imaging are nonspecific.
- Conservative treatment can alleviate the symptom and allow gradual return to athletic activities for both os trigonum syndrome and FHL stenosing tenosynovitis. If these measures fail, surgical excision is recommended.
- Both open and arthroscopic techniques are effective, but advantages of arthroscopy include (1) minimizing surgical injury and less scarring, (2) less immediate postoperative pain, (3) minimal overall morbidity, and (4) earlier return to activities.
- Impaired sensation from nerve injury is the most common surgical complication of both arthroscopic and open techniques. Nevertheless, most of the patients had resolution of nerve symptoms within 1 year.

INTRODUCTION

Os Trigonum

The os trigonum originates from a separate cartilaginous center that develops in the embryo during the second month of human gestation.[1] It appears at the posterior border of the talus as a secondary ossification center in early childhood and

[a] Department of Orthopaedics and Rehabilitation, University of Iowa Hospital and Clinics, 200 Hawkins Drive, Iowa City, IA 52242, USA; [b] Department of Orthopaedics, Phramongkutklao Hospital and College of Medicine, 315 Ratchawithi Road, Bangkok 10400, Thailand; [c] Department of Orthopaedics, University of North Carolina School of Medicine, 3147 Bioinformatics Building, 130 Mason Farm Road, Chapel Hill, NC 27514, USA
* Corresponding author.
E-mail address: phinit-phisitkul@uiowa.edu

Clin Sports Med 34 (2015) 741–759
http://dx.doi.org/10.1016/j.csm.2015.06.005
0278-5919/15/$ – see front matter © 2015 Elsevier Inc. All rights reserved.
sportsmed.theclinics.com

subsequently fuses through endochondral ossification with a cartilaginous synchondrosis to the posterior talus between age 7 and 11 years in girls and 11 and 13 years in boys.[2,3]

The os trigonum unites with the posterior aspect of the talus forming the posterolateral (PL) talar process, often called the Stieda process[4] or trigonal process,[5] at approximately 1 year after its appearance[3] (**Fig. 1**A).

Failure of fusion of the secondary ossification center is reported to occur in 1.7% to 49% of the general population.[6-9] The result is a separate ossicle connected to the talus by a fibrocartilagenous synchondrosis at the PL aspect of the talus and is referred to as the os trigonum.[3,10]

The cause and pathoanatomy of the os trigonum syndrome, initially reported by Rosenmuller in 1804,[11,12] have not been adequately described in the literature.[13] Shepherd and Moullin believed that the os trigonum originated from a nonunion of a fracture of the PL or trigonal process of the talus.[3,13,14] On the contrary, Steida and Turner believed that it originated from a failure of the ossific nucleus fusion, leaving a synchondrosis between the talus and the os trigonum.[2,13,15] Most patients with an os trigonum are actually asymptomatic and present with just incidentally abnormal radiographic findings.[10] Acute fracture of the Stieda process or the synchondrosis of the os trigonum is a rare condition, and only a few cases of this fracture have been reported in the literature.[10,16-21]

Often called posterior ankle impingement syndrome,[22] the syndrome is synonymous with the terms posterior talar compression syndrome,[11] os trigonum syndrome,[23,24] posterior ankle block,[2,25] nutcracker-type impingement,[26,27] and posterior tibiotalar impingement syndrome.[28]

Repeated forceful plantar flexion of the ankle joint is a well-known cause of os trigonum syndrome,[17] and it can cause pain posterior to the ankle joint.[11,13] It has been described in dancers, especially ballet dancers, and gymnasts, with a higher frequency than in the normal population.[29] It is more frequently bilateral than unilateral[30] and is more predominantly symptomatic in men than in women.[8,13]

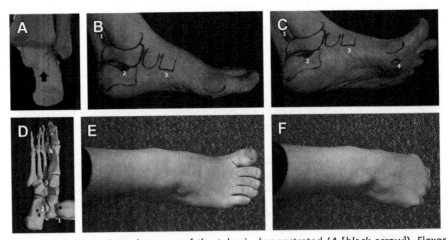

Fig. 1. A Stieda or trigonal process of the talus is demonstrated (*A* [*black arrow*]). Flexor hallucis longus can be palpated at posterior malleolus (*B–D*, [1]), inferior and medial to the sustentaculum tali (*B–D*, [2]), inferior to the medial cuneiform (*B–D*, [3]), and underneath the intersesamoid ligament (*C, D*, [4]). Patient can make a squeaking or crackling sound by dorsiflexion and plantarflexion of the first MTP joint when ankle joint is in full flexion (*E, F*).

Flexor Hallucis Longus

FHL stenosing tenosynovitis is caused by chronic entrapment of the FHL tendon inside its sheath.[31] A low-lying FHL muscle belly, rubbing against the os trigonum, and incongruity of maximum plantarflexion and dorsiflexion of the ankle joint and great toe can cause compression and lead to synovitis, hypertrophy, nodules, and partial tears of the FHL tendon.[31] The most common location of tenosynovitis is within the fibrous-osseous tunnel posterior to the medial malleolus; however, it can occur along the master knot of Henry or beneath the intersesamoid ligament.[31–33]

FHL tenosynovitis is typically ascribed to the female ballet dancers[22,34,35]; however, it can be seen in patients with os trigonum syndrome; forceful plantarflexion activities such as soccer, downhill running, swimming, ice skating, and gymnastics; and flexor digitorum accessorius longus.[34–40] It is a part of the os trigonum or posterior ankle impingement syndrome.[31]

ANATOMY
Os Trigonum

The os trigonum is one of the largest and most common accessory ossicles in the ankle and foot region.[6,10,41] As its name suggests, the shape is triangular, with anterior, inferior, and posterior surfaces; however, it can be oval or rounded and variable in size.[3,42–44] (**Fig. 2**A–D). It is about 10 mm in length and height; this may vary especially if it is bipartite or multipartite (see **Fig. 2**A, B; **Fig. 3**H).

The anterior surface is usually crescentic, accommodating a porous defect at the synchondrosis.[8,43] The margin of the os trigonum can be smooth or serrated.[43]

The anterior surface connects with the lateral tubercle by a fibrous or cartilaginous synchondrosis[43] (see **Fig. 2**D). The inferior surface may articulate with the calcaneus at the posterior facet of the subtalar joint (see **Fig. 2**B; **Fig. 4**A, C, D). The posterior surface is the nonarticular portion (see **Figs. 2**A and **4**E); however, capsuloligamentous structures, particularly posterior talofibular and posterior talocalcaneal ligaments, attach in this area.[43] The lateral part of the os trigonum and trigonal process receive fibers from the posterior talofibular ligament, whereas the medial part lies with the thick and fibrous tendon sheath of the FHL.[42,43]

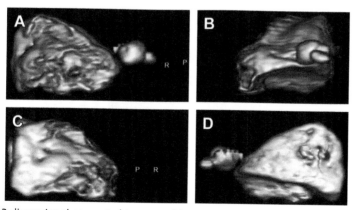

Fig. 2. A 3-dimensional computed tomographic reconstruction images show 360° views of bony anatomy of the os trigonum. The shape of the os trigonum is triangular with anterior (*D*) and posterior (*A, C*) nonarticular surface and inferior articular surface articulated to the calcaneus (*B*). P, posterior; R, right side.

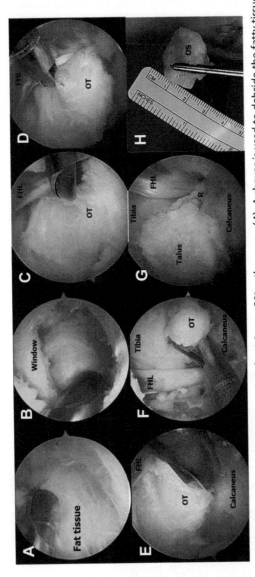

Fig. 3. A fatty tissue plane is demonstrated after inserting the 4.0-mm, 30° arthroscope (*A*). A shaver is used to debride the fatty tissue anteriorly until the os trigonum is identified, and it is used to create space or window for the procedure (*B*). Once the FHL tendon is identified, the shaver is placed and moved in the superior and inferior directions to the os trigonum (OT) with turning the cutting surface laterally to prevent injury to the neurovascular structures and FHL tendon (*C*). The os trigonum is shown after adequate debridement (*D*); the small os trigonum can be removed by shaver and burr (*E*), but the large os trigonum can be removed by using scissors to release soft tissue connecting the os trigonum to the posterior talus (*F*). Posterior surface of the talus is shown after complete debridement, and all sharp edges are round and smooth by the burr and shaver (*G*). A 2-cm os trigonum (OS) is demonstrated after it was removed from the PL portal (*H*). R, FHL retinaculum.

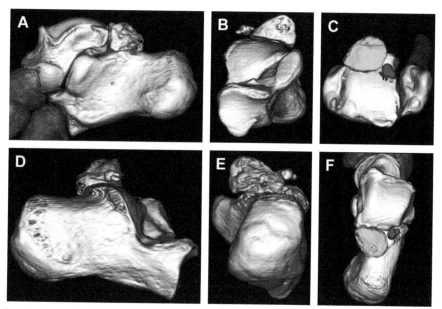

Fig. 4. Three-dimensional computed tomographic reconstruction images of the ankle demonstrate 360° of os trigonum with relationship to the calcaneus, tibia, and talus (*A–F*). A medial surface of the os trigonum (*A*), lateral surface of os trigonum (*D*), anterior surface of os trigonum (*B*), posterior surface of os trigonum (*E*), superior surface of os trigonum (*F*), and inferior surface of os trigonum (*C*) are demonstrated.

Flexor Hallucis Longus

The FHL originates from the posterior aspect of the fibula and interosseous membrane. It runs distally underneath the flexor retinaculum and within the tendon sheath, which attaches to the posterior talus and calcaneus forming a fibro-osseous tunnel.[37] The tendon lies medial to the os trigonum in the groove between the medial and lateral tubercle of the talus.[43]

The FHL runs distally and medially to the groove on the plantar surface of the sustentaculum tali, and it crosses dorsal to the flexor digitorum longus with a complex interconnection, the so-called knot of Henry, which occurs in the midfoot at the level of the first tarsometatarsal joint. The tendon then runs underneath the intersesamoid ligament and inserts at the plantar surface of the distal phalanx of the great toe.[45,46]

The blood supply to the FHL arises from the posterior tibial and medial plantar arteries, whereas the tibial nerve provides innervation to the muscle.[37]

The primary function of the FHL is as an active plantarflexor at the first metatarsophalangeal (MTP) and hallux interphalangeal joints and as the primary restraint to passive dorsiflexion at the first MTP joint.[37]

Dorsiflexion of the first MTP and ankle joints can increase the distal excursion of the FHL up to 25 mm and increase the tension on the interconnecting bands at the knot of Henry.[37]

PATHOLOGY
Os Trigonum Syndrome

Although rare, os trigonum syndrome may be the result of acute trauma or chronic repetitive injury that leads to a fracture of the Stieda process, cartilaginous synchondrosis disruption, os trigonum fracture, or an avulsion injury of the posterior talofibular ligament.[27] It can occur in both the athletic and nonathletic population.[3,13,27,47] Acute hyperplantarflexion injury and chronic repetitive or overuse injuries by forceful plantarflexion of the ankle joint are the typical mechanism of the os trigonum syndrome.[3,19,43] The talus rotates in the plantarflexed position, and the os trigonum or trigonal process is compressed between the posterior tibial plafond and calcaneus.[48] A united trigonal process has the capability to produce symptoms that are the same as a nonunited os trigonum.[43]

In the case of acute fracture, a long PL process (trigonal or Stieda process) can abut against the posterior malleolus and cause fracture of the trigonal process or damage of the synchondrosis of the os trigonum after forceful plantarflexion or axial loading.[14,20,47] However, excessive dorsiflexion may also cause an avulsion fracture of the lateral tubercle by increasing tension on the posterior talofibular ligament.[26] Strenuous and sport activities that force the ankle into plantar flexion such as ballet, dance, judo, football, basketball, running, and soccer were reported as the causes of trigonal process fracture,[17,19] which has been termed as Shepherd fracture.[14]

In overuse or chronic repeated plantar flexion, bone and soft tissue are compressed between the posterior malleolus and calcaneus. Bony protrusion superior to posterior articular facet of the talus can block full rotation of the talus in the ankle mortise during plantar flexion.[25] When this occurs, the posterior capsule and synovial tissue are squeezed between the 2 bony surfaces, and these soft-tissue structures are thought to be the sources of pain.[25] As pressure continues, swelling develops, followed by inflammatory change with eventual thickening and fibrosis; associated flexor hallucis longus tenosynovitis may develop.

Flexor Hallucis Longus Stenosing Tenosynovitis

The tendon of FHL is at risk of impingement because it travels in its sheath and groove, which is covered with the retinaculum between the medial and lateral tubercles of the talus. This exposure may cause or aggravate the symptoms of FHL tenosynovitis.[37] Impingement can occur at the flexor sheath posterior to medial malleolus, the entrance to the fibro-osseous tunnel, the knot of Henry, and the intersesamoid ligament.[46] When significant nodular change or hypertrophy appears in the FHL tendon, the excursion can be limited because of these 3 restriction points and may causes triggering or limitation of motion of the great toe.[22,37,49] However, when nodularity or hypertrophy part is moved proximal to the restricted fibro-osseous area by maximum plantar flexion of the ankle, dorsiflexion of the first MTP joint is restored, the so-called pseudo–hallux rigidus.[22,34,49]

In a ballet dancer, forced hyperplantarflexion of the ankle, particularly en pointe, may cause direct compression of the FHL through kinking of the tendon where it enters the fibro-osseous tunnel and lead to painful tenosynovitis.[22,35,37]

PATIENT HISTORY AND CLINICAL PRESENTATION

The routine history when evaluating a patient with posterior ankle impingement should include age, sex, occupation, sports activities, and mechanism of the injury.

In acute fracture of the PL process or disruption of the synchondrosis of os trigonum, the patients should report a hyperplantarflexion injury mechanism of the ankle joint.

For os trigonum syndrome, patients usually complain of pain that is located posteromedially[50,51]; however, it can be located posterolaterally[11,52] or diffusely posterior at the ankle joint.[53]

In FHL tenosynovitis, patients may report discomfort on the great toe[46] as well as at the posteromedial (PM) ankle; however, patients can present with plantar heel pain, plantar midfoot pain, pain at the first MTP joint, or multiple locations of pain.[21,22,37,40] Some patients may be presented with stiffness of the first MTP joint particularly in dorsiflexion, and some individuals may notice a crackling or squeaking sound. When FHL tenosynovitis appears at the level of the sesamoids, patients can present with inability to actively plantarflex the hallux at the interphalangeal joint.[33,54]

Pain is reproduced when weight bearing and aggravated by increasing ankle plantarflexion or during push-off. Pain is usually relieved with rest from plantarflexion activities; however, some patients may have periodic pain after ceasing activity.[19,27]

PHYSICAL EXAMINATION
Os Trigonum

The os trigonum may be palpated at the PL joint line of the ankle joint, and soft-tissue swelling may be found in this area.[29] Point of maximum tenderness or crepitus can be palpated on the posterior aspect of the ankle joint, posterior to the lateral malleolus.[10,22] In addition, pain is reproduced when the ankle was in maximum plantarflexion, the so-called nutcracker sign.[48] Ecchymosis may be present in front of the Achilles tendon insertion in a patient with acute fracture.[21]

Ankle range of motion, especially plantar flexion of the ankle, may be decreased in a patient with either acute fracture or chronic repetitive injury of the os trigonum.[27,55]

In the chronic stage, range of motion of the great toe hallux may be decreased because of the fibrosis of the FHL tendon in the fibro-osseous canal between the medial and lateral tubercles. Dorsiflexion of the hallux with the ankle fully dorsiflexed and the knee fully extended usually produces pain symptoms.[56]

Establishing the diagnosis of os trigonum syndrome can usually be made on clinical evaluation alone, but, if necessary, diagnostic injection can be performed by injection of local anesthetic at the posterior of ankle joint. This injection can relieve the painful symptoms; however, the maximum ankle range of motion does not change after injection.[29]

Flexor Hallucis Longus

The FHL can be palpated in 4 different locations.

- PM ankle joint (see **Fig. 1**B–D), the distal extent of the muscle belly can be palpated by moving the hallux up and down in ankle neutral position.[37]
- Sustentaculum tali (see **Fig. 1**B–D), it can be palpated inferior to the bone ridge of the sustentaculum.[37]
- Knot of Henry (see **Fig. 1**B–D), it can be palpated inferior to the medial cuneiform.[37]
- First MTP joint (see **Fig. 1**C, D), it can be palpated between the sesamoid bones.[37]

In FHL tenosynovitis, dorsiflexion of the MTP joint when the ankle is dorsiflexed (FHL stretch test) may be limited because of restriction of FHL excursion, but MTP joint motion is restored with plantarflexion of the ankle joint.[22,37,49]

Some patients can produce a squeaking or crackling sound at the back of the ankle in full flexion when they dorsiflex and plantarflex the first MTP joint (see **Fig. 1**E, F).

DIFFERENTIAL DIAGNOSIS
Os Trigonum

The differential diagnosis for posterior ankle pain includes associated fracture of the posterior malleolus, talus, or calcaneus; osteochondral lesion of the talus and tibia; talocalcaneal coalition and ganglion cyst; Achilles tendon rupture/avulsion, Achilles tendinitis, and Haglund deformity[56]; FHL and posterior tibial tendinitis or tendinopathy[22,29]; and peroneal tendon subluxation/dislocation.[56]

RADIOLOGY AND INVESTIGATION

The os trigonum can be visualized radiographically on a lateral view of the foot (**Fig. 5**A, B, D, E). A predisposition to impingement is indicated by a prominent PL process of the talus (Stieda process) or os trigonum (see **Fig. 5**B, D, E), prominence of the posterior malleolus of the tibia, and prominence of the posterior process of the calcaneus (see **Fig. 5**D).[43] Acute fracture can be defined by a jagged fracture edge of the posterior process of the talus.[50]

Lateral radiography of the foot in full plantarflexion at the ankle may be used to demonstrate the os trigonum or Stieda process impinged against the posterior malleolus.[56]

A 3-dimensional computed tomographic reconstruction scan can provide the details of the bony structure of the os trigonum, the relationship of the os trigonum to the tibia, talus, and calcaneus (see **Fig. 4**A–F), and pathology such as fracture or cystic change in the os trigonum (see **Fig. 5**C, F).

Technetium 99 scanning has been used because a symptomatic acute os trigonum fracture or chronic nonunion of os trigonum fracture can show intense focal uptake, whereas a negative scan excludes the fracture.[30,50]

MRI can identify the abnormality manifests as bone marrow edema, a fracture line, or fluid in the synchondrosis or osteoarthritis of the joint between the os trigonum and

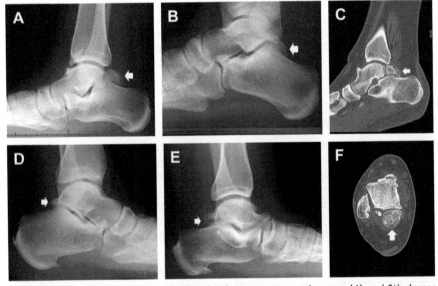

Fig. 5. Lateral views of the foot radiography demonstrate os trigonum (*A*) and Stieda process (*B, D, E* [*arrow*]). The sagittal and coronal views of the computed tomographic scan demonstrate large os trigonum posterior to the talus (*C, F* [*arrow*]) and prominence of the posterior process of calcaneus (*A, B, E*).

calcaneus[43] (**Fig. 6**A–F). MRI can also evaluate an associated FHL pathology, which can alter the planned surgical approach[43] (see **Fig. 6**C, F).

THERAPEUTIC OPTIONS AND SURGICAL TECHNIQUES
Nonsurgical Treatment

Rest, ice, oral nonsteroidal anti-inflammatory drugs, bracing, casting, and discontinuing activities that aggravate symptoms by forced hyperplantarflexion of the ankle joint should initially be recommended to provide relief of symptoms.[26,29,57] In FHL tenosynovitis, stretching exercises of the FHL tendon should be considered in the initial treatment.[37] Physical therapy consists of icing, massage, ultrasound therapy, whirlpool, and massage and can be performed to relieve acute inflammation while increasing range of motion and strength.[58]

Diagnostic injection can be obtained using 1% or 2% lidocaine injected into the posterior aspect of the talus for a goal of temporary pain relief.[11,44] Single or double-shot local steroid injection under fluoroscopic or ultrasound guidance can help relieve symptoms and predict the outcome of excisional surgery.[59]

Surgical Technique

Approach
Open surgery Failure of a 3- to 6-month period of conservative treatment is an indication for surgical treatment. Both PL and PM open approaches have been reported as a

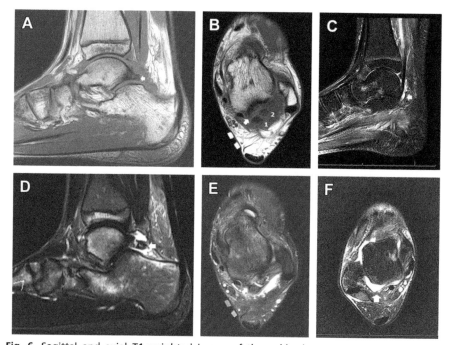

Fig. 6. Sagittal and axial T1-weighted image of the ankle demonstrates os trigonum (A [*white arrow*], B [1, 2]), and T2-weighted image of the ankle demonstrates 2 pieces of os trigonum connected with the posterior talus with synchondrosis (B, E [*white arrow*]). Sagittal and axial T2-weighted image of ankle MRI in patient with FHL stenosing tenosynovitis demonstrates fluid around the flexor hallucis longus tendon (C, F [*white arrow*]). Sagittal T2-weighted image of ankle MRI demonstrates fracture of Stieda process (D [*arrow*]).

successful technique for treatment of patients with os trigonum syndrome. The PL approach is usually recommended only for excision of os trigonum or PL process because there are no major neurovascular structures in this area except the sural nerve. However, the PM approach is preferred if bony impingement is accompanied by pathology in the neurovascular bundle or FHL tendon.

Posterolateral approach The patient is placed in the supine position with proximal thigh tourniquet on the affected leg. A 4- to 5-cm straight incision is made posterior to the lateral malleolus and medial to the peroneal tendons. Soft tissues are carefully dissected, and the sural nerve is identified to avoid injury to its branches. Then the posterior capsule of the ankle joint is identified and subsequently incised in line with the skin incision. The os trigonum is identified and removed using a rongeur forceps or an osteotome. The rasp is used to smooth the remaining bone, with bone wax subsequently applied to control the bleeding on the raw surface of PL process of the talus. Then the soft tissues and skin are irrigated, and skin is closed by nonabsorbable suture.

Posteromedial approach The patient is placed in the supine position and pneumatic tourniquet applied on the thigh. A curvilinear incision is made centered approximately 1 cm posterior to the medial malleolus and approximately 8 to 10 cm in length. Soft tissues are carefully dissected to avoid injury to the superficial branches of the tibial nerve. The flexor retinaculum is identified and released, and the flexor tendons and neurovascular bundle are identified, mobilized, and gently retracted for exposure. Thereafter, the resection is completed in a manner similar to the PL approach.

Alternatively, the patient is placed with the affected limb in external rotation. An incision is made approximately 1 cm anterior to the medial aspect of the Achilles tendon. Following incision of the skin, blunt dissection is directed anterolaterally toward the FHL. The FHL sheath is identified and released, ensuring that the muscle belly of the FHL is visualized before release. The tibial nerve does not require mobilization and retraction with this exposure in most instances. The FHL is then gently retracted medially with excision of the os trigonum as previously described.

Arthroscopic approach

Positioning The advantages of the arthroscopic approach over the open approaches are minimizing of surgical injury and less scarring, less postoperative pain, minimal morbidity, and earlier return to activities.[23]

Arthroscopic os trigonum excision can be performed from either a lateral or a posterior approach.[23,60–67] The authors prefer prone over lateral decubitus position because it provides a more direct approach to the os trigonum, decreases the risk of instrument skiving off toward the neurovascular bundles, and simultaneously allows performance of the procedure for FHL pathology.

The patient is placed in the prone position with proximal thigh tourniquet and standard padding (**Fig. 7**A, C). The foot is just beyond the end of the bed, allowing dorsiflexion of the ankle joint by leaning of surgeon's body forward (see **Fig. 7**D).

Portals Anatomic landmark and associated structures are the medial and lateral malleoli, superior aspect of calcaneal tuberosity, Achilles tendon, medial neurovascular structures, and sural nerve (see **Fig. 7**B).

PM and PL portals are located on either side of the Achilles tendon at approximately 15 mm above the superior aspect of the calcaneal tuberosity (see **Fig. 7**B).

The PL portal (see **Fig. 7**B) is established with a 5-mm vertical skin incision next to the lateral border of the Achilles tendon (see **Fig. 7**B), and thereafter, a blunt dissection

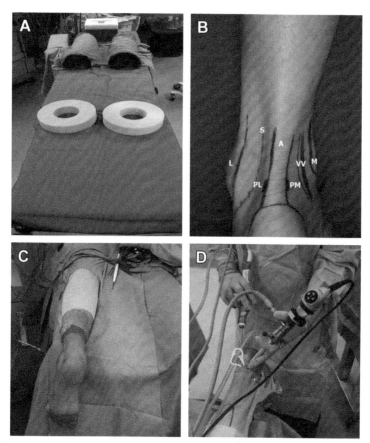

Fig. 7. Standard posterior ankle arthroscopy is demonstrated (*A*), and patient is placed in the prone position with thigh tourniquet and the foot is at the end of the bed (*C*). Surface anatomy shows posterolateral (PL), posteromedial (PM), Achilles tendon (*A*), medial malleolus (M), lateral malleolus (L), sural nerve (S), and tibial nerve and vessels (VV) (*B*). A 4.0-mm, 30° arthroscope is inserted in the PL portal, the shaver is inserted in the PM portal, and the surgeon can dorsiflex the ankle joint by leaning the surgeon's body forward (*D*).

is performed with a curved hemostat toward the second toe. The PM portal (see **Fig. 7**B) is subsequently established at the same level just medial to the medial border of the Achilles tendon, followed by blunt dissection with a curved hemostat directed toward the PL portal.

Once both portals are created, a 4-mm sheath with a blunt trochar is introduced into the PL portal, followed by a 4-mm, 30° arthroscope. Thereafter, a 4-mm shaver is introduced into the PM portal, and triangulation of both instruments is performed until the tip of the shaver is seen on the video monitor from the camera (see **Fig. 7**D).

Soft-tissue debridement Initial debridement is performed to remove a small portion of the posterior ankle fatty tissue (see **Fig. 3**A), creating a working space for arthroscopic maneuvering (see **Fig. 3**B).

The os trigonum is identified as the first osseous structure encountered. The FHL is then identified by carefully dissecting soft tissue on the plane cephalad to the os trigonum medially (see **Fig. 3**C).

When the FHL is identified by observing its excursion during manipulation of the first MTP joint, it can be used as an important boundary for protection of the neurovascular bundle (see **Fig. 3**D). One must not dissect on the PM side of the FHL where the neurovascular structures are located. Peroneocalcaneus internus muscle, false FHL, may mimic the FHL, leading to an incorrect plain of dissection and potential neurovascular injuries. Limitation of tendon gliding on manipulation of the great toe MTP joint may suggest the presence of this rare anatomic variant.

All soft tissues circumferentially around the os trigonum, including retinaculum of the FHL medially and posterior talofibular ligament laterally, are debrided and released thoroughly using the shaver and arthroscopic scissors (see **Fig. 3**D, F).

Excision of os trigonum or posterior lateral process The synchondrosis of the os trigonum can be visualized with the arthroscope and palpated by a probe or Freer elevator from the superior aspect. The Freer elevator can be used to lever and crack the synchondrosis by levering it superiorly or inferiorly to the os trigonum. Then a grasper or hemostat is inserted, and the os trigonum can be removed as a whole piece (see **Fig. 3**H) or piecemeal by a shaver or a burr (see **Fig. 3**E).

In cases with a prominent trigonal process, a burr can be used to remove the posterior aspect of the talus until absence of impingement on maximum plantarflexion.

After the os trigonum is removed, the posterior process of the talus should be examined and contoured so that no bony prominence compresses or irritates the FHL tendon (see **Fig. 3**G).

Flexor hallucis longus debridement and retinaculum and fibro-osseous tunnel release The FHL can be clearly examined by maximum plantarflexion and maximum dorsiflexion of the ankle joint and great toe after the os trigonum has been removed (**Fig. 8**A).

Impingement of the FHL musculotendinous junction to the fibro-osseous tunnel may be seen (see **Fig. 8**C).

Synovitis, fraying, and partial tear of the FHL tendon can be debrided and removed using a shaver; however, if a tear is greater than 50%, open FHL repair is indicated.

The FHL retinaculum (see **Fig. 8**B) and fibro-osseous tunnel of the FHL (see **Fig. 8**F) can be released to decompress the constricted FHL using arthroscopic or Metzenbaum scissors (see **Fig. 8**D, E).

After adequate release of the fibro-osseous tunnel, the FHL should be moved with no impingement during maximum dorsiflexion and plantarflexion of the ankle joint (see **Fig. 8**G, H).

Evaluation of associated lesion The posterior aspect of the ankle and subtalar joint can be evaluated through the same PL and PM portals (**Fig. 9**A). Synovitis or thickening of the intermalleolar ligament can be debrided. Loose bodies posterior to the ankle and subtalar joint can be removed if present.

Anterior draw of the ankle joint allows space in the posterior ankle joint (see **Fig. 9**B–D). Intra-articular views of the ankle joint are best achieved with a 2.7-mm arthroscope. The subtalar joint can be readily examined from the posterior approach (see **Fig. 9**E, F).

Postoperative Protocol

Portals are closed by a 3-0 nonabsorbable suture, and standard dressing is applied. The patient is instructed to be weight bearing as tolerated in a CAM walking boot for 2 weeks, removing the boot to do range-of-motion exercises of the ankle joint and the great toe. After 2-week follow-up, patients can wean off the boot and transition to

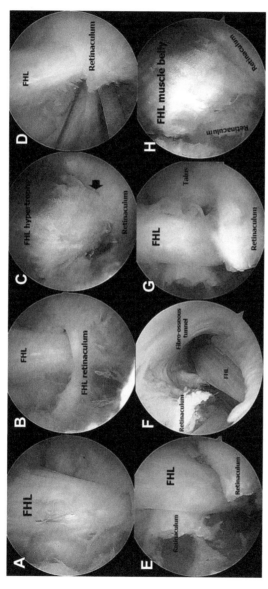

Fig. 8. The FHL and its retinaculum are shown after completely removing the os trigonum (A, B). The impingement of the FHL is demonstrated at the fibro-osseous tunnel when the ankle joint is fully dorsiflexed (C [black arrow]). A Metzenbaum scissors is inserted to the PM portal, and the retinaculum is cut in the vertical direction (D). After complete release of the retinaculum (E), the fibro-osseous tunnel is visualized by deeply advancing the 4.0-mm, 30° arthroscope into the tunnel behind the FHL (F). Full range of motion of FHL is required to confirm that there is no impingement after complete release of the FHL retinaculum and fibro-osseous tunnel (G, H).

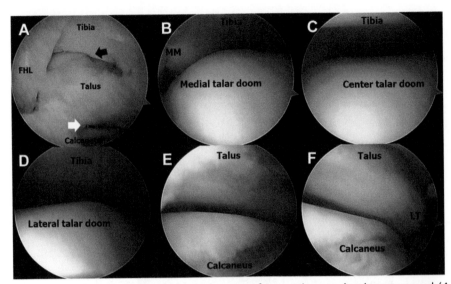

Fig. 9. The ankle and subtalar joint can be seen after os trigonum has been removed (*A* [*white arrow*: ankle joint; *black arrow*: subtalar joint]). After performing the anterior draw, the ankle joint can be examined and evaluated for associated pathology, medial talar dome, and medial tibia plafond (*B*); center of talar dome and center of tibial plafond (*C*); and lateral talar dome and lateral tibial plafond (*D*). The subtalar joint and lateral process of talus (LT) can be evaluated for associated pathology (*E*, *F*).

regular shoes. Physical therapy for FHL and ankle strengthening and range of motion exercises can be started.

CLINICAL OUTCOMES
Os Trigonum

Conservative treatment may help alleviate the symptom and allow for gradual return to less demanding athletic activities[68]; however, symptoms often recurred after return to higher level of activities.[29] The success rate is approximately 60% to 84% after 4 to 6 months of conservative treatment as reported in the literature.[26,32,58]

The success rate of corticosteroid injection varies (range, 29%–100%).[26,58,59] Temporary pain relief can delay surgery in professional or collegiate athletes[69] and confirm diagnosis as a planning step for surgical excision.[59] However, corticosteroid injection should not be encouraged in blind technique nor should multiple injections in a short period be given because of the risk of FHL or Achilles tendon rupture or skin and soft-tissue hypotrophy.[56]

Arthroscopic approaches in prone and supine positions have been reported to be an effective technique for treatment of patients with os trigonum syndrome. Previous reports in the literature showed good to excellent outcomes[70] and significant improvement of American Orthopaedic Foot and Ankle Society (AOFAS) score (average AOFAS score of 85.9–99.0 points at final follow-up)[23,60–63,65,66,70–72] and visual analog scale (VAS) (average improvement of VAS of 4.9/10 at final follow-up)[62] postoperatively. Average time to return to sports or activities was 5.9 weeks to 5.8 months.[23,60–63,65,66,70–72]

Open excision of the os trigonum through PM or PL approaches were effective and safe in the patients with os trigonum syndrome.[29,73] Previous studies reported significant improvement of AOFAS scores, and average AOFAS scores were

87.6 to 100.0 points at the final postoperative visit.[13,23,57,74] Average time to return to sports and activities was 3 to 5.7 months.[13,23]

Flexor Hallucis Longus

In FHL stenosing tenosynovitis, conservative treatment in severe cases may yield full recovery at 1 year after injury; however, recurrence of symptoms is common.[75] The success rate is approximately 46% to 64%,[37] and 13% of these patients have a longitudinal tear of the FHL tendon.[40]

Debridement of the FHL tendon and release of the retinaculum and fibro-osseous tunnel through the PM approach or arthroscopically has been reported to be an effective method for the treatment of patients with stenosing tenosynovitis of the FHL. Studies have shown 85.2% to 90.0% patient satisfaction after open surgery[22,40] and 80% patient satisfaction after arthroscopic approach.[31]

The mean improvement of VAS at the final follow-up was 5.5[2] and the mean improvement of AOFAS scores was 89.9 points in the arthroscopic approach,[31,60] whereas no outcomes scores were reported in studies using the open approach. Reportedly, 81.1% to 100%[18,35] and 81% to 100%[31,60] of patients can return to previous activities and sports[18,35] after FHL release in open and arthroscopic approaches, respectively. Average time to return to activities is 12 to 25 weeks[18,35,40] in the open approach and 6 to 8 weeks in the arthroscopic approach.[46,60]

COMPLICATIONS AND CONCERNS
Complications

Improper PL portal location and poor placement of instruments in the arthroscopic approach as well as overzealous dissection and retraction in open PL approach can cause injury to the sural nerve. Sural nerve injury was reported at a rate of 3.4% to 8.3% in the arthroscopic approach[23,60,62,65,71,72] and 6.3% to 19.5% in the open approach.[13,23] In addition, superficial peroneal nerve injury at the anterolateral portal was reported 9.1% using supine position; however, all cases of injury spontaneously resolved.[76]

Arthroscopic debridement medially to the FHL or posteromedial open approach can cause injury to the posterior tibial artery/vein and the tibial nerve. Tibial nerve injury was reported at a rate of 6.7% in the open approach[29] and 11.1% in the arthroscopic approach[31]; however, all patients fully recovered within 1 year after surgery.[29]

In posterior arthroscopic debridement using the supine position, a potential hazard is injury to the calcaneofibular ligament or peroneal tendons while making the centrolateral portal.[66]

Superficial wound infection was reported in 3.3% to 6.7%[29,62] and deep wound infection in 3.3% from the arthroscopic approach,[62] whereas only superficial wound infection was reported in 2.4% from the open approach. Ankle stiffness was reported in 6.7% and triggering of the hallux in 3.7% from the arthroscopic approach; there are no such reports in series involving the open approach.[31,72]

Concerns

Comprehensive understanding of the anatomy of the posterior ankle, portal setup, and instrument placement are crucial steps for preventing injury to important structures of the posterior ankle.

Injury to the PM neurovascular structures should be avoided, and strictly working lateral to the FHL tendon prevents this injury. Failure to recognize anatomic variations may lead to iatrogenic injuries.

Careful and judicious technique allows successful debridement and osseous excision, as adjacent structures, such as the FHL tendon and articular cartilage of the ankle and subtalar joints, can be damaged during os trigonum debridement.

REFERENCES

1. Bardeleben K. Tarsus and carpus. J Anat Physiol 1885;19:509–10.
2. Grogan DP, Walling AK, Ogden JA. Anatomy of the os trigonum. J Pediatr Orthop 1990;10:618–22.
3. McDougall A. The os trigonum. J Bone Joint Surg Br 1955;37-B:257–65.
4. Stieda L. Ueber secundare fusswurselkochen. Archiv Fur Anatomie, Physiologie, under Wissenshcaftliche Medicine. 1869. p. 108.
5. Sarrafian SK. Anatomy of the foot and ankle: descriptive, topographic, functional. Philadelphia: Lippincott; 1983.
6. Bizarro AH. On sesamoid and supernumerary bones of the limbs. J Anat 1921;55: 256–68.
7. Burman MS, Lapidus PW. The functional disturbances caused by the inconstant bones and sesamoids of the foot. Arch Surg 1931;22:936–75.
8. Mann RW, Owsley DW. Os trigonum. Variation of a common accessory ossicle of the talus. J Am Podiatr Med Assoc 1990;80:536–9.
9. Salyers SG, Fu FH. Posterior ankle impingement syndrome in a ballet dancer. Orthop Consult 1989;10:9–12.
10. Kose O, Okan AN, Durakbasa MO, et al. Fracture of the os trigonum: a case report. J Orthop Surg 2006;14:354–6.
11. Brodsky AE, Khalil MA. Talar compression syndrome. Am J Sports Med 1986;14: 472–6.
12. Rosenmuller JC. De non nullis musculorum corporis humani varietatibus. Leipzig (Germany): Klaubarthia; 1804.
13. Abramowitz Y, Wollstein R, Barzilay Y, et al. Outcome of resection of a symptomatic os trigonum. J Bone Joint Surg Am 2003;85-A:1051–7.
14. Shepherd FJ. A hitherto undescribed fracture of the astragalus. J Anat Physiol 1882;17:79–81.
15. Turner W. A secondary astragalus in the human foot. J Anat Physiol 1882;17: 82–3.
16. Anwar R, Nicholl JE. Non-union of a fractured os trigonum. Injury 2005;36: 267–70.
17. Escobedo EM, MacDonald TL, Hunter JC. Acute fracture of the os trigonum. Emerg Radiol 2006;13:139–41.
18. Hamilton WG, Geppert MJ, Thompson FM. Pain in the posterior aspect of the ankle in dancers. Differential diagnosis and operative treatment. J Bone Joint Surg Am 1996;78:1491–500.
19. Ihle CL, Cochran RM. Fracture of the fused os trigonum. Am J Sports Med 1982; 10:47–50.
20. Mouhsine E, Djahangiri A, Garofalo R. Fracture of the non fused os trigonum, a rare cause of hindfoot pain. A case report and review of the literature. Chir Organi Mov 2004;89:171–5.
21. Meisenbach R. Fracture of the os trigonum: report of two cases. JAMA 1927;89: 199–200.
22. Hamilton WG. Stenosing tenosynovitis of the flexor hallucis longus tendon and posterior impingement upon the os trigonum in ballet dancers. Foot Ankle 1982;3:74–80.

23. Guo QW, Hu YL, Jiao C, et al. Open versus endoscopic excision of a symptomatic os trigonum: a comparative study of 41 cases. Arthroscopy 2010;26:384–90.
24. Moeller FA. The os trigonum syndrome. J Am Podiatry Assoc 1973;63:491–501.
25. Howse AJ. Posterior block of the ankle joint in dancers. Foot Ankle 1982;3:81–4.
26. Hedrick MR, McBryde AM. Posterior ankle impingement. Foot Ankle Int 1994;15:2–8.
27. Nault ML, Kocher MS, Micheli LJ. Os trigonum syndrome. J Am Acad Orthopaedic Surgeons 2014;22:545–53.
28. Kleiger B. The posterior tibiotalar impingement syndrome in dancers. Bull Hosp Jt Dis Orthop Inst 1987;47:203–10.
29. Marotta JJ, Micheli LJ. Os trigonum impingement in dancers. Am J Sports Med 1992;20:533–6.
30. Lawson JP. Symptomatic radiographic variants in extremities. Radiology 1985;157:625–31.
31. Corte-Real NM, Moreira RM, Guerra-Pinto F. Arthroscopic treatment of tenosynovitis of the flexor hallucis longus tendon. Foot Ankle Int 2012;33:1108–12.
32. Albisetti W, Ometti M, Pascale V, et al. Clinical evaluation and treatment of posterior impingement in dancers. Am J Phys Med Rehabil 2009;88:349–54.
33. Sanhudo JA. Stenosing tenosynovitis of the flexor hallucis longus tendon at the sesamoid area. Foot Ankle Int 2002;23:801–3.
34. Hardaker WT Jr, Margello S, Goldner JL. Foot and ankle injuries in theatrical dancers. Foot Ankle 1985;6:59–69.
35. Kolettis GJ, Micheli LJ, Klein JD. Release of the flexor hallucis longus tendon in ballet dancers. J Bone Joint Surg Am 1996;78:1386–90.
36. Eberle CF, Moran B, Gleason T. The accessory flexor digitorum longus as a cause of flexor hallucis syndrome. Foot Ankle Int 2002;23:51–5.
37. Michelson J, Dunn L. Tenosynovitis of the flexor hallucis longus: a clinical study of the spectrum of presentation and treatment. Foot Ankle Int 2005;26:291–303.
38. Nathan H, Gloobe H, Yosipovitch Z. Flexor digitorum accessorius longus. Clin Orthop Relat Res 1975;(113):158–61.
39. Ogut T, Ayhan E. Hindfoot endoscopy for accessory flexor digitorum longus and flexor hallucis longus tenosynovitis. Foot Ankle Surg 2011;17:e7–9.
40. Sammarco GJ, Cooper PS. Flexor hallucis longus tendon injury in dancers and nondancers. Foot Ankle Int 1998;19:356–62.
41. Mellado JM, Ramos A, Salvado E, et al. Accessory ossicles and sesamoid bones of the ankle and foot: imaging findings, clinical significance and differential diagnosis. Eur Radiol 2003;13(Suppl 6):L164–77.
42. Davies MB. The os trigonum syndrome. Foot 2004;14:119–23.
43. Karasick D, Schweitzer ME. The os trigonum syndrome: imaging features. AJR Am J Roentgenol 1996;166:125–9.
44. Quirk R. Talar compression syndrome in dancers. Foot Ankle 1982;3:65–8.
45. O'Sullivan E, Carare-Nnadi R, Greenslade J, et al. Clinical significance of variations in the interconnections between flexor digitorum longus and flexor hallucis longus in the region of the knot of Henry. Clin Anat 2005;18:121–5.
46. Theodoropoulos JS, Wolin PM, Taylor DW. Arthroscopic release of flexor hallucis longus tendon using modified posteromedial and posterolateral portals in the supine position. Foot 2009;19:218–21.
47. Maquirriain J. Posterior ankle impingement syndrome. J Am Acad Orthop Surg 2005;13:365–71.
48. Schubert JM, Adler DC. Talar fractures. In: Banks AS, Downey MS, Martin DE, editors. McGlamry's comprehensive textbook of foot and ankle surgery. Volume I, 3rd edition. Philadelphia: Lippincott Williams and Wilkins; 2001. p. 1871–4.

49. Hamilton WG. Foot and ankle injuries in dancers. Clin Sports Med 1988;7:143–73.
50. Johnson RP, Collier BD, Carrera GF. The os trigonum syndrome: use of bone scan in the diagnosis. J Trauma 1984;24:761–4.
51. Maffulli N, Lepore L, Francobandiera C. Traumatic lesions of some accessory bones of the foot in sports activity. J Am Podiatr Med Assoc 1990;80:86–90.
52. Wenig JA. Os trigonum syndrome. J Am Podiatr Med Assoc 1990;80:278–82.
53. Martin BF. Posterior triangle pain: the os trigonum. J Foot Surg 1989;28:312–8.
54. Gould N. Stenosing tenosynovitis of the flexor hallucis longus tendon at the great toe. Foot Ankle 1981;2:46–8.
55. Paulos LE, Johnson CL, Noyes FR. Posterior compartment fractures of the ankle. A commonly missed athletic injury. Am J Sports Med 1983;11:439–43.
56. Blake RL, Lallas PJ, Ferguson H. The os trigonum syndrome. A literature review. J Am Podiatr Med Assoc 1992;82:154–61.
57. Rogers J, Dijkstra P, McCourt P, et al. Posterior ankle impingement syndrome: a clinical review with reference to horizontal jump athletes. Acta Orthop Belg 2010; 76:572–9.
58. Mouhsine E, Crevoisier X, Leyvraz PF, et al. Post-traumatic overload or acute syndrome of the os trigonum: a possible cause of posterior ankle impingement. Knee Surg Sports Traumatol Arthrosc 2004;12:250–3.
59. Jones DM, Saltzman CL, El-Khoury G. The diagnosis of the os trigonum syndrome with a fluoroscopically controlled injection of local anesthetic. Iowa Orthop J 1999;19:122–6.
60. Ahn JH, Kim YC, Kim HY. Arthroscopic versus posterior endoscopic excision of a symptomatic os trigonum: a retrospective cohort study. Am J Sports Med 2013; 41:1082–9.
61. Calder JD, Sexton SA, Pearce CJ. Return to training and playing after posterior ankle arthroscopy for posterior impingement in elite professional soccer. Am J Sports Med 2010;38:120–4.
62. Galla M, Lobenhoffer P. Technique and results of arthroscopic treatment of posterior ankle impingement. Foot Ankle Surg 2011;17:79–84.
63. Horibe S, Kita K, Natsu-ume T, et al. A novel technique of arthroscopic excision of a symptomatic os trigonum. Arthroscopy 2008;24:121.e1–4.
64. Lee KB, Kim KH, Lee JJ. Posterior arthroscopic excision of bilateral posterior bony impingement syndrome of the ankle: a case report. Knee Surg Sports Traumatol Arthrosc 2008;16:396–9.
65. Noguchi H, Ishii Y, Takeda M, et al. Arthroscopic excision of posterior ankle bony impingement for early return to the field: short-term results. Foot Ankle Int 2010; 31:398–403.
66. Park CH, Kim SY, Kim JR, et al. Arthroscopic excision of a symptomatic os trigonum in a lateral decubitus position. Foot Ankle Int 2013;34:990–4.
67. van Dijk CN, Scholten PE, Krips R. A 2-portal endoscopic approach for diagnosis and treatment of posterior ankle pathology. Arthroscopy 2000;16:871–6.
68. Rathur S, Clifford PD, Chapman CB. Posterior ankle impingement: os trigonum syndrome. Am J Orthop 2009;38:252–3.
69. Mitchell MJ, Bielecki D, Bergman AG, et al. Localization of specific joint causing hindfoot pain: value of injecting local anesthetics into individual joints during arthrography. AJR Am J Roentgenol 1995;164:1473–6.
70. Willits K, Sonneveld H, Amendola A, et al. Outcome of posterior ankle arthroscopy for hindfoot impingement. Arthroscopy 2008;24:196–202.
71. Ogut T, Ayhan E, Irgit K, et al. Endoscopic treatment of posterior ankle pain. Knee Surg Sports Traumatol Arthrosc 2011;19:1355–61.

72. Tey M, Monllau JC, Centenera JM, et al. Benefits of arthroscopic tuberculoplasty in posterior ankle impingement syndrome. Knee Surg Sports Traumatol Arthrosc 2007;15:1235–9.

73. Wredmark T, Carlstedt CA, Bauer H, et al. Os trigonum syndrome: a clinical entity in ballet dancers. Foot Ankle 1991;11:404–6.

74. de Landevoisin ES, Jacopin S, Glard Y, et al. Surgical treatment of the symptomatic os trigonum in children. Orthop Traumatol Surg Res 2009;95:159–63.

75. Norris RN. Common foot and ankle injuries in dancers. In: Teoksessa Solomon R, Solomon J, Cerny M, editors. Preventing dance injuries. Champaign (IL): Human Kinetics; 2005. p. 39–51.

76. Marumoto JM, Ferkel RD. Arthroscopic excision of the os trigonum: a new technique with preliminary clinical results. Foot Ankle Int 1997;18:777–84.

Stage I and II Posterior Tibial Tendon Dysfunction

Return to Running?

Norman Espinosa, MD*, Marc A. Maurer, MD

KEYWORDS

• Flatfoot • Tibial • Tendon • Dysfunction • Treatment

KEY POINTS

- Posterior tibial tendon (PTT) dysfunction can be a difficult entity to treat in the athletic population.
- Understanding the deformity components allows the physician to maximize nonoperative intervention with orthotics and physical therapy.
- Not all patients improve with nonoperative treatment, and surgical intervention can be successful in minimizing symptoms.
- Although return to full athletic activity is not universally possible, an active lifestyle is possible for many after surgical reconstruction.

INTRODUCTION

PTT dysfunction is a common pathology in daily orthopedic practice. However, there is no universal agreement regarding the optimal treatment of this clinical, sometimes debilitating, problem. There are many satisfactory treatment strategies available, making it difficult to prefer one over the others. The art is to select not only a proper but also individual solution to help the patient to improve. During decision making, the surgeon needs to figure out whether to consider conservative measures or embark on surgery. Surgical decision making itself depends on the stage of disease, amount of deformity, and flexibility. Sometimes, this process is complicated by the fact that the disease has a continuous progression from one stage to another and that certain stages cannot clearly be defined by any classification system.

This article focuses on stage I and II PTT dysfunction.

Institute for Foot and Ankle Reconstruction Zurich, Kappelistrasse 7, Zurich 8002, Switzerland
* Corresponding author.
E-mail address: espinosa@fussinstitut.ch

Clin Sports Med 34 (2015) 761–768
http://dx.doi.org/10.1016/j.csm.2015.06.012
0278-5919/15/$ – see front matter © 2015 Elsevier Inc. All rights reserved.

DEFINITION OF STAGE I AND II POSTERIOR TIBIAL TENDON DYSFUNCTION

Stage I PTT dysfunction defines a simple tenosynovitis without deformity. The tendon is found inflamed or partially ruptured. There is almost no or only minimal deformity present at the hindfoot. The continuity of the tendon is preserved. Tendon power might be normal, and patients present with almost normal function of the PTT combined with slight discomfort during exertional stress.[1]

This stage is divided into 3 categories, including inflammatory disease (resulting from systemic disease, eg, rheumatoid arthritis), partial PTT tear with normal anatomy, and partial PTT tear with slight deformity. The last represents a border-line stage with a continuum into stage II disease.

Stage II PTT dysfunction is defined by the presence of PTT rupture as confirmed by clinical assessment and imaging. This stage is divided into 5 categories that are important to distinguish because they have an impact on surgical decision making.[2]

II A: Hindfoot valgus: The disease reveals a flexible hindfoot valgus that can be manually reduced to neutral with a varying degree of forefoot supination.

II B: Flexible forefoot supination: The same characteristics apply as seen for IIA but with a remarkable amount of forefoot supination. The forefoot supination is flexible. With plantarflexion of the ankle the forefoot supination reduces to neutral. It is thought that gastrocnemius contracture leads to the forefoot supination.

II C: Fixed forefoot supination: This stage includes a fixed frontal plane deformity at the forefoot due to adaptive alterations of the anatomy due to longstanding hindfoot valgus deformity. When reducing the hindfoot into neutral while plantarflexing the ankle joint, the forefoot supination persists.

II D: Forefoot abduction: Flexible hindfoot valgus combined with transversal tarsal joint abduction, that is, not only significant frontal plane but also transversal plane deformity.

II E: Medial ray instability: The same characteristics as seen in stage II A apply for this type of disease. However, instability of the medial column is present. This instability can take place at any location on the medial ray (talonavicular, naviculocuneiform, metatarsocuneiform joint). During stance phase, the incompetent medial ray is pushed dorsally while getting less loaded than the lateral rays resulting in foot pronation.

CLINICAL ASSESSMENT

The patient is examined barefoot both during walking and in a standing position. It is important to visualize the thigh and to examine all lower limb axes. The alignment of legs and hindfoot is evaluated. The goal of clinical evaluation is to obtain a detailed appreciation of the deformity type. Leg, hindfoot, midfoot, and forefoot deformities should be checked and assessed to estimate the rigidity and potential of possible correction. Throughout the clinical evaluation particular attention is paid to signs of concomitant pathologies, such as subfibular ankle impingement, peroneal tendon irritation, and contracture of calf muscles.

Inspection

Hindfoot alignment is observed during stance and includes inspection of soft-tissue conditions, for example, atrophy. Measurement of hindfoot alignment is performed while looking at the patient from behind. The angle between the long axis of the leg and the axis of the calcaneous is measured. Normal values range from 0° neutral to 5° valgus.[3]

The examiner could look whether a too many toes sign is present: When examining the patient from the back, the visibility of the medial and lateral toes indicates the presence of hindfoot valgus. The height of the medial longitudinal arch and the amount of first ray plantarflexion are noted, and special attention is paid on the position of the forefoot and midfoot under varus and valgus stress as well as pronation and supination. Analysis of gait and distribution of callosities at the plantar aspect may reveal dynamic components and could indicate regions that are overloaded.[4]

Palpation

During palpation, special attention is paid to tender spots along the course of the PTT and spring ligament complex. The examiner is able to assess any flexibility or rigidity of deformity while trying to reduce manually the heel under the tibia. In addition, it is of value to examine the medial and lateral ligament complexes around the ankle as well as the joint lines of the ankle and subtalar, Chopart, and Lisfranc joints. Tenderness along the peroneal tendons may indicate a subfibular impingement due to excessive hindfoot valgus with consecutive tendinopathy or partial rupture and needs specific imaging, for example, MRI.

Function and Specific Tests

Range of motion at the ankle and subtalar and Chopart joints is assessed. To assess the contribution of a short gastrocnemius-soleus complex, the so-called Silferskjöld test is performed. It is important to rule out shortening of the Achilles tendon and contractures of the triceps surae as they may play an important role in correcting the hindfoot and determining whether additional surgery should be performed.

The single-heel rise test assesses the dynamic function of the PTT.[5] If the patient cannot stand on his or her tiptoes, the test is seen as positive, indicating dysfunction of the PTT. Finally, the examination is completed with neurologic examination for sensation and reflexes. Bilateral absence of Achilles tendon reflexes may indicate the presence of peripheral neuropathy and requires additional neurologic examinations.

RADIOGRAPHIC ASSESSMENT
Conventional Radiography

Standard anteroposterior and lateral radiographs of the ankle under weight-bearing conditions are obtained. In addition, the authors recommend hindfoot alignment or long axial views to measure the amount of valgus deformity.[6,7] To rule out adjacent joint arthritis, dorsoplantar and lateral radiographs of the foot are obtained. On the lateral view of the foot, flatfoot deformity can be measured using different angles. Most commonly, the talus-first metatarsal (Meary) and talocalcaneal angles are assessed to describe the deformity. On the mortise view, the congruency of the ankle joint can be judged and any subfibular impingement suspected. On the dorsoplantar view, the talus-first metatarsal angle can be measured. In case of forefoot abduction the angle becomes wider. In addition, the talus coverage angle helps to assess the abduction of the forefoot too. Midfoot arthritis or posttraumatic Lisfranc joint deformity can mimic the clinical appearance of stage II PTT dysfunction. If the apex of the deformity is noted to be at the tarsometatarsal joints with preservation of the alignment of the talonavicular joint, surgical correction is focused at the midfoot; most commonly, a realignment midfoot fusion is required. In the case of midfoot driving flatfoot, the algorithms discussed in this article do not apply.

Hindfoot Assessment

Saltzman and el-Khoury[8] introduced the hindfoot view, a modification of the Cobey view. Its superiority to visual judgment of hindfoot alignment and its correlation to pedobarographic load distributions after total ankle replacement have been confirmed. In addition, the hindfoot view has proven good to excellent intraobserver reliability. But interobserver reliability is low and clearly surpassed when using a long axial view only.[6] One of the drawbacks of the hindfoot view is its susceptibility to rotatory malpositioning of the foot. Thus, the measurements obtained with the hindfoot view have to be interpreted with caution. A far more reliable angle measurement can be done when using the long axial view or the medial and lateral borders of the calcaneus.[6]

Although preoperative assessment of hindfoot alignment under weight-bearing conditions is done in a standardized manner, there is no technique available to do so under non–weight-bearing conditions, such as during surgery. Min and Sanders[9] described varus-valgus referencing relative to the medial process of the posterior calcaneal tuberosity in the unloaded Mortise view. Its usefulness and feasibility will be the subject of future research.

Advanced Imaging

MRI and computed tomography allow precise 3-dimensional depiction of the bones and soft tissues. Therefore, they are mainly indicated for the evaluation of the medial ligamentous complex, spring ligament, PTT, and concomitant pathology such as peroneal tendinopathy, osteochondral lesions, or osteoarthritis. Ultrasonography is a quick and cost-effective means to assess disorders of the PTT. In a study by Nallamshetty and colleagues,[10] MRI and ultrasound imaging of the PTT have been found to be concordant in most cases investigated. However, the sensitivity of MRI is still superior. Ultrasound imaging is operator dependent but allows assessment of the PTT, the spring ligament, and tibiotalar and medial midfoot ligaments.

CONSERVATIVE TREATMENT

In patients with slight deformity or minor symptoms, nonoperative treatment can offer a viable strategy to help improve the condition. There are many treatment options available combining medication, cryotherapy, physical therapy, footwear modifications, and orthoses. In athletes, a cross-training design shoe provides good support of the longitudinal arch while allowing lateral motion activities and providing better hindfoot control. Orthoses may work well in patients with stage I PTT dysfunction. Alvarez and colleagues[11] published a protocol including the use of an orthosis together with high-repetition exercise program, aggressive plantarflexion activities, and stretching of the gastrocnemius and soleus muscles. After 4 months of treatment, 87% of patients reported a successful subjective and functional outcome. In contrast, Kulig and colleagues[12] presented a progressive eccentric tendon-loading and calf-stretching program with orthoses. All individuals treated by this program reported improvement regarding symptoms and function. Although each patient's foot is unique, the orthotic should be prescribed with hindfoot inversion and arch support. In the cases of fixed forefoot supination, addition of a medial forefoot wedge is important to support the forefoot during stance. Patients with a gastrocnemius contracture can also be treated with a heel lift to reduce the strain on the PTT. This wedge can be built into the custom orthotic, or an over-the-counter 0.25- to 0.5-in (0.6- to 1.2-cm) wedge may be used. In their daily shoe wear, avoidance of flat shoes is important to minimize strain on the PTT. Physical therapy can be initiated focusing on stretching of the gastrocnemius and PTT. Gastrocnemius stretching should be performed in athletic shoes with the orthotic in place to decrease strain across the hindfoot during exercise.

Those patients who are not able to fit in commercially available athletic or comfort footwear are candidates for custom-made shoes. Steb and Marzano[13] published a remarkable review article on the topic of nonoperative measures in flatfoot deformity. The authors suggest the readers to read this article for further information.

SURGICAL DECISION MAKING

When conservative measures fail (usually after a trial of 3–6 months), surgical treatment should be considered. Flatfoot deformity is a progressive disease. As long as there are healthy joints present, it is worth to use a joint-preserving technique to restore anatomy, to relieve pain, and to improve function.

Stage I Posterior Tibial Tendon Dysfunction

Surgical treatment in patients with stage I PTT dysfunction encompasses tenosynovectomy and debridement. Teasdall and Johnson[5] reported on the results in 19 patients. Of these, 14 patients (74%) reported complete relief of pain, 3 (16%) reported minor pain, 1 had moderate pain, and 1 continued to suffer severe pain. Sixteen patients (84%) felt much better and were able to perform a single-heel rise, indicating restored function of the PTT. Two patients did not benefit from the treatment and moved on to receive a subtalar fusion. This procedure was done mainly because of progressive deformity and pain. Although open surgery might be an option, endoscopic approaches have begun to evolve. Chow and colleagues[14] suggested tendoscopic debridement for stage I PTT dysfunction to avoid wound problems, to reduce pain, and to prevent scar formation.

Khazen and Khazen[15] reported the detailed technique of tendoscopy as a minimally invasive procedure to achieve synovectomy with promising results. Patients resumed work at 10 weeks and sports after 6 months. In these cases, careful inspection for a concomitant gastrocnemius contracture is important, and it should be released if noted to minimize the risk of recurrence.

Stage II Posterior Tibial Tendon Dysfunction

Selection of treatment depends on the type of stage II deformity. The authors base their decision on whether a mainly coronal plane or transversal plane deformity is present. Sometimes, and this is usually the case, the differences are distinct, and combinations of both may be present. Therefore, the apex of deformity should be sought to define the proper treatment strategy.

Flexible hindfoot valgus, no forefoot abduction

In patients with a flexible hindfoot valgus but no forefoot abduction, the authors prefer a simple medial sliding calcaneal osteotomy in conjunction with a transfer of the flexor digitorum longus (FDL) tendon. The osteotomy is effective and redirects forces transmitted through the Achilles tendon while moving the vector from eversion into inversion.[16] The calcaneus is approached through a lateral skin incision over the lateral wall of the calcaneus. The osteotomy is performed by means of an oscillating saw. In general, the tuberosity of the calcaneus is shifted medially by approximately 10 mm and then fixed with one or two 6.5-/7.3-mm screws. The use of a calcaneal osteotomy alone has shown to be insufficient to correct the whole flatfoot deformity. The authors almost always combine an osteotomy together with a transfer of the FDL tendon. The PTT is approached through a medial approach and its sheath opened. Any frayed tendon is debrided. The FDL tendon lies directly underneath the PTT and can be approached through the same incision. At the same time, an inspection of the spring ligament is performed. In case of rupture, the spring ligament can be reinserted by using suture anchors, which are placed into the navicular bone. The FDL is not detached. It is simply sutured onto the insertion of the PTT at the level of the navicular tuberosity. By doing so, the same lever arm of the PTT is used for the FDL transfer. The authors have discontinued the classic transfer technique rerouting the tendon through the navicular bone. The rest of the FDL is then sutured side to side to the PTT to reinforce the tendon.

Flexible hindfoot valgus, flexible forefoot supination
The same principle for osseous correction applies in these patients. However, as gastrocnemius contracture is thought to cause some of the forefoot supination, the authors may add, depending on intraoperative findings, a gastrocnemius release. The release can be done through a classic medial approach at the calf or proximal-medial.

Flexible hindfoot valgus, fixed forefoot supination
In case of fixed forefoot supination, the medial ray needs to be lowered to the ground to provide a competent base for stand. To achieve a lowering of the medial ray, the authors prefer the Cotton osteotomy (plantarflexion osteotomy of the medial cuneiform), which is performed through a dorsal approach.[17] After vertical osteotomy of the medial cuneiform, the bone is spread and filled with an autologous or allogenic allograft. At times there is need to secure the construct with a small plate, which is placed dorsally. In case of degenerative disease at the first TMT-I joint or additional hypermobility of the first ray, the authors add a modified Lapidus procedure.[18–21]

Flexible hindfoot valgus, forefoot abduction
In the practice of the authors this is the most common deformity found. A flatfoot deformity is always a 3-dimensional deformity and needs specific attention. In case of forefoot abduction, the authors prefer the lateral column lengthening (LCL) procedure.

According to Hentges and colleagues,[22] the LCL procedure reduces the inversion demand on PTT, reduces the Achilles force required to achieve heel rise, adducts and plantarflexes the midfoot in relation to the hindfoot, and creates a bowstringing effect that restores the longitudinal arch. After the anterior calcaneal osteotomy, an allograft bone is inserted to fill the gap. A study showed that allograft bone was safe and effective for LCL.[23] However, alternatively, autologous iliac crest graft can be used. Fixation is performed by using a 3.5-mm screw or a little plate placed laterally to the osteotomy.

Hintermann and colleagues[24] reported excellent results in 12 of 14 patients who underwent LCL for the treatment of PTT dysfunction. Oh and colleagues[25] showed similar results in adolescents and young adults, with a high number of patients resuming their original sports activities. All patients in that study received a combination of a medial sliding calcaneal osteotomy and LCL and FDL transfer. When performing an LCL, one must be careful not to overcorrect the deformity, as this results in hindfoot stiffness, lateral border foot pain, and decreased functional outcomes. Use of a trial when performing the osteotomy allows the surgeon to balance the amount of correction while ensuring that appropriate hindfoot motion is retained. The surgeon should err on the side of undercorrection to ensure appropriate hindfoot motion.

Medial ray instability
In case of simple medial ray instability due to hypermobility at the TMT-I joint, the authors perform a modified Lapidus procedure. However, in case of severe instability of the medial ray involving the TMT-I, naviculocuneiform, and talonavicular joints, extended (medial plate) or selected fusions (Miller procedure) may be needed to create a stable medial column.[26]

SUMMARY

Stage I and II PTT dysfunction can successfully be addressed by conservative and operative measures. The first-line treatment consists of nonoperative measures, with a high probability to return to sports activities.

Not much evidence is available in the literature regarding the return to sports after surgical treatment of stage II PTT dysfunction. However, there are reports revealing promising results. The authors conclude that running might be possible even after complex reconstructions of the flexible flatfoot deformity.

REFERENCES

1. Myerson M. Reconstructive foot and ankle surgery. Philadelphia: Elsevier-Saunders; 2005.
2. Bluman EM, Myerson MS. Stage IV posterior tibial tendon rupture. Foot Ankle Clin 2007;12(2):341–62, viii.
3. Iossi M, Johnson JE, McCormick JJ, et al. Short-term radiographic analysis of operative correction of adult acquired flatfoot deformity. Foot Ankle Int 2013; 34(6):781–91.
4. Perry J, Schoneberger B. Gait analysis: normal and pathological function. Thorofare (NJ): Slack Inc; 1992.
5. Teasdall RD, Johnson KA. Surgical treatment of stage I posterior tibial tendon dysfunction. Foot Ankle Int 1994;15(12):646–8.
6. Buck FM, Hoffmann A, Mamisch-Saupe N, et al. Hindfoot alignment measurements: rotation-stability of measurement techniques on hindfoot alignment view and long axial view radiographs. AJR Am J Roentgenol 2011;197(3):578–82.
7. Reilingh ML, Beimers L, Tuijthof GJ, et al. Measuring hindfoot alignment radiographically: the long axial view is more reliable than the hindfoot alignment view. Skeletal Radiol 2010;39(11):1103–8.
8. Saltzman CL, el-Khoury GY. The hindfoot alignment view. Foot Ankle Int 1995; 16(9):572–6.
9. Min W, Sanders R. The use of the mortise view of the ankle to determine hindfoot alignment: technique tip. Foot Ankle Int 2010;31(9):823–7.
10. Nallamshetty L, Nazarian LN, Schweitzer ME, et al. Evaluation of posterior tibial pathology: comparison of sonography and MR imaging. Skeletal Radiol 2005; 34(7):375–80.
11. Alvarez RG, Marini A, Schmitt C, et al. Stage I and II posterior tibial tendon dysfunction by a structured nonoperative management protocol: an orthosis and exercise program. Foot Ankle Int 2006;27(1):2–8.
12. Kulig K, Burnfield JM, Reischl S, et al. Effect of foot orthoses on tibialis posterior activation in persons with pes planus. Med Sci Sports Exerc 2005;37(1):24–9.
13. Steb HS, Marzano R. Conservative management of posterior tibial tendon dysfunction, subtalar joint complex, and pes planus deformity. Clin Podiatr Med Surg 1999;16(3):439–51.
14. Chow HT, Chan KB, Lui TH. Tendoscopic debridement for stage I posterior tibial tendon dysfunction. Knee Surg Sports Traumatol Arthrosc 2005;13(8):695–8.
15. Khazen G, Khazen C. Tendoscopy in stage I posterior tibial tendon dysfunction. Foot Ankle Clin 2012;17(3):399–406.
16. Chan JY, Williams BR, Nair P, et al. The contribution of medializing calcaneal osteotomy on hindfoot alignment in the reconstruction of the stage II adult acquired flatfoot deformity. Foot Ankle Int 2013;34(2):159–66.

17. Hirose CB, Johnson JE. Plantarflexion opening wedge medial cuneiform osteotomy for correction of fixed forefoot varus associated with flatfoot deformity. Foot Ankle Int 2004;25(8):568–74.
18. Young NJ, Zelen CM. New techniques and alternative fixation for the lapidus arthrodesis. Clin Podiatr Med Surg 2013;30(3):423–34.
19. Sorensen MD, Hyer CF, Berlet GC. Results of lapidus arthrodesis and locked plating with early weight bearing. Foot Ankle Spec 2009;2(5):227–33.
20. Sangeorzan BJ, Hansen ST Jr. Modified Lapidus procedure for hallux valgus. Foot Ankle 1989;9(6):262–6.
21. Maguire W. The Lapidus procedure for hallux valgus. J Bone Joint Surg Br 1973; 55:221.
22. Hentges MJ, Moore KR, Catanzariti AR, et al. Procedure selection for the flexible adult acquired flatfoot deformity. Clin Podiatr Med Surg 2014;31(3):363–79.
23. Dolan CM, Henning JA, Anderson JG, et al. Randomized prospective study comparing tri-cortical iliac crest autograft to allograft in the lateral column lengthening component for operative correction of adult acquired flatfoot deformity. Foot Ankle Int 2007;28(1):8–12.
24. Hintermann B, Valderrabano V, Kundert HP. Lengthening of the lateral column and reconstruction of the medial soft tissue for treatment of acquired flatfoot deformity associated with insufficiency of the posterior tibial tendon. Foot Ankle Int 1999;20(10):622–9.
25. Oh I, Williams BR, Ellis SJ, et al. Reconstruction of the symptomatic idiopathic flatfoot in adolescents and young adults. Foot Ankle Int 2011;32(3):225–32.
26. Cohen BE, Ogden F. Medial column procedures in the acquired flatfoot deformity. Foot Ankle Clin 2007;12(2):287–99, vi.

Stress Fractures of the Foot

Munier Hossain, FRCS (Orth), MSc (Orth Eng), MSc (Oxon)[a],
Juliet Clutton, MBBS, MRCS[a], Mark Ridgewell, MBBS, FFSEM, MSc (SEM)[b],
Kathleen Lyons, MBBS[b], Anthony Perera, MBChb, MFSEM, FRCS (Orth)[a,b,*]

KEYWORDS

- Stress fracture • Navicular • Metatarsal • Sports injury • Biological therapy

KEY POINTS

- Stress fractures are common in athletes.
- A high index of suspicion is appropriate and early investigation may prevent progression to frank fractures.
- Both navicular and fifth metatarsal (MT) stress fractures are considered high-risk fractures where early surgery may be more beneficial.
- There is limited evidence at present for biological treatment of stress fractures but biological agents may be useful adjuncts.
- Identification and alleviation of risk factors are essential parts of management of stress fractures.

INTRODUCTION

Stress fractures were first reported in military recruits but are not uncommon in athletes whose lower limbs are subjected to frequent submaximal loading. All bones of the lower extremity can sustain stress fractures but navicular and fifth MT fractures are at high risk of delayed union and nonunion.[1] Lack of appropriate diagnosis and conservative management of these injuries in the past have not always yielded satisfactory results.[2] A high index of suspicion, however, along with early investigation and proactive management that includes surgery where necessary can give good results and early resumption of physical activity.[2,3]

STRESS FRACTURE OF THE NAVICULAR
Pertinent Anatomy

The navicular bone is extensively covered by articular cartilage. The area available for blood supply is, therefore, limited and the navicular receives its blood supply via the dorsalis pedis and the posterior tibial arteries; these enter the bone via the dorsal

[a] Cardiff Regional Foot and Ankle Unit, University Hospital of Wales, Cardiff CF14 4XW, UK;
[b] Sports Medicine Department, Spire Cardiff Hospital, Croescadarn Road, Cardiff CF23 8XL, UK
* Corresponding author. Cardiff Regional Foot and Ankle Unit, University Hospital of Wales, Cardiff CF14 4XW, UK.
E-mail address: footandanklesurgery@gmail.com

Clin Sports Med 34 (2015) 769–790
http://dx.doi.org/10.1016/j.csm.2015.06.011
0278-5919/15/$ – see front matter © 2015 Elsevier Inc. All rights reserved.

sportsmed.theclinics.com

and plantar surfaces and the insertion of the tibialis posterior tendon. The vascular network branches out medially and laterally but the central third is relatively avascular. This area has been described as a watershed area and is the site most vulnerable to stress fractures and nounion.[4]

Biomechanics

The navicular bone is the link between the midfoot and the hindfoot. It is also the keystone of the medial longitudinal arch and anatomically related to the head of talus as well as the anterior process of the calcaneus. This anatomic proximity results in a coupling of movement between the talonavicular and the subtalar joint. A mobile talonavicular joint is critical for normal functioning of the subtalar joint. Therefore, a navicular stress fracture, if not treated appropriately, not only results in collapse of the medial longitudinal arch but also causes loss of supination.[5,6]

The navicular bone is maximally compressed during foot strike between the proximally located talar head and the distally located first and second metatarsocuneiform (MTC) joints. The navicular bone experiences maximum compressive forces during the end of the stance phase when the forefoot becomes loaded. Because of the unequal distribution of compressive forces between the first and the second MTC joints, maximum sheer stress is borne at the central third of navicular at the junction between the first and the second MTC joints.[7] This is also the watershed area of blood supply and, therefore, the most vulnerable to stress fractures. Therefore, fractures are more likely in track and field athletes and sprinters or jumpers in particular who engage in forceful push-off.

Risk Factors

Pes cavus, limited ankle dorsiflexion, restricted subtalar motion, short first MT, long second MT, and metatarsus adductus have all been proposed as predisposing factors for navicular stress fracture[7] (**Table 1**). The theory is that if ankle dorsiflexion is limited, the midfoot tends to compensate with a larger excursion, and this increased motion may result in navicular impingement in dorsiflexion. There is no compelling evidence implicating any of these anatomic factors.

Clinical Assessment

It is useful to have a high index of suspicion because clinical signs may be limited. In many of the reported series, delay in diagnosis was common and attributed to initial nonspecific and/or mild symptoms.[4] Patients typically present with activity-related dorsal or occasionally nonspecific pain that abates at rest. There may not be any obvious swelling or bruise. Pain may be aggravated on standing on tiptoes. In cases of late presentation, symptoms likely are more severe and can affect activities of daily living. In late stage there may be pain and tenderness over the dorsum of the navicular between the tendons of tibialis anterior and extensor hallucis longus. This area

Table 1 High- and low-risk stress fractures (foot and ankle)—summary of risk factors	
High Risk	**Low Risk**
Navicular	Calcaneus
Fifth MT	Cuboid
Medial malleolus	Cuneiform
Talus	Lateral malleolus
Sesamoid	

corresponds to the central third of the navicular and has been termed, *the N spot.*[3] Ankle strength and range of motion are likely normal. Patients may have a cavovarus foot and this should be specifically assessed. Although there is no clear evidence implicating this deformity in navicular stress fracture, a cavovarus foot is a relatively rigid structure and does not absorb the impact of weight bearing as well as a normal foot. Therefore, identification of this deformity and appropriate orthotic support and/or surgery are likely to prove beneficial for the athlete. As in any other sports-related injury, training issues like faulty technique, incorrect equipment, and overuse should also be carefully ruled out.

Investigations

Radiograph

The initial tool for investigation should be weight-bearing anteroposterior, lateral, and oblique views of the foot. Radiographs, however, may not show any obvious injury (**Fig. 1A**). There are 2 reasons for this low sensitivity. First, navicular stress fractures occur in the sagittal plane and involve the central third. It is difficult to get x-ray beams truly perpendicular to the fracture plane with normal radiologic views (see **Fig. 1A**). Besides, most of these fractures are incomplete and do not involve the plantar cortex and, therefore, are not visible until osteoclastic resorption has taken place (see **Fig. 1B**).[4] As such, if radiographs are negative and suspicions remain, further imaging is recommended.[4] Bone, Computed Tomography (CT), or MRI scan can be performed. There is no clear superiority of one investigation over another and each has its advantages.

Bone scan

Bone scan has high sensitivity but is nonspecific and should be not used as a first-line investigation; however, it can be helpful when CT and MRI fail to demonstrate a clear diagnosis.

CT scan

CT scan can delineate fracture lines accurately but requires thin slices and should be performed through the plane of the talonavicular joint. With early CT scans it was not uncommon for stress fractures to be missed; however, with modern scanners at 0.625 mm, this is now a reliable modality (see **Fig. 1C**). Saxena and colleagues[8] proposed a CT-based classification system based on the fracture pattern (**Box 1**). The stress fracture is best visualized on the coronal reformatted images.

CT scan can also be used to monitor healing. Clinical union, however, often precedes signs of radiologic union. The first radiologic sign of healing is dorsal cortical proliferation and can be seen as early as 6 weeks after injury (**Fig. 2**). Bony healing should be consolidated by 3 to 4 months but abnormalities like a medullary cyst or cortical notching may be persistent even after complete fracture healing.[9]

MRI scan

MRI scan is better at detecting bone edema and stress reaction before an impending fracture but is inferior to CT in identifying a stress fracture. When a stress fracture is suspected, the initial imaging modality should be CT to visualize the fracture line. If the CT does not demonstrate a fracture, an MRI is the next appropriate imaging modality to determine if a stress reaction has occurred (discussed later).

Differential Diagnosis

a. Navicular stress reaction (NSR): a stress reaction rather than a stress fracture is said to be present when a patient presents with identical symptoms and has similar changes in bone scan and MRI but no obvious fracture line in a CT scan. The

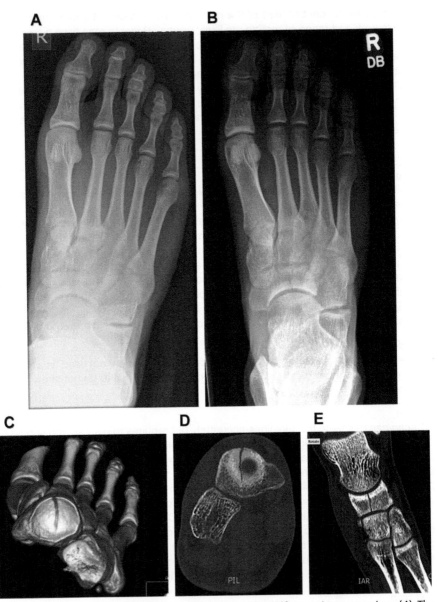

Fig. 1. An 18-year-old professional rugby player with midfoot pain on running. (*A*) The initial radiographs do not show any navicular injury. (*B*) Late films show the fracture line as resorption occurs. (*C–E*) The fracture line is clearly evident on the CT scan.

observed bony changes may be attempted bone remodeling in response to stress and a precursor to a frank stress fracture.[7] A regime of non–weight-bearing mobilization and gradual return to activities may prevent patients presenting with NSR progress to frank stress fracture.[4]

b. Osteochondritis dissecans: this condition is often confused with a stress fracture or a stress reaction. It usually affects the central third of the navicular just like a stress

Box 1
Classification of navicular stress fracture from Saxena and colleagues

Type 1: fracture involves dorsal cortex only

Type 2: fracture extends from dorsum onto the navicular body

Type 3: complete bicortical disruption.

From Saxena A, Fullem B, Hannaford D. Results of treatment of 22 navicular stress fractures and a new proposed radiographic classification system. J Foot Ankle Surg 2000:39(2);98.

injury and is most likely traumatic in etiology. In the authors' experience this typically affects athletes in their late teens to 20s although occasionally is seen beyond that age.

Unlike a stress injury, it presents with a cartilage injury, usually at the junction of the middle and medial thirds. This can lead to cyst formation just below the articular surface and occasionally there are several smaller cysts around it on the CT scan and a halo of high signal on the MRI denoting a more active lesion. Sometimes fragmentation is seen.

This lesion starts dorsally and proximally and heads distally but does not extend plantarward (**Fig. 3**). The other major difference is that in the senior authors' experience (KL and AP) it does not progress into a stress fracture. It is often self-limiting with conservative treatment (injection, rest, support, and activity modification) and if

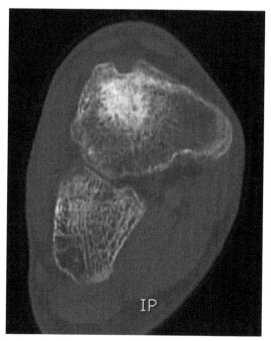

Fig. 2. Healing navicular stress fracture in a 19-year-old male rugby player; the fracture line has filled in and there is a dorsal cortical proliferation typical of this condition.

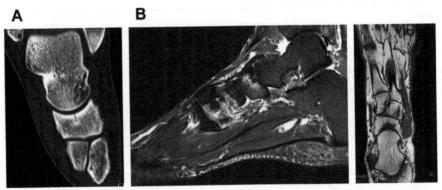

Fig. 3. (A) Early osteochondritis dissecans in a 17-year-old female athlete. (B) Late-stage chronic osteochondritis dissecans that was found on MRI in a 41-year-old man who presented with a recent-onset plantar fascia tear. Despite the extensive size of the lesion and the chronicity of the cyst (as evidenced by the sclerosis and lack of edema), there has been no plantar extension. A bone scan or single-photon emission CT scan can be used if there is a question about how active this lesion is. If indicated, surgery would be in the form of grafting from above rather than screw fixation.

surgery is required bone grafting rather than fixation is usually successful with a high return to play even in elite athletes. If the articular damage is significant, then the prognosis for return to play is poor.

Therapeutic Options and/or Surgical Technique

There is limited good-quality evidence in the literature and general disagreement regarding the best treatment options. No clear guidelines can, therefore, be produced. Stress fractures of the lower extremity, however, have been divided into high- and low-risk groups that predict the possible risk of progression to delayed and/or nonunion and guide management.[1]

Small retrospective case series comparing surgery with conservative treatment did not find any difference in outcome between the 2 modes of treatment. These were not controlled trials, however, and the treatment groups were not equal. Additionally, these series had small sample sizes that may not have been adequately powered to detect a treatment difference. Published literature is also rife with incomplete reporting, lack of validated outcome tools, and no clear indication of follow-up length. Several investigators performed meta-analyses of different treatment options and concluded that a non–weight-bearing cast is the treatment of choice for incomplete fractures or complete but nondisplaced fractures.[10–12] The investigators found limited weight bearing of limited use and advised against it as an initial treatment option; 6 to 8 weeks of non–weight-bearing mobilization is recommended. If there is no tenderness after 6 to 8 weeks, patients can be allowed to start rehabilitation and plan gradual return to sports (**Box 2**).

Saxena and colleagues[8] suggested a treatment algorithm based on their proposed fracture classification. They advised nonoperative treatment of type 1 fractures and surgery for type 2 and 3 fractures. Other investigators have suggested that elite athletes with type 1 fracture may benefit from surgery with earlier return to sports. There is limited evidence to support the assertion that primary surgery may help athletes return to sports early and/or reduce the rate of refractures. A recent article, however, from Jacob and Paterson[13] showed promising results of primary surgery and early

---

Box 2
Recommended non–weight-bearing regime from de Clercq and colleagues

0 To 6 wk: non–weight bear

6 To 8 wk: weight bear as able in removable cast

8 To 10 wk: weight bear out of cast, resistive strengthening exercise, light jogging

10 To 12 wk: full running, sport-specific training

Greater than 12 wk: full return to sports

Patients progress to the next stage only if they remain asymptomatic.

From de Clercq PFG, Bevernage BD, Leemrijse T. Stress fracture of the navicular bone. Acta Orthop Belg 2008;74(6):725–34.

---

weight bearing in a small series of athletes, although 7 of 11 of those were incomplete fractures.[13] This study used a single lag screw and postoperatively allowed weight bearing as tolerated. This is the practice of the senior author (AP) and the results have been similar, with a low rate of complications; thus, there is lower threshold for surgery in elite athletes although a period of conservative management ought to be trialed first and a noninvasive bone stimulator may be used.

Surgery is the treatment of choice for displaced fractures, delayed union, or nonunion.[14] Surgery is performed via either the percutaneous or the open approach.[4] Two commonest approaches have been described: longitudinal incision between the tendons of tibialis anterior and tibialis posterior or more dorsally just medial to the neurovascular bundle.[15] Any sclerotic bone should be removed and the gap impacted with bone graft and the fracture stabilized with 2 screws. Both parallel and cross-screw configurations have been described. Exact trajectory of the screws depends on the site of the fracture but 2 partially threaded, parallel, cannulated screws placed lateral to medial are most likely to gain maximum bony purchase. The first screw should be sited proximal and dorsal and the second screw distal and plantar to not interfere with each other. Because of the shape of the navicular, it is imperative to confirm with fluoroscopy that the screws do not violate the joint. The authors' preferred technique is to use iliac crest bone graft (either cancellous graft or aspirate). Because of the difficulty of achieving anatomic reduction, Hsu and Lee[16] recently advocated the use of intraoperative CT scan. This may be a useful technique in difficult cases.

Postoperatively patients should be kept non–weight bearing for 6 to 8 weeks and rehabilitation commenced thereafter. A CT scan should be performed to confirm bony healing before athletes are allowed to resume sports. Again hyperbaric oxygen or a noninvasive bone stimulator can be useful in elite athletes given the long period of recovery, although there are few data to support its use.

Clinical Outcomes

Clinical outcome depends on the severity of the fracture.[17] The more severe the fracture the longer it takes for the navicular to heal. On average it takes 4 months for a fracture to be united and 5 months before athletes are able to return to sports.[12] Data from small series with medium term follow-up suggest that up to 50% of patients may not be able to return to the same level of sports after a stress fracture.[2] Many patients continue to complain of pain and remain tender over the N spot despite showing signs of radiologic healing. There is limited evidence to suggest that pain and tenderness may be marginally more common after surgery.[18] Because of the risk of nonunion and delayed union, some investigators have suggested a repeat CT/MRI and radiologic signs of healed fracture before athletes are allowed to return to sports.[4]

Complications and Concerns

Complications of navicular stress fracture include delayed union, nonunion, refracture, persistent pain, and degenerative arthritis. Because of the heterogeneity of cases and treatment given it is difficult to calculate the true rate of complications. This seems further complicated by the findings of some series that have demonstrated persistent tenderness and/or CT scan changes despite clinical evidence of union.[11,18] Nonunion rate seems low, however, whether patients are treated conservatively with non–weight-bearing immobilization or with surgery. Management of nonunion is difficult and prone to failure. Toren and colleagues[19] in a recent report described talonavicular and naviculocuneiform arthrodesis augmented by vascularized scapular free bone graft. Saxena and Fullem's[17] series suggest that up to 25% of patients may progress to delayed union.

METATARSAL STRESS FRACTURES

MT stress fractures are common among athletes. Stress fractures of the second or the fifth MT are more common than the rest. Both acute and stress fractures are common in the fifth MT but the presentation as well as location differs. Because of the unique anatomy and differing function it is conventional to group MT fractures into fractures of the medial column (first MT), central column (second–third MT), and the lateral column (fourth–fifth MT).

Anatomy

The 5 MT bones are not of uniform shape. The first MT is the stoutest and bears maximum weight. The first MT bears approximately one-third of the total body weight. Any displacement of the first MT is poorly tolerated and results in loss of normal weight-bearing function. The second MT is the longest and sustains the greatest stresses during normal weight bearing. The second tarso-MT joint (TMT) is a stable joint and affords little movement. Consequently the second MT is the least mobile of all MT.

The MT bones have strong ligamentous attachments to each other and to the tarsal and phalangeal bones proximally as well as distally. The MT heads are united by deep transverse MT ligaments that bind them together. Because of this arrangement, isolated fractures usually do not displace significantly.

Deforming forces for MT fractures include the flexor digotorum longus and the intrinsic muscles. They pull the distal fragment to plantar flexion so that the MT head is displaced plantar and proximal. If left unreduced, the resulting deformity can increase localized loading and result in metatarsalgia and intractable plantar keratosis. Stress fractures, however, usually do not show much displacement.

Both the fourth and the fifth MTs are strongly attached to the cuboid. They are subject to traction stress and may, therefore, be prone to delayed healing. The fifth MT also articulates with the fourth MT medially. The base of the fifth MT gives attachment to the tendons of the peroneus brevis (PB) and the peroneus tertius (PT) on the dorsal surface and the plantar aponeurosis (PA) on the plantar surface. PB is attached to the tuberosity.[20] The dorsal surface of the fifth MT base receives PT insertion that extends along the dorsal surface of the shaft for some variable distance.[21]

The proximal diaphysis of the fifth MT is supplied by a short recurrent single nutrient artery. The tuberosity of the fifth MT is supplied by numerous metaphyseal arteries. A watershed area exists between these 2 sources of blood supply and is located at the proximal metadiaphyseal junction distal to the tuberosity. This area is prone to delayed and/or nonunion after a stress fracture.

Biomechanics

The foot shape has been divided into 3 types: the Egyptian foot is the most common type and is characterized by a longer great toe; the Greek foot has a longer second toe; and the square foot has relatively equal toes. Maestro and colleagues[22] proposed the concept of a harmonious foot shape and argued that MT length was an important factor in determining forefoot load distribution during weight bearing. They described forefoot movement in relation to a fixed second MT bone and argued that goal of surgery should be to restore MT parabola (**Fig. 4**). There is no clear evidence, however, of any relation between MT length and stress fracture. A recent study found that MT length did not correlate with peak plantar loading pressure.[23,24]

A study investigating loading conditions of the lesser MT found that maximum stress occurred within 3 to 4 cm of the proximal end of the lesser MT. This area generally corresponds to the typical location of stress fracture.[25] Although the first MT fracture is typically found proximally, the second to fourth MTs usually fracture in midshaft or more distally. The second MT is subjected to the highest bending stress and is most prone to stress fractures. Women may be more prone to this injury because they have a higher middle forefoot loading than men.

Although the MT heads are located at the same plane distally, the bases are stacked proximally, forming the transverse arch. The apex of this proximal transverse arch is formed by the base of the second MT. The MTs are all flexed distally and contribute to the longitudinal arch on the sagittal plane. Because of the relative height of the bases of the first and the fifth MTs, the height of the medial longitudinal arch is more pronounced than the lateral longitudinal arch. The PA supports the longitudinal arch of the foot. It elevates and depresses the arch by the windlass and the reverse windlass mechanism respectively. PA has an effect on modulating forefoot stress. Sectioning of the PA increases MT strain on weight bearing to 100% of normal values.

Risk Factors

Risk factors for MT stress fractures generally are divided into several categories (**Box 3**).

Clinical Assessment

Patients may present acutely with a complaint of sudden aggravation of chronic pain and inability to weight bear or with a long history of dull aching pain aggravated by

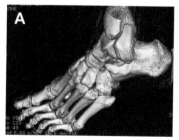
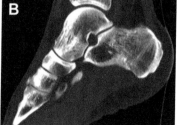

Fig. 4. (*A*) 3-D reconstruction shows that the periosteal reaction is all dorsal on this stress fracture of the MT. (*B*) The sagittal section of the same injury shows the resultant dorsal injury and slight dorsal elevation at the fracture site.

Box 3
Summary of risk factors for metatarsal stress fracture

General factors

  Female gender

Metabolic

  Hormonal imbalance, absence of regular menstruation

  Female athlete triad

Anorexia

Occupation

  Athlete: any sports involving repetitive jumping, cutting, landing, long distance running; ballet dance; tennis; basketball

  Military personnel

Training related

  Sudden increase in intensity or duration of training

  Poor physical conditioning

  Training on hard surface

  Poor footwear

Local factors

  Bony abnormalities

    Ankle varus, hindfoot varus, and forefoot supination can all increase the stress on the lateral forefoot and the fourth/fifth MT.

    Metatarsus adductus is a risk factor for both fourth and fifth MT stress fractures.

    Reduced bone density

  Soft tissue abnormalities

    Muscle imbalance especially gastrocnemus contracture.

  Poor blood supply

    Pes planus also increases local strain.

    Muscle fatigue increases local strain and may contribute to stress fracture of the MT.

---

physical activity. Late presenters may also develop a limp. Swelling may not be present initially but point tenderness, if present, is said to be diagnostic. Depending on the time of presentation swelling, ecchymosis and palpable callus may also be present.

A thorough history should be taken to elicit any possible risk factors and, if present, threshold for investigation should be low. Clinical examination should be systematic and specifically assess gait, hindfoot alignment, any deformity, flexibility of deformity, tendo Achilles tightness, range of motion of ankle, and callosity at the lateral border.

First Metatarsal Stress Fracture

First MT stress fractures are rare. There are reports of proximal base stress fracture that healed with conservative management.[26]

Second to Third Metatarsal Stress Fracture

The most common area for these fractures is just proximal to the MT neck. More proximal fractures at the base, however, have been reported in ballet dancers as well as athletes.[27] Distal fractures usually have a good prognosis and heal well with conservative management. Proximal fractures, on the other hand, are at high risk of delayed and nonunion (**Fig. 5**). A case-control study found that those with proximal fracture are more likely to have a short first toe, tibialis anterior tightness, and low bone mass and experience multiple fractures.[28] Extreme plantar flexion, as practiced by ballet dancers, may increase the risk of proximal fractures.

Fourth to Fifth Metatarsal Stress Fracture

Proximal fourth MT stress fracture occurring at the metadiaphyseal junction behaves similar to fifth MT stress fractures and is prone to delayed union.[29] More distal fractures are also reported that are more amenable to conservative management.[30]

Patients with cavus foot are especially at risk of fifth MT stress fracture. Lee and colleagues[31] found an association between elevated calcaneal pitch and fifth MT fractures in athletes. Both acute and stress fractures are common in fifth MT but the presentation as well as the site differs. The eponymous term, Jones fracture, has given rise to widespread confusion in the literature between an acute fracture and a stress fracture. It may be best to discontinue use of eponymous terms and describe fractures according to anatomic site because stress fractures of the fifth MT have a typical presentation and most importantly they occur at a specific site (**Fig. 6**). Logan and colleagues[32] proposed a simplified classification system that may be of use especially to define the site of the stress fracture (**Box 4**). According to this classification, a Jones fracture is a type III injury and a stress fracture is a type IV injury. Typical stress fracture of the fifth MT occurs more distal to the site of the

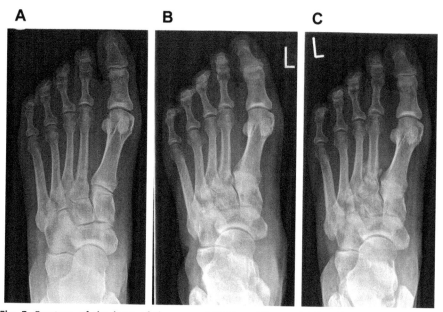

A   **B**   **C**

Fig. 5. Fracture of the base of the second MT in a 36-year-old female marathon runner. (*A*) At first presentation, the fracture line is visible at the base; this area is difficult to off-load and can be associated with nonunion or, in this case (*B*, *C*), with delayed union characterized but a significant callus reaction.

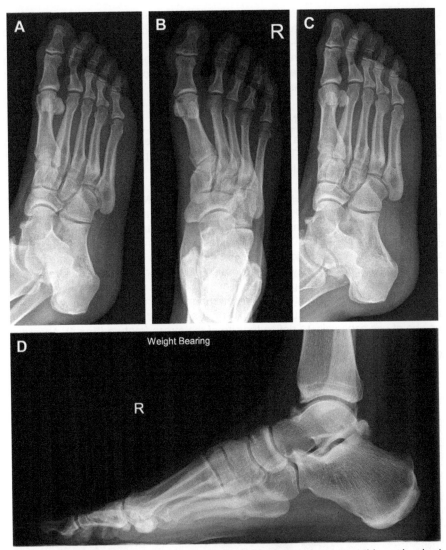

Fig. 6. A 28-year-old male soccer player. (*A, B*) The fracture line is just visible at the classic site on the oblique view but not on the DP view. (*C*) As it heals, there is first resorption at the fracture site (*D*) and then cortical healing and remodeling.

Jones fracture. Type III fractures also have a tendency to go into delayed and nonunion but they are not typically stress fractures. Also, there may be some overlap in anatomic site of the injury. Clinical assessment and x-ray examination, however, should be able to differentiate between the 2. A stress fracture has a prodromal history and may have risk factors, and radiograph shows changes typical of stress fracture rather than a clean radiolucent line of an acute fracture. Torg and colleagues[33] divide fifth MT stress fractures into 3 types (**Box 5**). Surgery is recommended for types 2 and 3.

Box 4
Classification of fifth metatarsal fracture from Logan and colleagues

Type I: at the junction of extra- and intra-articular parts of the tuberosity

Type II: at the proximal fourth–fifth intermetatarsal joint

Type III: at the distal fourth–fifth intermetatarsal joint

Type IV: more distally in the diaphysis

From Logan AJ, Dabke H, Finlay D, et al. Fifth metatarsal base fractures: a simple classification. Foot Ankle Surg 2007;13(1):30–4.

Investigation

Vitamin D

There is a growing awareness of the importance of the role of vitamin D, with multiple studies showing that it is frequently low in fracture patients, particularly in Northern Europe. In the senior author's experience, in a series of 30 consecutive fifth MT fractures, including cases of acute trauma as well as stress fractures, 25% had marked deficiency and 40% had insufficiency. All patients should be tested for this because even some elite and international-level athletes were found to have hypovitaminosis, some among the lowest levels.[34]

Radiograph

Radiographs should include weight-bearing AP, lateral, and oblique views of the foot. Early radiograph may not show any changes but a periosteal reaction is seen in the subacute stage with abundant callus formation in late stage. The radiographs can be repeated after 2 weeks and the healing reaction may be seen but approximately half of MT stress fractures never have clear changes on the plain films. Periosteal reaction is uncommon in the first MT, which instead usually shows linear sclerosis.

Ultrasound

Ultrasound is generally the most easily accessible modality for further investigation; most professional teams have access to an ultrasound scan and fortunately it can be extremely sensitive and helpful in diagnosing early stress reaction. The periosteal reaction and edema can be identified in cases where radiographs may be normal because the stress reaction generally commences dorsally (**Fig. 7**).

Box 5
Classification for fifth metatarsal stress fractures from Torg and colleagues

Type 1: periosteal reaction, early stress fracture

Type 2: widened fracture line and intramedullary sclerosis, delayed union

Type 3: complete obliteration on intramedullary canal, established nonunion.

From Torg JS, Balduini FC, Zelko RR, et al. Fractures of the base of the fifth metatarsal distal to the tuberosity. Classification and guidelines for non-surgical and surgical management. J Bone Joint Surg Am 1984;66(2):209–14.

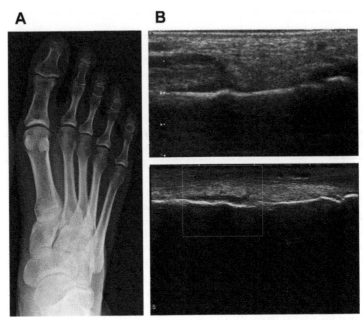

Fig. 7. A second MT stress fracture in 28-year-old female triathlete. (*A*) Despite the classic presenting features, the radiographs do not show any obvious pathology. (*B*) An ultrasound performed on the same day shows peristeal elevation and thickening and also dorsal cortical irregularity.

MRI

MRI is helpful especially in early cases and may reveal bony edema before a fracture becomes evident (**Fig. 8**). Major[35] has reported that early MRI-revealed bony changes may also allow preventive measures to be taken to prevent development of a frank stress fracture. This can have a critical role in managing players at risk.

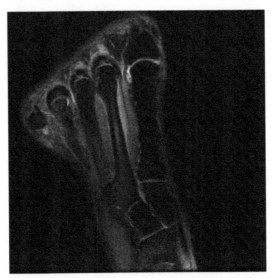

Fig. 8. A 31-year-old soccer player with early mild and vague forefoot pains; an MRI showed a prefracture bone reaction that was managed conservatively.

Bone scan

Bone scan is helpful when a radiograph is negative but clinical suspicion remains. Bone scan shows changes in early phase of injury. It is positive in all 3 phases in case of stress fracture in contrast to soft tissue injury, which is only positive in the first phase.

Treatment

Conservative treatment is the mainstay of treatment of MT stress fractures. Initial treatment is conservative with activity modification until symptoms subside. Romani and colleagues[36] have recommended a detailed 3-phase rehabilitation program that takes into account the physiology of stress fracture repair.

Phase I: this phase lasts from 1 to 3 weeks. The emphasis of this phase is to remove stress, control pain, and allow bone to commence healing with angiogenesis and periosteal and osteocyte maturation. Limited weight bearing with crutches is recommended. Patients can be provided with a hard sole shoe, off-the-shelf walker boot, or a short leg walking cast. Ice massage may help improve swelling. Patients who have delayed union may benefit from a period of immobilization in a non–weight-bearing cast. Patients should be allowed to gradually increase weight bearing from partial to full weight bearing as tolerated. Lower extremity conditioning exercises are also recommended at this stage. These include towel toe curl, ankle isometrics, and so forth. This phase is taken to be completed when normal activities become pain-free.

Phase II: this phase lasts for 2 to 3 weeks after resolution of pain. The focus of this stage is general conditioning and strengthening specific to the injured extremity. Ice compression is continued, pool training should progress from walking to jogging, and wobble board exercise can also include weight bearing. The aim of this phase is to be able to fully weight bear without pain for at least 30 minutes 3 times a week.

Phase III: activities at this stage aim to allow gradual remodeling of the bone. This phase alternates with 2 weeks of gradually increasing stress followed by a week of rest. It is thought that alternating between stress and rest helps the osteocytes and periosteum to mature quicker at this stage. Patients are allowed running and functional activities and progress to plyometrics.

Surgery

Surgery is mainly proposed for delayed union or nonunion. It is useful to consider surgery, however, as the primary treatment of high-risk fractures that are more prone to delayed union, especially in athletes wishing to return to activity sooner. Open reduction and internal fixation are recommended. Bone graft is not required for surgical fixation of an acute fracture and is generally recommended for management of delayed union and nonunion. Because of concerns regarding nonunion, however, some investigators have elected to augment acute fracture fixation with bone graft and have reported earlier return to sports.

Fifth MT: surgery is recommended for Torg types II and III fractures.[33] Logan and colleagues,[32] however, advised primary surgery for stress fractures displaced more than 2 mm. Intramedullary screw fixation augmented with autologous bone graft may give better results compared with screw fixation alone. A partially threaded cannulated screw is technically easier to insert. There are reports of headless compression screw fixation as well but this is not widely favored.[37] A minimum diameter of 4 mm is recommended but Tsukada and colleagues[38] recommended the largest diameter screw should be inserted that fits the width of the medullary canal. The screw should remain intramedullary and avoid the cuboid or the fourth/fifth intermetatarsal joint. The screw tip should avoid contact with the dorsal cortex to avoid risk of stress fracture. The proximal fifth MT has a dorsal convex curvature that is pronounced in some patients. In these cases the screw should be sited more dorsal and aimed toward the sole of the foot to align the screw as closely as possible to the bone axis.[38] The CT study of Ochenjele and colleagues[39] demonstrated that for a majority of patients (male and female), the narrowest point of the shaft was 5 mm and, therefore, recommended using a 5-mm screw. Furthermore, they were able to show that the average straight segment was 50 mm from the base and that using a screw of 50 mm or less in length would avoid having an impact on the cortex at the bow.

Patients are kept non–weight bearing in the postoperative period. A controlled ankle movement walker boot may be a better option than a cast to offload the fifth MT postoperatively.[40]

Complications

Both delayed union and nonunion can complicate MT stress fractures after conservative management as well as after surgical fixation. Therefore, several investigators recommend adjuvant bone grafting at the time of surgical fixation of acute stress fractures.[37] Investigators have also advised against earlier resumption of sports after surgery to reduce the risk of delayed and/or nonunion but there are not enough data to support their claim. Recurrent fracture is also a risk especially if risk factors are not recognized and treated. Earlier return to sports is a risk factor for recurrent fracture and functional bracing or orthotics may be useful to reduce the risk. Lee and colleagues[41] proposed "plantar gap" as a prognostic factor for time to union as well as nonunion after tension band wiring of fifth MT stress fracture.

Plantar gap is the distance between the fracture margins on the plantar lateral side of the fifth MT bone and is best viewed on an oblique radiograph of the foot. The same investigators also found that patients with high body mass index and a protruding fifth MT had high risk of recurrent fracture.[42]

STRESS FRACTURE OF THE CALCANEUS

The clinical features are generally straightforward; typically, a distance runner presents with resting pain. Bone health is often an issue, particularly in female runners with the terrible triad, and vitamin D may be low. Radiographs can be helpful but either CT scan (**Figs. 9** and **10**) or MRI is reliable.

Treatment with rest, immobilization, and graduated return to sport is reliable.

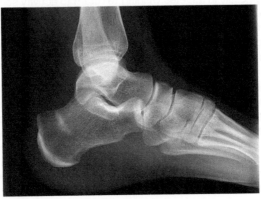

Fig. 9. Plain film radiograph of a 23-year-old male elite runner with a calcaneal stress fracture.

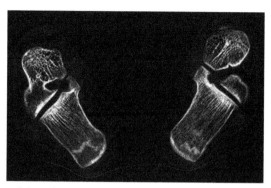

Fig. 10. CT imaging of the calcaneal stress fracture shows that this commences dorsolaterally although it can extend the whole way medially and inferiorly as it deteriorates.

OTHER STRESS FRACTURES

In the authors' experience, stress fractures of the cuboid are almost invariably only seen in female athletes, primarily runners. Surprisingly, a cavus foot pattern is not always present; generally, the foot is mobile and this may be the etiologic factor. Conservative treatment is reliable although orthotics may be required.

Stress fracture of the sesamoid usually affects the medial bone. The foot presents with rest pain and swelling and it is uncomfortable to walk without cushioned footwear or orthotics. Radiographs are difficult to interpret and CT is scan is the most useful modality. If conservative treatment with rest, boot, orthotics, and possibly injections has failed, then partial sesamoidectomy is the surgery of choice. Athletes must be warned, however, that return to play is expected but difficult to predict, particularly in barefoot sports.

GENERAL PRINCIPLES OF TREATMENT OF FOOT AND ANKLE STRESS FRACTURES

A stress fracture occurs when the mechanical forces outweigh the biological abilities of the bone. It is, therefore, essential to ensure that the forces are minimized and the biology is optimized.

Biomechanical Therapy for Stress Fractures

Rest and activity modification are key components in the treatment of a stress fracture. They can be a challenge in athletes in-season and one must work closely with the therapists, trainer, player, agent, and so forth so that everyone is on board with the treatment goals and criteria for return to play. Sometimes this may mean complete rest, even non–weight bearing, for a period; however, it is essential to consider cross-training, such as cycling, rowing, and swimming, to maintain cardiovascular fitness and lower limb strength. It may be possible to continue to run but to alter the nature of the training, mixing the program, type of surface, and so forth. An antigravity treadmill or even hydrotherapy can be used to get a player running with a reduced impact on the foot.

Abnormal loading may occur in the presence of abnormal alignment that requires orthotic correction and shock absorption, although these are perhaps most useful in prevention rather than treatment. It can also occur in the presence of normal alignment, for instance, due to a muscle imbalance, in particular, a tight gastrocnemius or due to the running style. These need careful evaluation and management but that these may be factors that allowed an athlete to excel prior to injury.

Biological Therapy for Management of Stress Fractures

Several adjuvant treatments strategies, such as bone morphogenic protein (BMP), shock wave therapy (SWT), low-intensity pulsed ultrasound therapy (LIPUS), teriparatide, electromagnetic stimulation, and hyperbaric oxygen have been recommended in the literature to enhance fracture healing. On review of the literature, it is difficult to make a firm conclusion on their effectiveness because of the heterogeneity of patient population and the interventions offered as well as different outcome measures considered. Some have used them as adjuvant to surgical therapy and others have used them for delayed union or nonunion. Where biological therapy has been used as adjuvant to surgical treatment, autograft remains the gold standard. In addition, most of the published reports are of case series rather than controlled trials. There are often animal data as well as physiologic explanations, however, regarding their effectiveness. Evidence base at present is not strong and it may be best to decide on their application on an individual basis rather than take a blanket approach on their effectiveness. Many of these modalities have little or no evidence for use in foot and ankle stress fractures, for instance, bisphosphonates, hyperbaric oxygen, electromagnetic stimulation, and low-level laser treatment, although they are in use in elite sports.[43]

Shock wave therapy

SWT acts by up-regulating proteins essential for angiogenesis and by increasing the local concentration of growth factors. Several case series have been published showing satisfactory healing and earlier return to sports after SWT treatment after established nonunion of chronic stress fractures of the lower extremity.[44,45] There is no high-quality evidence, however, supporting these results.

Low-intensity pulsed ultrasound therapy

LIPUS has been proposed as another mode of treatment of management of nonunion or delayed union. A recent systematic review concluded, however, that LIPUS management did not reduce the time to return to work for nonoperatively treated stress fractures.[46]

Electrical stimulation

Electrical stimulation (ES) therapy is provided via several modes: direct current, capacitative coupling, inductive coupling, and pulsed electromagnetic field. Although there is some difference in how these modes work, in general, there is evidence that endochondral bone formation may be appropriately stimulated by application of an electromagnetic field. Laboratory specimens demonstrated enhanced cell proliferation, calcification, and increased mechanical strength when stimulated with electrical current. They may also stimulate growth factor expression. Several studies have reported improved bone healing using ES for nonunions. There is little evidence, however, for their use in stress fractures. Beck and colleagues[47] found that ES did not accelerate healing in tibial stress fracture compared with placebo. The investigators claimed that there was a trend for quicker healing in more severe stress fractures. Post hoc subgroup analyses of this nature, however, require careful validation that is lacking at present.

Bone morphogenic protein

There is also an interest in use of BMP to augment fracture healing. BMPs belong to transforming growth factor β superfamily proteins and act as osteoinductive agents. Several BMPs have been isolated. Both BMP2 and BMP7 have been in wide use and also subjected to clinical trials. Results of the BMP-2 Evaluation in Surgery for Tibial Trauma trial supported the use of BMP for management of open tibial fractures.[48] There is, however, no evidence to support its use in stress fractures.

Teriparatide

Teriparatide is a bone anabolic agent that is approved for management of osteoporosis. It is a recombinant human parathyroid hormone analogue. It stimulates new bone formation by stimulating osteoblasts. Results of a randomized controlled trail found that teriparatide shortened the time to fracture healing compared with placebo.[49] There have been case reports of earlier healing of stress fractures using teriparatide but no controlled trials as yet.[50]

SUMMARY

Navicular stress fracture is more likely in athletes who are involved in sports that require explosive push-off. It is important to have a high index of suspicion for timely diagnosis because delays are common. Symptoms may be vague and nonspecific and fracture may not be visible on initial radiograph. Incomplete and undisplaced fractures should initially be treated with non–weight-bearing immobilization for 6 to 8 weeks. Surgery is the treatment of choice for displaced fractures or nonunion. Immediate percutaneous surgery and early weight bearing seem a promising alternative to prolong immobilization but further studies are needed.

Natural history and the risk factors of MT stress fractures are now better understood. Therefore, a high index of suspicion as well as early investigation and appropriate management can give satisfactory functional outcome. Primary surgery combined with autologous bone graft may be a suitable management option for athletes wishing to return to sports early.[51,52] Evidence for management is not strong; therefore, before planning management it is good practice to conduct a thorough discussion of risk-benefit ratio with patients and make a shared decision. Risk of recurrence can be reduced by identifying and managing risk factors. There is fair-quality evidence from randomized controlled trials that supplementation of vitamin D and calcium reduced the rate of stress fractures among female navy recruits.[53] Biological therapy may also turn out to be a promising treatment strategy but remains unproved at present.

REFERENCES

1. Mayer SW, Joyner PW, Almekinders LC, et al. Stress fractures of the foot and ankle in athletes. Sports Health 2014;6(6):481–91.
2. Burne SG, Mahoney CM, Forster BB, et al. Tarsal navicular stress injury: long-term outcome and clinicoradiological correlation using both computed tomography and magnetic resonance imaging. Am J Sports Med 2005;33(12):1875–81.
3. de Clercq PFG, Beverage BD, Leemrijse T. Stress fracture of the navicular bone. Acta Orthop Belg 2008;74(6):725–34.
4. Mann JA, Pedowitz DI. Evaluation and treatment of navicular stress fractures, including nonunions, revision surgery, and persistent pain after treatment. Foot Ankle Clin 2009;14(2):187–204.
5. Kapandji IA. The physiology of the joints: annotated diagrams of the mechanics of the human joints. 2nd edition. London: Churchill Livingstone; 1970.
6. van Langelaan EJ. A kinematical analysis of the tarsal joints. An X-ray photogrammetric study. Acta Orthop Scand Suppl 1983;204:1–269.

7. Lee S, Anderson RB. Stress fractures of the tarsal navicular. Foot Ankle Clin 2004; 9(1):85–104.

8. Saxena A, Fullem B, Hannaford D. Results of treatment of 22 navicular stress fractures and a new proposed radiographic classification system. J Foot Ankle Surg 2000;39(2):96–103.

9. Tuthill HL, Finkelstein ER, Sanchez AM, et al. Imaging of tarsal navicular disorders: a pictorial review. Foot Ankle Spec 2014;7(3):211–25.

10. Fowler JR, Gaughan JP, Boden BP, et al. The non-surgical and surgical treatment of tarsal navicular stress fractures. Sports Med 2011;41(8):613–9.

11. Khan KM, Fuller PJ, Brukner PD, et al. Outcome of conservative and surgical management of navicular stress fracture in athletes. Eighty-six cases proven with computerized tomography. Am J Sports Med 1992;20(6):657–66.

12. Torg JS, Moyer J, Gaughan JP, et al. Management of tarsal navicular stress fractures: conservative versus surgical treatment: a meta-analysis. Am J Sports Med 2010;38(5):1048–53.

13. Jacob KM, Paterson RS. Navicular stress fractures treated with minimally invasive fixation. Indian J Orthop 2013;47(6):598–601.

14. Fitch KD, Blackwell JB, Gilmour WN. Operation for non-union of stress fracture of the tarsal navicular. J Bone Joint Surg Br 1989;71(1):105–10.

15. Choi LE, Chou LB. Surgical treatment of tarsal navicular stress fractures. Oper Tech Sports Med 2006;14(4):248–51.

16. Hsu AR, Lee S. Evaluation of tarsal navicular stress fracture fixation using intraoperative O-arm computed tomography. Foot Ankle Spec 2014;7(6):515–21.

17. Saxena A, Fullem B. Navicular stress fractures: a prospective study on athletes. Foot Ankle Int 2006;27(11):917–21.

18. Potter NJ, Brukner PD, Makdissi M, et al. Navicular stress fractures: outcomes of surgical and conservative management. Br J Sports Med 2006;40(8):692–5 [discussion: 695].

19. Toren AJ, Hahn DB, Brown WC, et al. Vascularized scapular free bone graft after nofnunion of a tarsal navicular stress fracture: a case report. J Foot Ankle Surg 2013;52(2):221–6.

20. DeVries JG, Taefi E, Bussewitz BW, et al. The fifth metatarsal base: anatomic evaluation regarding fracture mechanism and treatment algorithms. J Foot Ankle Surg 2015;54(1):94–8.

21. Landorf KB. Fifth metatarsal fractures are not all the same: proximal diaphyseal fractures are prone to delayed healing. Foot 1998;8(1):38–45.

22. Maestro M, Besse JL, Ragusa M, et al. Forefoot morphotype study and planning method for forefoot osteotomy. Foot Ankle Clin 2003;8(4):695–710.

23. Davidson G, Pizzari T, Mayes S. The influence of second toe and metatarsal length on stress fractures at the base of the second metatarsal in classical dancers. Foot Ankle Int 2007;28(10):1082–6.

24. Kaipel M, Krapf D, Wyss C. Metatarsal length does not correlate with maximal peak pressure and maximal force. Clin Orthop Relat Res 2011;469(4):1161–6.

25. Arangio GA, Beam H, Kowalczyk G, et al. Analysis of stress in the metatarsals. Foot Ankle Surg 1998;4:123–8.

26. Harato K, Ozaki M, Sakurai A, et al. Stress fracture of the first metatarsal after total knee arthroplasty: two case reports using gait analysis. Knee 2014;21(1): 328–31.

27. Watson HI, O'Donnell B, Hopper GP, et al. Proximal base stress fracture of the second metatarsal in a Highland dancer. BMJ Case Rep 2013;2013 [pii: bcr2013010284].

28. Chuckpaiwong B, Cook C, Pietrobon R, et al. Second metatarsal stress fracture in sport: comparative risk factors between proximal and non-proximal locations. Br J Sports Med 2007;41(8):510–4.

29. Saxena A, Krisdakumtorn T, Erickson S. Proximal fourth metatarsal injuries in athletes: similarity to proximal fifth metatarsal injury. Foot Ankle Int 2001;22(7):603–8.

30. Rongstad KM, Tueting J, Rongstad M, et al. Fourth metatarsal base stress fractures in athletes: a case series. Foot Ankle Int 2013;34(7):962–8.

31. Lee KT, Kim KC, Park YU, et al. Radiographic evaluation of foot structure following fifth metatarsal stress fracture. Foot Ankle Int 2011;32(8):796–801.

32. Logan AJ, Dabke H, Finlay D, et al. Fifth metatarsal base fractures: a simple classification. Foot Ankle Surg 2007;13(1):30–4.

33. Torg JS, Balduini FC, Zelko RR, et al. Fractures of the base of the fifth metatarsal distal to the tuberosity. Classification and guidelines for non-surgical and surgical management. J Bone Joint Surg Am 1984;66(2):209–14.

34. Clutton J, Perera A. (n.d.). Insufficiency and Deficiency of Vitamin D in patients with Fractures of the Fifth Metatarsal.

35. Major NM. Role of MRI in prevention of metatarsal stress fractures in collegiate basketball players. AJR Am J Roentgenol 2006;186(1):255–8.

36. Romani WA, Gieck JH, Perrin DH, et al. Mechanisms and management of stress fractures in physically active persons. J Athl Train 2002;37(3):306–14.

37. Nagao M, Saita Y, Kameda S, et al. Headless compression screw fixation of jones fractures: an outcomes study in Japanese athletes. Am J Sports Med 2012; 40(11):2578–82.

38. Tsukada S, Ikeda H, Seki Y, et al. Intramedullary screw fixation with bone autografting to treat proximal fifth metatarsal metaphyseal-diaphyseal fracture in athletes: a case series. Sports Med Arthrosc Rehabil Ther Technol 2012;4(1):25.

39. Ochenjele G, Ho B, Switaj PJ, et al. Radiographic study of the fifth metatarsal for optimal intramedullary screw fixation of Jones fracture. Foot Ankle Int 2015;36(3): 293–301.

40. Hunt KJ, Goeb Y, Esparza R, et al. Site-specific loading at the fifth metatarsal base in rehabilitative devices: implications for Jones fracture treatment. PM R 2014;6(11):1022–9 [quiz: 1029].

41. Lee KT, Park YU, Jegal H, et al. Prognostic classification of fifth metatarsal stress fracture using plantar gap. Foot Ankle Int 2013;34(5):691–6.

42. Lee KT, Park YU, Jegal H, et al. Factors associated with recurrent fifth metatarsal stress fracture. Foot Ankle Int 2013;34(12):1645–53.

43. Graham EM, Burns J, Hiller CE, et al. Management for common lower leg stress fractures in athletes. Phys Ther Rev 2015;20(1):29–41.

44. Moretti B, Notarnicola A, Garofalo R, et al. Shock waves in the treatment of stress fractures. Ultrasound Med Biol 2009;35(6):1042–9.

45. Furia JP, Rompe JD, Cacchio A, et al. Shock wave therapy as a treatment of nonunions, avascular necrosis, and delayed healing of stress fractures. Foot Ankle Clin 2010;15(4):651–62.

46. Busse JW, Kaur J, Mollon B, et al. Low intensity pulsed ultrasonography for fractures: systematic review of randomised controlled trials. BMJ 2009;338:b351.

47. Beck BR, Matheson GO, Bergman G, et al. Do capacitively coupled electric fields accelerate tibial stress fracture healing? A randomized controlled trial. Am J Sports Med 2008;36(3):545–53.

48. Alt V, Donell ST, Chhabra A, et al. A health economic analysis of the use of rhBMP-2 in Gustilo-Anderson grade III open tibial fractures for the UK, Germany, and France. Injury 2009;40(12):1269–75.

49. Aspenberg P, Genant HK, Johansson T, et al. Teriparatide for acceleration of fracture repair in humans: a prospective, randomized, double-blind study of 102 postmenopausal women with distal radial fractures. J Bone Miner Res 2010; 25(2):404–14.

50. Raghavan P, Christofides E. Role of teriparatide in accelerating metatarsal stress fracture healing: a case series and review of literature. Clin Med Insights Endocrinol Diabetes 2012;5(5):39–45.

51. Ekstrand J, van Dijk CN. Fifth metatarsal fractures among male professional footballers: a potential career-ending disease. Br J Sports Med 2013;47(12):754–8.

52. Mallee WH, Weel H, van Dijk CN, et al. Surgical versus conservative treatment for high-risk stress fractures of the lower leg (anterior tibial cortex, navicular and fifth metatarsal base): a systematic review. Br J Sports Med 2015;49(6):370–6.

53. Lappe J, Cullen D, Haynatzki G, et al. Calcium and vitamin d supplementation decreases incidence of stress fractures in female navy recruits. J Bone Miner Res 2008;23(5):741–9.

Entrapment Neuropathies of the Foot and Ankle

Eric Ferkel, MD[a],*, William Hodges Davis, MD[b], John Kent Ellington, MD[b]

KEYWORDS

- Jogger's foot • Tarsal tunnel syndrome • Lateral plantar nerve entrapment
- Morton neuroma in athletes • Superficial and deep peroneal nerve entrapment

KEY POINTS

- Posterior tarsal tunnel syndrome is the result of compression of the posterior tibial nerve.
- Anterior tarsal tunnel syndrome (entrapment of the deep peroneal nerve) typically presents with pain radiating to the first dorsal web space.
- Distal tarsal tunnel syndrome results from entrapment of the first branch of the lateral plantar nerve and is often misdiagnosed initially as plantar fasciitis.
- Medial plantar nerve compression is seen most often in running athletes, typically with pain radiating to the medial arch.
- Morton neuroma is often seen in athletes who place their metatarsal arches repetitively in excessive hyperextension.

TARSAL TUNNEL SYNDROME
Introduction: Nature of the Problem

Posterior tarsal tunnel syndrome is a compression of the posterior tibial nerve and its associated branches that occurs within the tarsal tunnel, a fibro-osseous space that is defined by the medial malleolus (superiorly), tibia (anterior border), posterior process of the talus (posterior border), calcaneus (lateral border), abductor hallucis (inferior border), and the flexor retinaculum (laciniate ligament), which lays over the tibial nerve to create an enclosed space. The contents of the tunnel include the posterior tibial nerve, the posterior tibialis, the flexor halluces longus, the flexor digitorum longus, and the posterior tibial artery/vein. Recently, it has been described that there are 3 well-defined fascial septae (medial, lateral, and intermediate), in addition to the flexor retinaculum and the abductor hallucis, as potential sites of compression.[1] The

[a] Southern California Orthopaedic Institute, 6815 Noble Avenue, Van Nuys, CA 91405, USA;
[b] OrthoCarolina Foot and Ankle Institute, 2001 Vail Avenue, #200B, Charlotte, NC 28207, USA
* Corresponding author.
E-mail address: eferkel@scoi.com

Clin Sports Med 34 (2015) 791–801
http://dx.doi.org/10.1016/j.csm.2015.06.002
0278-5919/15/$ – see front matter © 2015 Elsevier Inc. All rights reserved.

posterior tibial nerve is a branch of the sciatic nerve that divides into the medial calcaneal nerve and the lateral plantar nerve (LPN) and medial plantar nerve (MPN).

Tarsal tunnel contents
- Posterior tibial nerve
- The posterior tibialis
- The flexor hallucis longus
- The flexor digitorum longus
- Posterior tibial artery/vein

The syndrome was initially described Kopell and Thompson[2] in 1960, and is an uncommon diagnosis in athletes, although a slightly higher predominance is seen in women.[3]

Typically the tibial nerve is entrapped within the tarsal canal because of trauma and repetitive stress in runners and soccer players, and hyperpronation and poor running mechanics can predispose athletes to entrapment. Compression can also occur by space-occupying masses, such as ganglion cysts, tumors, or accessory musculature. Multiples sites of entrapment can create a double-crush phenomenon that, when it radiates proximally, is known as the Valleix phenomenon.

Symptoms

- Burning, tingling, and shooting pain along the heel and medial aspect of the ankle
- Increase in symptoms with standing, walking, or running
- Evaluate for ankle instability, which can also contribute to tarsal tunnel syndrome in running athletes

MRI can be a helpful way of identifying the pathologic cause of symptoms. In one study, MRIs found the symptomatic mass in 88% of patients presenting with clinical signs of tarsal tunnel syndrome.[4]

Therapeutic Options and/or Surgical Technique

Nonoperative management

- Immobilization
- Oral and topical nonsteroidal antiinflammatory drugs (NSAIDs), compounding creams
- Orthotics
- Tricyclic antidepressants, gabapentin, pregabalin
- Steroid injections

Operative management

With the patient supine with a thigh tourniquet, an incision of 5 to 7 cm is made along the posteromedial aspect of the ankle from just proximal to the medial malleolus extending distally along the course of the nerve, gently curving anteriorly at the LPN. It is important to protect the medial calcaneal nerve. Sharply release the retinacula and, if necessary, remove any space-occupying mass. Be sure to release any arterial vascular leash that may indent on the nerve or create scar tissue surrounding the nerve. Trace the posterior tibial nerve distal to the MPN and LPN branches if required and the fascia of the abductor hallucis, both superficial and deep, to prevent any source of further compression.

Clinical Outcomes

Tarsal tunnel release surgery has had mixed results regarding postoperative improvement. Gondring and colleagues[5] reported an 85% improvement in clinical findings (Tinel sign and nerve conduction velocity [NCV]); however, only 51% of their patients reported symptom relief. Sammarco and Chang[6] reported that patients' American Orthopaedic Foot and Ankle Society scores improved from 61 out of 100 to 80 out of 100 postoperatively. Cimino[7] reported 91% improvement and 69% resolution of symptoms with only 2% recurrence.

Complications and Concerns

Gould describes failure to be less than 5%, and that initial releases often fail because of failure to control hemostasis, which leads to scarring and neuritis or nerve damage from lack of anatomic knowledge. He states that revision results were often worse.[8–11] Dr Gould also reported 63% good to excellent results using a vein wrap in revision surgeries.

ANTERIOR TARSAL TUNNEL SYNDROME/DEEP PERONEAL NERVE ENTRAPMENT
Introduction: Nature of the Problem

Anterior tarsal tunnel syndrome, also known as deep peroneal nerve (DPN) entrapment, was first described by Kopell and Thompson[2] as compression of the DPN:

- Along the superior border of the inferior extensor retinaculum at the ankle joint
- Beneath the extensor halluces longus (EHL)[2]

The nerve can also be compressed because of:

- Osteophytes from the talonavicular (TN), navicular-cuneiform (NC), or tarsal-metatarsal (TMT) joint.
- Entrapment by an os intermetatarseum in athletes[12,13]
- Entrapment from ice skate or ski boot wear, swelling, fractures, high-heeled or tight-fitting running shoes
- Chronic osteophytes from kicking sports, such as soccer or martial arts[14,15]

Borders of anterior tarsal tunnel

- Superficial: inferior extensor retinaculum
- Lateral: lateral malleolus
- Medial: medial malleolus
- Deep: talonavicular joint capsule

Contents of anterior tarsal tunnel

- Dorsalis pedis artery and vein
- DPN
- Peroneus tertius
- Tibialis anterior
- Extensor hallucis longus
- Extensor digitorum longus

Schon and Baxter[15] observed compression of the nerve from athletes using metal bars to hold their feet when doing sit-ups or from keeping their keys beneath the tongues of their running shoes. It is important to rule out exertional anterior compartment syndrome or common peroneal nerve entrapment as a cause of the transient numbness. The nerve can also experience a traction injury caused by chronic ankle instability and ankle sprains.

The DPN travels between the extensor digitorum longus (EDL) and tibialis anterior and distally between the EDL and EHL just proximal to the ankle before dividing into the lateral and medial branches, typically 1.3 cm proximal to the ankle joint. The lateral branch, usually the smaller of the two, innervates the extensor digitorum brevis (EDB) and the TMT and metatarsophalangeal joint (MTP) joints. The medial branch, which lies just medial to the dorsalis pedis, travels to the first dorsal web space, delivering sensation to the area, and has a dorsomedial cutaneous branch to the second toe and a dorsolateral cutaneous branch to the hallux. Entrapment of the medial branch can occur from the extensor hallucis brevis (EHB) as it travels over the nerve at the first and second TMT joints.[14]

Patients typically present with pain along the dorsum of the foot with intermittent numbness radiating to the first dorsal web space. The EDB can be weak or atrophied and the practitioner may be able to elicit a Tinel sign by percussing over the superior and inferior retinaculum along the DPN, leading to tingling over the first dorsal web space of the foot. Patients may also complain of aching and tightness along the ankle joint or numbness at the first dorsal web space when the ankle is placed in plantar flexion with the toe extended. Electromyography and NCV tests should be ordered to confirm the diagnosis and location of the entrapment. Weight-bearing radiographs of the foot and ankle can assist in identifying osteophytes that may be contributing to the entrapment.

Surgical management

- Preoperative identification of the entrapment and its location
- At the inferior extensor retinaculum, incise over the anterior ankle and release approximately half of the retinaculum
- Continue with neurolysis of the DPN
- Remove any osteophytes at the superior talus or along the TN, NC, or TMT joints
- Resect the EDB as it crosses over the nerve
- If the retinaculum was lengthened, then close in a lengthened position

Nonoperative management

- Shoe-wear modification
- Custom orthotics or padding[16]
- Topical compound creams
- NSAIDs, gabapentin
- Corticosteroid and lidocaine injection to the site of entrapment[17]
- If ankle instability is the cause, physical therapy can assist with pain relief and strengthening

Clinical Outcomes

Dellon[19] studied 20 nerves in 18 patients who had surgery to release entrapment of the DPN's sensory branch over the dorsum of the foot. They observed excellent results in 60% of these patients, good results in 20%, and no improvement in 20% by 26 months after surgery.[18–20]

Complications and Concerns

Complications include nerve injury or EHB wasting in late-stage presentation.

DISTAL TARSAL TUNNEL SYNDROME/FIRST BRANCH OF LATERAL PLANTAR NERVE
Introduction: Nature of the Problem

Distal tarsal tunnel syndrome results from compression of the first branch of the LPN (sometimes called the Baxter nerve). This syndrome is a commonly encountered, but often misdiagnosed, cause of neuropathy in runners, ballerinas,[21] and gymnasts[22] and should be in the differential for heel pain in the athletic population. Other diagnoses to consider at the time of presentation include plantar fasciitis, fat pad atrophy, apophysitis, and calcaneal stress fracture. The MPN, a mixed sensory and motor nerve, travels below the abductor hallucis and flexor digitorum brevis and above the quadratus plantae along the medial border of the calcaneus. The nerve, which innervates the abductor digiti quinti, flexor digitorum brevis, and quadratus plantae, can become compressed as it travels between the fascia of the abductor hallucis longus and the medial border of the quadratus plantae muscle.

Athletes often present with chronic medial heel pain that occurs with brisk walking or running, worse in the morning and when getting going, making it difficult to differentiate it from plantar fasciitis. Patients typically describe point tenderness approximately 5 cm anterior to the posterior border of the heel where the plantar and medial skin intersects.[15,23] Burning pain and tingling are often described as radiating along the plantar aspect of the foot laterally and are reproduced with a positive Tinel along the nerve's course deep to the abductor hallucis. It is important to distinguish this medially sided pain from plantar fasciitis, which is typically more plantar; however, there can be concomitant compression of the LPN with plantar fasciitis. MRI has been shown to be nonspecific,[24] but electrodiagnostic studies can be helpful in confirming the diagnosis.[23]

Causes of compression

- Hypermobile pronated feet[25]
- Abductor hallucis or quadratus plantae hypertrophy
- Accessory musculature
- Stretching and tethering of the LPN in a running athlete, most often in a cavus-type foot[26]

Therapeutic Options and/or Surgical Technique
Nonoperative

NSAIDs, rest, ice massage, physical therapy, or steroid injections. Orthotics to assist in correcting over pronation or heel pads can assist in conservative therapy, which should be attempted for at least 12 to 20 months.

Surgical management

The authors prefer open surgical management; however, Lui[27,28] described endoscopic release of the first branch of the LPN.

- Supine with thigh tourniquet.
- Curvilinear incision made just distal to the posterior medial malleolus extending to the plantar aspect of the foot, centering on the first branch of the LPN (**Fig. 1**).
- Divide the superficial fascia of the abductor hallucis and expose the muscle belly, then retract it distally to expose the deep fascia (**Fig. 2**).
- Release the deep fascia then retract the muscle proximally and finish the release of the deep fascia to ensure that the nerve is no longer compressed. Remove a small portion of the deep fascia and expose the plantar fascia (**Fig. 3**).
- Transect the medial 50% of the plantar fascia under direct visualization.
- Irrigate and close, and place in a splint for 2 weeks on crutches, followed by walking boot for 4 weeks.

Clinical Outcomes

Approximately 90% of patients improve with nonoperative management.[29] Watson and colleagues[29] reported an 88% good to excellent rating after surgical intervention and a 93% level of satisfaction with the surgery. Baxter and Pfeffer[30] showed 89% good to excellent results with 83% of their patients experiencing complete resolution of their pain.

Complications and concerns

- Wound dehiscence
- Deep vein thrombosis
- Nerve injury

Watson and colleagues[29] noted that 52% of the patients required at least 6 months to reach maximum improvement and that 8 to 12 months to improvement is what is discussed in preoperative counseling.[29]

MEDIAL PLANTAR NERVE (JOGGER'S FOOT)
Introduction: Nature of the Problem

MPN entrapment is classically described in runners, typically with hyperpronation and excessive heel valgus, presenting as radiating pain along the medial arch, and is usually worse with exercise.[3,31,32] Examination finds maximal tenderness and Tinel sign along the abductor hallucis with dysesthesia along the plantar aspect of the first and second toes, and symptoms can be made worse with heel rise or eversion of the foot, which tightens the abductor hallucis. MRI is not mandatory, but it can assist in showing abnormal signal intensity or fatty atrophy in the abductor hallucis or flexor hallucis brevis, consistent with denervation. A diagnostic nerve block at the site of the entrapment often assists in confirming the diagnosis.[23,32]

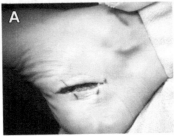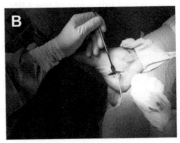

Fig. 1. (*A, B*) Exposure along the plantar medial aspect of the foot, approx. 3 to 5 cm in length.

Entrapment of MPN locations

- Direct compression where the flexor digitorum longus and flexor hallucis longus cross along the plantar surface (knot of Henry)
- External compression through the medial arch from orthotics[33]

Therapeutic Options and/or Surgical Technique

Nonoperative management includes therapy, NSAIDs, rest, injections, removing or modifying rigid orthosis, and physical therapy to assist in training modification.

Surgical intervention involves making an incision of 4 to 8 cm along the plantar aspect of the talonavicular joint and releasing the superficial and deep fascia of the abductor hallucis, followed by exposing the knot of Henry to release the calcaneonavicular ligament.

Clinical Outcomes

Little recurrence has been seen with a MPN release.[34]

SUPERFICIAL PERONEAL NERVE ENTRAPMENT
Introduction: Nature of the Problem

Superficial peroneal nerve (SPN) entrapment is a dynamic entrapment of the SPN as the nerve exits the deep crural fascia. The SPN courses in the lateral compartment, between the peroneus longus and brevis, exiting the fascia approximately 13 cm from the tip of the fibula.[35] Entrapment occurs in various athletic groups, including runners and hockey, tennis, and soccer players,[32,36] typically resulting from chronic ankle sprain (tethering of the nerve during forced inversion and plantarflexion),[37] ganglion cysts, direct trauma, muscle herniation, or mass effect from swelling or tumors (lipomas, schwannomas).[15,38,39] It is a separate entity from exertional compartment syndrome.

It is imperative to rule out spinal involvement, and evaluate for common peroneal nerve entrapment at the fibular head. Nerve conduction studies can help, but are neither conclusive nor exclusionary.[3] MRI can assist in identifying facial defects or nerve compression mass effect lesions.

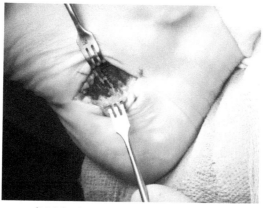

Fig. 2. Dividing the superficial fascia to expose the abductor hallucis muscle belly.

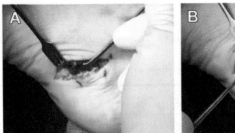
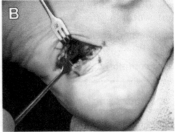

Fig. 3. (A, B) After exposing the muscle belly, the muscle is retracted distally to expose the deep fascia, which should be released to provide complete decompression of the LPN.

Symptoms include:

- Pain, tingling, numbness over the dorsum of the foot
- Tinel along the exiting point of the nerve[40,41] while the foot is plantar flexed
- Direct pressure with the foot everted and dorsiflexed against resistance
- Passive plantar flexion and inversion

Therapeutic Options and/or Surgical Technique

Nonoperative management

- Lidocaine/Marcaine injection (can be diagnostic and therapeutic)
- Physical therapy, focusing on peroneal strengthening
- Lateral forefoot wedge to reduce varus thrust

Surgical management

- Patient is lateral decubitus or supine
- Incision is anterior to the preoperative Tinel (marked in preoperative area)
- Incise fascia to release SPN (**Fig. 4**)
- Perform only a single-layer closure

Clinical Outcomes

Fasciotomy and neurolysis were shown by Styf[41] to obtain 80% relief in athletes; however, in only half of the cases, athletes were completely satisfied.[40,41]

Complications and Concerns

There is risk of injury to the neurovascular bundle as well as recurrence. Recurrence should be managed with repeat exploration and consideration for transection and burial into bone.[42]

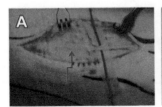
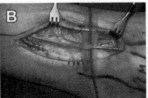
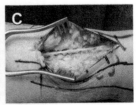

Fig. 4. (A) Superficial fascia tethering in the SPN (Arrow). (B, C) SPN after release from its compressing fascia.

MORTON NEUROMA
Introduction: Nature of the Problem

Initially described by Civinni in 1835, Thomas Morton, in 1876, mistakenly wrote about pain related to a fourth MTP joint and relief from resection of the fourth metatarsal head.[43] Morton neuroma is an entrapment neuropathy, not a primary neuroma, and can be accurately described as interdigital neuralgia from perineural fibirosis.[3] The condition most commonly affects women (10 times more often than men), most likely because of a narrow shoebox that causes traction of the interdigital nerve. It is observed in runners and dancers (specifically in the demi-pointe position in ballerinas), typically caused by hyperextension at the MTP joints and repetitive trauma to the metatarsals.[44] These stresses can lead to increased swelling of the bursa causing greater compression of the interdigital nerve and thickening of the intermetatarsal ligament.

MRI is not usually necessary and diagnosis can be made on clinical examination.

Clinical examination

- Pain, tingling, and numbness at the web space
- Shooting electrical shock to the tip of the toes from the web space
- Mulder click with pain
- Mini-Lachman test to evaluate for MTP joint instability[45]

Therapeutic Options and/or Surgical Technique
Conservative management

- Shoe-wear modification or inserts to reduced pressure beneath metatarsal heads
- Lidocaine/steroid injection to web space
- Alcohol sclerosing therapy has shown mixed results in the literature,[43,46] but, when combined with ultrasonography guidance, symptom relief is improved[47,48]

Surgical management

- Supine with ankle tourniquet
- Dorsal approach (recent study has shown no difference in dorsal or plantar approach[49]) over the web space with care to avoid injury to the dorsal digital nerves
- Place lamina spreader to put strain on the transverse intermetatarsal ligament to assist with its release, and expose and remove the interdigital nerve and its accompanying neuroma, which should be sent for histologic examination

Clinical Outcomes

Multiple studies have shown 70% to 85% improvement after surgery.[3]

Complications and Concerns

Web-space atrophy from multiple steroid injections can lead to increased joint instability and wound problems.

REFERENCES

1. Singh G, Kumar VP. Neuroanatomical basis for the tarsal tunnel syndrome. Foot Ankle Int 2012;33(6):513–8.

2. Kopell HP, Thompson WA. Peripheral entrapment neuropathies of the lower extremity. N Engl J Med 1960;262:56–60.
3. Espinosa N. Peripheral nerve entrapment around the foot and ankle. In: Miller MD, Thompson SR, DeLee J, et al, editors. DeLee & Drez's orthopaedic sports medicine: principles and practice. 4th edition. Philadelphia: Elsivier/Saunders; 2014. p. 1351–68.
4. Frey C, Kerr R. Magnetic resonance imaging and the evaluation of tarsal tunnel syndrome. Foot Ankle 1993;14(3):159–64.
5. Gondring WH, Shields B, Wenger S. An outcomes analysis of surgical treatment of tarsal tunnel syndrome. Foot Ankle Int 2003;24(7):545–50.
6. Sammarco GJ, Chang L. Outcome of surgical treatment of tarsal tunnel syndrome. Foot Ankle Int 2003;24(2):125–31.
7. Cimino WR. Tarsal tunnel syndrome: review of the literature. Foot Ankle 1990;11(1):47–52.
8. DiGiovanni BF, Abuzzahab FS Jr, Gould JS. Plantar fascia release with proximal and distal tarsal tunnel release: a surgical approach to chronic, disabling plantar fasciitis with associated nerve pain. Tech Foot Ankle Surg 2003;2(4):254–61.
9. Gould JS. Tarsal tunnel syndrome. Foot Ankle Clin 2011;16(2):275–86.
10. Gould JS. The failed tarsal tunnel release. Foot Ankle Clin 2011;16(2):287–93.
11. Gould JS. Recurrent tarsal tunnel syndrome. Foot Ankle Clin 2014;19(3):451–67.
12. Noguchi M, Iwata Y, Miura K, et al. A painful os intermetatarseum in a soccer player: a case report. Foot Ankle Int 2000;21(12):1040–2.
13. Nakasa T, Fukuhara K, Adachi N, et al. Painful os intermetatarseum in athletes: report of four cases and review of the literature. Arch Orthop Trauma Surg 2007;127(4):261–4.
14. Melendez MM, Glickman LT, Dellon AL. Peroneal nerve compression in figure skaters. Clin Res Foot Ankle 2013;1:102.
15. Schon LC, Baxter DE. Neuropathies of the foot and ankle in athletes. Clin Sports Med 1990;9(2):489–509.
16. Hirose CB, McGarvey WC. Peripheral nerve entrapments. Foot Ankle Clin 2004;9(2):255–69.
17. Gessini L, Jandolo B, Pietrangeli A. The anterior tarsal syndrome. Report of four cases. J Bone Joint Surg Am 1984;66(5):786–7.
18. Murphy PC, Baxter DE. Nerve entrapment of the foot and ankle in runners. Clin Sports Med 1985;4(4):753–63.
19. Dellon AL. Deep peroneal nerve entrapment on the dorsum of the foot. Foot Ankle 1990;11(2):73–80.
20. Baumhauer JF, Nawoczenski DA, DiGiovanni BF, et al. Ankle pain and peroneal tendon pathology. Clin Sports Med 2004;23(1):21–34.
21. McCrory P, Bell S, Bradshaw C. Nerve entrapments of the lower leg, ankle and foot in sport. Sports Med 2002;32(6):371–91.
22. Fredericson M. Lateral plantar nerve entrapment in a competitive gymnast. Clin J Sport Med 2001;11(2):111–4.
23. Schon LC, Glennon TP, Baxter DE. Heel pain syndrome: electrodiagnostic support for nerve entrapment. Foot Ankle 1993;14(3):129–35.
24. Recht MP, Grooff P, Ilaslan H, et al. Selective atrophy of the abductor digiti quinti: an MRI study. AJR Am J Roentgenol 2007;189(3):W123–7.
25. Radin EL. Tarsal tunnel syndrome. Clin Orthop Relat Res 1983;181:167–70.
26. Baxter DE, Thigpen CM. Heel pain–operative results. Foot Ankle 1984;5(1):16–25.
27. Lui T. Endoscopic decompression of the first branch of the lateral plantar nerve. Arch Orthop Trauma Surg 2007;127(9):859–61.

28. Lui TH. Arthroscopy and endoscopy of the foot and ankle: indications for new techniques. Arthroscopy 2007;23(8):889–902.
29. Watson TS, Anderson RB, Davis WH, et al. Distal tarsal tunnel release with partial plantar fasciotomy for chronic heel pain: an outcome analysis. Foot Ankle Int 2002;23(6):530–7.
30. Baxter DE, Pfeffer GB. Treatment of chronic heel pain by surgical release of the first branch of the lateral plantar nerve. Clin Orthop Relat Res 1992;(279):229–36.
31. Rask MR. Medial plantar neurapraxia (jogger's foot): report of 3 cases. Clin Orthop Relat Res 1978;(134):193–5.
32. Schon LC, Reed MA. Disorders of the nerves. In: Coughlin MJ, Saltzman CL, Anderson RB, editors. Mann's surgery of the foot and ankle. 9th edition. Philadelphia: W.B. Saunders/Elsevier; 2014. p. 621–82.
33. Flanigan RM, DiGiovanni BF. Peripheral nerve entrapments of the lower leg, ankle, and foot. Foot Ankle Clin 2011;16(2):255–74.
34. Peck E, Finnoff JT, Smith J. Neuropathies in runners. Clin Sports Med 2010;29(3): 437–57.
35. Sarrafian SK, Kelikian AS. Sarrafian's anatomy of the foot and ankle: descriptive, topographic, functional. In: Kelikian AS, Sarrafian SK, editors. 3rd edition. Philadelphia; Baltimore (MD); New York; London; Buenos Aires (Argentina); Hong Kong (China); Sydney (Australia); Tokyo: Wolters Kluwer; Lippincott Williams & Wilkins; 2011. p. 390.
36. Schepsis AA, Fitzgerald M, Nicoletta R. Revision surgery for exertional anterior compartment syndrome of the lower leg: technique, findings, and results. Am J Sports Med 2005;33(7):1040–7.
37. Styf J, Morberg P. The superficial peroneal tunnel syndrome. Results of treatment by decompression. J Bone Joint Surg Br 1997;79(5):801–3.
38. Kernohan J, Levack B, Wilson JN. Entrapment of the superficial peroneal nerve. Three case reports. J Bone Joint Surg Br 1985;67(1):60–1.
39. Styf J. Diagnosis of exercise-induced pain in the anterior aspect of the lower leg. Am J Sports Med 1988;16(2):165–9.
40. Johnston EC, Howell SJ. Tension neuropathy of the superficial peroneal nerve: associated conditions and results of release. Foot Ankle Int 1999;20(9):576–82.
41. Styf J. Entrapment of the superficial peroneal nerve. Diagnosis and results of decompression. J Bone Joint Surg Br 1989;71(1):131–5.
42. Chiodo CP, Miller SD. Surgical treatment of superficial peroneal neuroma. Foot Ankle Int 2004;25(10):689–94.
43. Espinosa N, Seybold JD, Jankauskas L, et al. Alcohol sclerosing therapy is not an effective treatment for interdigital neuroma. Foot Ankle Int 2011;32(6):576–80.
44. Konstantine B. The treatment of Morton's neuroma, a significant cause of metatarsalgia for people who exercise. Int J Clin Med 2013;04(01):19–24.
45. Espinosa N, Brodsky JW, Maceira E. Metatarsalgia. J Am Acad Orthop Surg 2010;18(8):474–85.
46. Gurdezi S, White T, Ramesh P. Alcohol injection for Morton's neuroma: a five-year follow-up. Foot Ankle Int 2013;34(8):1064–7.
47. Pasquali C, Vulcano E, Novario R, et al. Ultrasound-guided alcohol injection for Morton's neuroma. Foot Ankle Int 2015;36(1):55–9.
48. Hughes RJ, Ali K, Jones H, et al. Treatment of Morton's neuroma with alcohol injection under sonographic guidance: follow-up of 101 cases. AJR Am J Roentgenol 2007;188(6):1535–9.
49. Akermark C, Crone H, Skoog A, et al. A prospective randomized controlled trial of plantar versus dorsal incisions for operative treatment of primary Morton's neuroma. Foot Ankle Int 2013;34(9):1198–204.

Index

Note: Page numbers of article titles are in **boldface** type.

Clin Sports Med 34 (2015) 803–809
http://dx.doi.org/10.1016/S0278-5919(15)00073-3
0278-5919/15/$ – see front matter © 2015 Elsevier Inc. All rights reserved.

sportsmed.theclinics.com

United States Postal Service

Statement of Ownership, Management, and Circulation
(All Periodicals Publications Except Requestor Publications)

1. Publication Title	2. Publication Number	3. Filing Date
Clinics in Sports Medicine	0 0 0 - 7 0 2	9/18/15

4. Issue Frequency	5. Number of Issues Published Annually	6. Annual Subscription Price
Jan, Apr, Jul, Oct	4	$340.00

7. Complete Mailing Address of Known Office of Publication (Not printer) (Street, city, county, state, and ZIP+4®)

Elsevier Inc.
360 Park Avenue South
New York, NY 10010-1710

Contact Person
Stephen R. Bushing
Telephone: (Include area code)
215-239-3688

8. Complete Mailing Address of Headquarters or General Business Office of Publisher (Not printer)

Elsevier Inc., 360 Park Avenue South, New York, NY 10010-1710

9. Full Names and Complete Mailing Addresses of Publisher, Editor, and Managing Editor (Do not leave blank)

Publisher (Name and complete mailing address)

Linda Belfus, Elsevier Inc., 1600 John F. Kennedy Blvd., Suite 1800, Philadelphia, PA 19103

Editor (Name and complete mailing address)

Jennifer Flynn-Briggs, Elsevier Inc., 1600 John F. Kennedy Blvd., Suite 1800, Philadelphia, PA 19103-2899

Managing Editor (Name and complete mailing address)

Adrianne Brigido, Elsevier Inc., 1600 John F. Kennedy Blvd., Suite 1800, Philadelphia, PA 19103-2899

10. Owner (Do not leave blank. If the publication is owned by a corporation, give the name and address of the corporation immediately followed by the names and addresses of all stockholders owning or holding 1 percent or more of the total amount of stock. If not owned by a corporation, give the names and addresses of the individual owners. If owned by a partnership or other unincorporated firm, give its name and address as well as those of each individual owner. If the publication is published by a nonprofit organization, give its name and address.)

Full Name	Complete Mailing Address
Wholly owned subsidiary of	1600 John F. Kennedy Blvd, Ste. 1800
Reed/Elsevier, US holdings	Philadelphia, PA 19103-2899

11. Known Bondholders, Mortgagees, and Other Security Holders Owning or Holding 1 Percent or More of Total Amount of Bonds, Mortgages, or Other Securities. If none, check box. ☐ None

Full Name	Complete Mailing Address
N/A	

12. Tax Status (For completion by nonprofit organizations authorized to mail at nonprofit rates) (Check one)
The purpose, function, and nonprofit status of this organization and the exempt status for federal income tax purposes:
☐ Has Not Changed During Preceding 12 Months
☐ Has Changed During Preceding 12 Months (Publisher must submit explanation of change with this statement)

PS Form 3526, July 2014 (Page 1 of 3 (Instructions Page 3)) PSN 7530-01-000-9931 PRIVACY NOTICE: See our Privacy policy in www.usps.com

13. Publication Title	14. Issue Date for Circulation Data Below
Clinics in Sports Medicine	July 2015

15. Extent and Nature of Circulation		Average No. Copies Each Issue During Preceding 12 Months	No. Copies of Single Issue Published Nearest to Filing Date
a. Total Number of Copies (Net press run)		590	518
b. Legitimate Paid and/or Requested Distribution (By Mail and Outside the Mail)	(1) Mailed Outside-County Paid/Requested Mail Subscriptions stated on PS Form 3541. (Include paid distribution above nominal rate, advertiser's proof copies and exchange copies)	294	252
	(2) Mailed In-County Paid/Requested Mail Subscriptions stated on PS Form 3541. (Include paid distribution above nominal rate, advertiser's proof copies and exchange copies)		
	(3) Paid Distribution Outside the Mails Including Sales Through Dealers And Carriers, Street Vendors, Counter Sales, and Other Paid Distribution Outside USPS®	69	74
	(4) Paid Distribution by Other Classes of Mail Through the USPS (e.g. First-Class Mail®)		
c. Total Paid and/or Requested Circulation (Sum of 15b (1), (2), (3), and (4)) ▲		363	326
d. Free or Nominal Rate Distribution (By Mail and Outside the Mail)	(1) Free or Nominal Rate Outside-County Copies included on PS Form 3541	83	77
	(2) Free or Nominal Rate In-County Copies Included on PS Form 3541		
	(3) Free or Nominal Rate Copies mailed at Other classes Through the USPS (e.g. First-Class Mail®)		
	(4) Free or Nominal Rate Distribution Outside the Mail (Carriers or Other means)		
e. Total Nonrequested Distribution (Sum of 15d (1), (2), (3) and (4))		83	77
f. Total Distribution (Sum of 15c and 15e) ▲		446	403
g. Copies not Distributed (See Instructions to publishers #4 (page #3)) ▲		144	115
h. Total (Sum of 15f and g) ▲		590	518
i. Percent Paid and/or Requested Circulation (15c divided by 15f times 100) ▲		81.39%	80.89%

* If you are claiming electronic copies go to line 16 on page 3. If you are not claiming Electronic copies, skip to line 17 on page 3.

16. Electronic Copy Circulation	Average No. Copies Each Issue During Preceding 12 Months	No. Copies of Single Issue Published Nearest to Filing Date
a. Paid Electronic Copies		
b. Total paid print Copies (Line 15c) + Paid Electronic copies (Line 16a)		
c. Total Print Distribution (Line 15f) + Paid Electronic Copies (Line 16a)		
d. Percent Paid (Both Print & Electronic copies) (16b divided by 16c X 100)		

☐ I certify that 50% of all my distributed copies (electronic and print) are paid above a nominal price

17. Publication of Statement of Ownership
If the publication is a general publication, publication of this statement is required. Will be printed in the October 2015 issue of this publication.

18. Signature and Title of Editor, Publisher, Business Manager, or Owner

Stephen R. Bushing – Inventory Distribution Coordinator

Date: September 18, 2015

I certify that all information furnished on this form is true and complete. I understand that anyone who furnishes false or misleading information on this form or who omits material or information requested on the form may be subject to criminal sanctions (including fines and imprisonment) and/or civil sanctions (including civil penalties).

PS Form 3526, July 2014 (Page 3 of 3)

Moving?

Make sure your subscription moves with you!

To notify us of your new address, find your **Clinics Account Number** (located on your mailing label above your name), and contact customer service at:

Email: journalscustomerservice-usa@elsevier.com

800-654-2452 (subscribers in the U.S. & Canada)
314-447-8871 (subscribers outside of the U.S. & Canada)

Fax number: 314-447-8029

Elsevier Health Sciences Division
Subscription Customer Service
3251 Riverport Lane
Maryland Heights, MO 63043

*To ensure uninterrupted delivery of your subscription, please notify us at least 4 weeks in advance of move.